PROSTATE CANCER

Acknowledgement
This project was supported by
the National Cancer Institute of the United States of America
under Grant No 5 R01-CA05096-17

UICC Technical Report Series - Volume 48

UICC Workshop on Prostatic Cancer
(1978 : Geneva)

Prostate Cancer

A Series of Workshops on the Biology of Human Cancer

Report No 9

Edited by Donald S. Coffey and John T. Isaacs

International Union Against Cancer
Union Internationale Contre le Cancer

Geneva 1979

THE UICC WORKSHOP ON PROSTATIC CANCER

Geneva, 23-26 October 1978

LIST OF PARTICIPANTS

Dr. Donald S. Coffey (Chairman)
Departments of Urology, Oncology
and Pharmacology
Johns Hopkins University
School of Medicine
725 North Wolfe Street
Baltimore, Md. 21205, USA

Dr. John T. Isaacs (Secretary)
Department of Pharmacology and
 Experimental Therapeutics
Johns Hopkins University
School of Medicine
725 North Wolfe Street
Baltimore, Md. 21205, USA

Dr. Nicholas Bruchovsky
Department of Medicine
Clinical Sciences Building
The University of Alberta
Edmonton, Alberta
T6G, 2G3, Canada

Dr. John Horton
Division of Oncology
Albany Medical College
45 New Scotland Avenue
Albany, New York 12208, USA

Dr. M. Krieg
University of Hamburg
Second Medical Clinic
Department of Clinical Chemistry
2000 Hamburg 20
Martinistrasse 52
West Germany

Dr. Ian P. Mainwaring
Department of Biochemistry
The University of Leeds
9 Hyde Terrace
Leeds LS2 9LS, England

Dr. John E. McNeal
Herrick Memorial Hospital
2001 Dwight Way
Berkeley, California 94704, USA

Dr. Hanspeter Rohr
Institut fur Pathologie
Schonbienstrasse 40
CH-4056 Basel, Switzerland

Dr. Isadore D. Rotkin
Department of Preventive Medicine
and Community Health
University of Illinois at the
 Medical Center
Chicago, Illinois 60090, USA

Dr. Avery Sandberg
Roswell Park Memorial Institute
660 Elm Street
Buffalo, New York 14203, USA

Dr. Fritz H. Schroeder
Institute of Urology
Erasmus Universiteit Rotterdam
P. O. Box 1738
Rotterdam, The Netherlands

Dr. A. Vermeulen
Section of Endocrinology
Academic Hospital
De Pintelaan, 135
B Ghent, Belgium

ISBN : 92-9018-048-X

CONTENTS

CHAIRMAN'S REPORT

The UICC Workshop on Prostatic Cancer was held in Geneva on October 23-26, 1978. The purpose of the meeting was two-fold: 1.) to provide an indepth discussion of the present status and future directions of research designed to develop new methods of controlling this form of cancer. The exchange of ideas between the twelve world leaders was both lively and rewarding. 2.) to provide a technical report that would be both thoughtful and challenging to other investigators who are studying this most difficult problem.

Chapter I provides a current review of the endocrinological factors believed to control normal prostatic growth and function. This overview presents diagrams of metabolic pathways which are included to assist the reader and also forms the background for much of the subsequent chapters.

Chapter II - Dr. John E. McNeal presents the details of his new concept of the anatomy of the human prostate. In the past there has been much confusion and conflict of opinions concerning the functional and anatomical areas of this gland. The new model is discussed in relation to the development of BPH and prostatic adenocarcinoma.

Chapter III - In the past, histopathological studies have been most difficult to analyze in a quantitative manner. The development of stereology has now advanced these quantitative measurements at both the light and electron microscopic levels. Dr. Hanspeter Rohr presents the basic fundamentals of stereology which is already provinding new insight into subcellular changes associated with human BPH. These changes are being correlated with those observed in experimentally induced canine BPH. These stereological studies have implicated specific stromal changes which require both estrogen and androgen for their full development.

Chapter IV - Dr. I. D. Rotkin provides a thoughtful review of the worldwide morbidity and mortality data for prostatic cancer. He summarizes our present knowledge concerning risk factors associated with this cancer. Dr. Rotkin proposes a new model for carcinogenesis in the human prostate that involves sexual behavior and development. He discusses the merits and limitations of the model and presents the data that were useful in developing this concept.

1

Chapter V - Hormones have always been prime suspects as etiological factors in the development of both BPH and prostatic cancer. What is the present evidence to support these claims? Dr. A. Vermeulen discusses the study of age related endocrine changes and how they are altered in BPH and prostatic carcinoma.

Chapter VI - Dr. M. Krieg discusses alteration in androgen metabolism and binding which are associated with abnormal growth of the human prostate.

Chapter VII - Dr. J. Isaacs analyzes factors regulating androgen levels within the normal prostates of animals. Methods are presented to study the natural constraint on normal prostatic growth. Relationships of tissue androgen levels to DNA synthesis are discussed and enzymatic pathways regulating androgen levels are analyzed.

Chapter VIII - Dr. W. I. P. Mainwaring reviews the present status of steroid receptor studies and how they are being used to study the regulation of chromatin function.

Chapter IX - What controls the involution of the prostate following androgen withdrawal and how is the process reversed? Dr. N. Bruchovsky discusses how androgen receptor dynamics are correlated with DNA content and growth of the human prostate.

Chapters X and XI - New methods are needed to study the human prostate under in vitro conditions. Dr. F. H. Schroeder analyzes the present state of the art of prostatic cell culture and Dr. A. Sandberg reviews organ culture techniques with an example of how these methods are utilized in drug studies.

Chapters XII and XIII - Recently new animal models of prostatic cancer have been evaluated and characterized. In these two chapters, Dr. J. Isaacs and Dr. N. Bruchovsky review the properties of these models and reveal how they have already provided new insight into the study of prostatic cancer. Particular emphasis is placed on hormonal induction and control of these cancers.

Chapter XIV - New approaches to therapy are being developed at both the experimental and conceptual levels. Many of these approaches are reviewed with an analysis of their possible advantages and limitations.

Chapter XV - Methods to evaluate human prostatic cancer have been formulated in several new cooperative studies. Dr. J. Horton discusses the merits of these systems and how they are being applied in new therapeutic trials. This is a most thoughtful and critical analysis of these cooperative studies and provides the reader with an update of the present status of these trials.

During the course of this Workshop much discussion focused on the specifics of each of these topics. Each participant was requested to provide an analysis of future research needs in their area of interest. They were encouraged to speculate on the developing trends and to propose new models where appropriate. It is our hope that the readers will share our thoughts and challenge them with new experiments and concepts. It is our belief that this major form of cancer has not attracted enough research interest from the scientific and clinical disciplines. We have therefore attempted to present these papers in a manner that might attract new investigators to this field.

The participants wish to thank Dr. J. F. DelaFresnaye and his staff of the UICC in Geneva for their skillful hosting of this conference. The chairman also wishes to thank Ms. Ruth Middleton and Ms. Mary Buedel for their assistance in preparing these manuscripts.

Donald S. Coffey
Chairman

In men over 40 years of age, the prostate gland is a favored site of infections and neoplastic growths. In a Norwegian study of 206 consecutive autopsies of men over 40 years of age, Harbitz and Haugen (29) reported an overall incidence of benign prostatic hyperplasia (BPH) of 81 percent. Evidence of carcinoma was observed in 34 percent (70/206), and these cases were almost all incidental, only four cases having been previously diagnosed as prostatic cancer. These recent reports of a high incidence of abnormal prostatic growth confirm many earlier studies of benign prostatic hyperplasia (19,60) as well as studies of the high incidence of latent prostatic adenocarcinoma (20,21,24,39). Many of these latent prostatic adenocarcinomas may grow very slowly or may never express clinical manifestations; however, prostatic adenocarcinoma is still the third leading cause of death from cancer. The figures for cancer mortality for males in the United States in 1973 were: lung, 59,187; colon and rectum, 22,709; prostate, 18,830; pancreas, 10,380; and stomach, 9,178 (54). There have been several reviews on the general topic of normal and abnormal growth of the prostate (7,12,26,28, 61,71). The common occurrence of prostatic disease, coupled with our lack of knowledge of many aspects of the biochemistry and physiology of the prostate is a major reason for undertaking more precise basic and clinical investigations. It is the purpose of this chapter to provide a current review of some of the basic concepts related to the function and control of growth of the prostate.

Factors Controlling Prostatic Growth

Endocrine and growth factors that are important in regulating the growth of the prostate gland are depicted in the schematic drawing of Figure 1.

Testicular Androgens:

The growth and function of the prostate is primarily dependent on androgenic stimulus. In the normal male, the major circulating androgen is testosterone, which is almost exclusively (more than 95 percent) of testicular origin (31, 37). Under normal physiologic conditions the Leydig cells of the testis are the major source of the testicular androgens. (For pathway see Figure 2.) The Leydig cells are stimulated by the gonadotropins (Primarily luteinizing hormone) to synthesize testosterone from acetate and cholesterol. The spermatic vein concentration of testosterone is 40 to 50 µg/100 ml and is approximately 75 times more concentrated than the level detected in the peripheral venous serum, which is approximately 600 ng of testosterone/100 ml. Other

---

*Donald S. Coffey

FIGURE 1

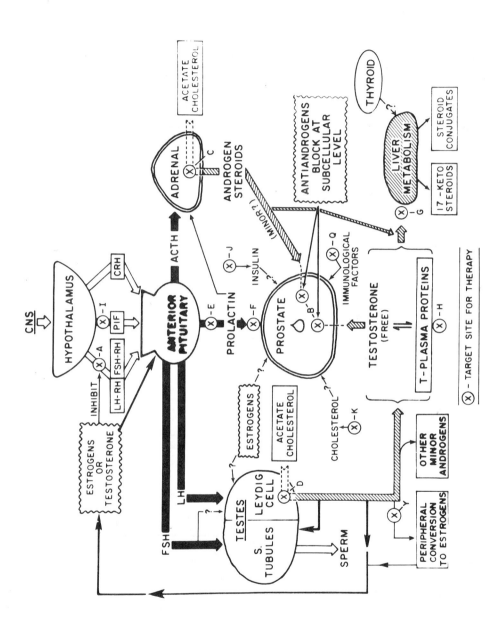

FIGURE 2

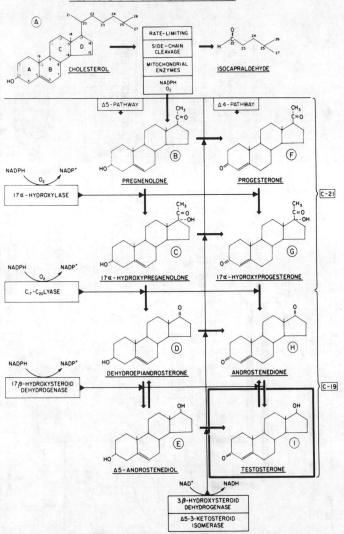

TESTOSTERONE SYNTHESIS IN TESTES

androgens also leave the testes by the spermatic vein, and these include androstanediol, androstendione, and dehydroepiandrosterone; however, the concentrations of these androgens are much lower than those of testosterone.

Testosterone in the plasma is primarily that synthesized by the testes, and although other steroids, such as androstenedione, can be converted by peripheral metabolism to testosterone, they probably account for less than 5 per cent of the overall production of plasma testosterone. The total testosterone that enters the plasma is referred to as the testosterone blood production rate and is determined from the product of the metabolic clearance rate and the mean concentration of testosterone in the plasma. The average testosterone production rate in normal adult males is 6 to 7 mg/day. The mean metabolic clearance rate for testosterone is around 1,000 liters per 24 hours and is related to the testosterone production rate.

The average testosterone concentration in the adult human male plasma is approximately 611 ng/100 ml $\pm$ 186 and is not remarkably related to age between 25 and 70 years, although it does decline gradually to approximately 500 ng/ 100 ml after 70 years of age.

It is recognized that plasma concentrations of testosterone can vary widely in an individual in any one day and may reflect both episodic and diurnal variations in the production rate of testosterone. In addition, longer cycles or periods have been observed if regular daily measurements are determined in the same patient for many weeks. In 12 subjects the average periodicity of the cycle varied from 8 to 30 days, with most cycles lasting 20 to 22 days (16). During these cycles the variation in the fluctuation of the testosterone level was 21 per cent.

The free testosterone (not protein bound) in the plasma is available for metabolism by the liver and intestines, primarily to the 17-ketosteroids, which are secreted in the urine as the conjugates of sulfuric acid and glucuronic acid. (See Fig. 3) The total 17-ketosteroids in the urine in adult males is from 4 to 25 mg/24 hours and is not an accurate index of testosterone production, since other steroids from the adrenals as well as nonandrogenic steroids can be metabolized to 17-ketosteroid forms. This is apparent since the daily production rate of testosterone averages only 6 to 7 mg/24 hours. Only small (25 to 160 µg/day) amounts of testosterone enter the urine without metabolism, and this represents less than 2 per cent of the daily testosterone production.

FIGURE 3

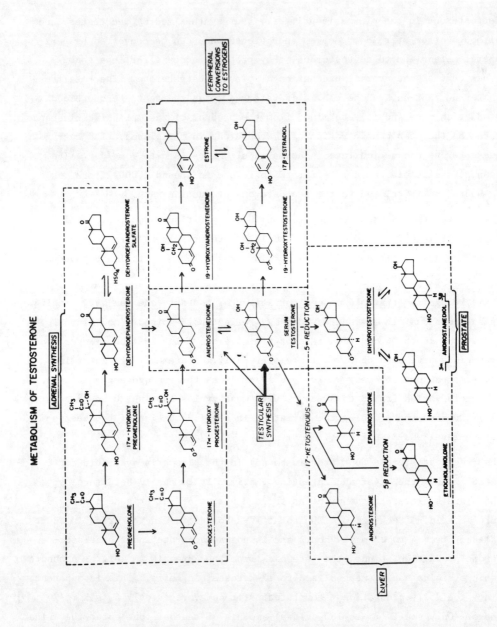

Although testosterone is the primary plasma androgen inducing growth of the prostate gland, it nevertheless appears to function as a prehormone in that the active form of the androgen in the prostate is a testosterone metabolite, dihydrotestosterone (9). Dihydrotestosterone can form in part, from peripheral conversion, which involves the reduction of the $\Delta 4$ double bond in testosterone through the enzymatic action of the 5α-reductase. This conversion can take place directly in the prostate and seminal vesicles. Dihydrotestosterone concentration in the plasma of normal men in very low, 56 ng $\pm$ 20/100 ml, in comparison to testosterone, which is 11-fold higher at approximately 611 ng/100 ml. In summary, although dihydrotestosterone is a potent androgen (1.5 to 2.5 times as potent as testosterone in most bioassay systems), its low plasma concentration and tight binding to plasma proteins diminishes its direct importance as a circulating androgen affecting prostate and seminal vesicle growth. In contrast, dihydrotestosterone is of paramount importance within the sex accessory tissue, where it is formed from testosterone. In sex accessory tissues dihydrotestosterone binds to critical receptors and becomes the major androgen regulating the cellular events of growth and differentiation.

The plasma levels of some important steroids are summarized in Table 1. These values are derived as averages from several combined sources (8,17,22, 67). The complete biologic importance of many of the different steroids circulating in the plasma has not been resolved.

Adrenal Androgens: (See Fig. 3) There is ample biologic evidence that under some conditions steroids secreted from the adrenal cortex can have an influence on the growth of the prostate. Virilism has been observed in humans with hyperfunction of the adrenal cortex associated with neoplasis or hyperplasia of the adrenal gland. However, the effect of adrenal androgens on the prostate in noncastrated adult male rats may not be significant, since adrenalectomy has very little effect on prostate size. Furthermore, following castration in animals, the prostate diminishes to a very small size (90 per cent reduction) without concomitant adrenalectomy. This small ventral prostate in the castrated rat can be reduced further by performing adrenalectomy (5) or hypophysectomy (62). It has been concluded similarly that the prostate of man does not restore itself following castration, indicating that adrenal androgens were insufficient to compensate for the loss of testicular function. While the androgens from the adrenal gland of castrated animals do not restore the size of the prostate gland, it is nevertheless clear that

9

TABLE 1   Plasma Levels of Steroids in Healthy Human Males

Common Name	Chemical Name	Plasma Concentration			Blood Production Rate (mg/day)	Relative Androgenicity Rat V.P. Assay
		NG/100 ML	MOLARITY	RELATIVE MOLARITY		
Testosterone	17β-hydroxy-4-androstene-3-one	611 ± 186	2.1×10^{-8}	100	6.6 ± 0.5	100
Dihydrotestosterone (DHT; Stanolone)	17β-hydroxy-5α-androstan-3-one	56 ± 20	1.9×10^{-9}	9	0.3 ± 0.06	181
5α-Androstane-3α,17β diol (3α-androstanediol)	5α-androstan-3α,17β-diol	14 ± 4	4.8×10^{-10}	2	0.2 ± 0.03	126
5α-Androstane-3β,17β diol (3β-androstanediol)	5α-androstan-3β,17β-diol	<2	$<7 \times 10^{-11}$	<0.3		18
Androstenediol	5-androstene-3β-17β-diol	161 ± 52	5.6×10^{-9}	26		0.21
Androsterone	3α-hydroxy-5α-androstan-17-one	54 ± 32	1.9×10^{-9}	9	0.28	53
Androstenedione	4-androstene-3,17 dione	150 ± 54	5.2×10^{-9}	25	1.4	39
Dehydroepiandrosterone (DHA)	3β-hydroxy-5-androstene-17-one	501 ± 98	1.7×10^{-8}	81	} 29	15
Dehydroepiandrosterone sulfate (DHAS)	17-oxo-5-androstene-3β-γ1-sulfate	135,925 ± 48,000	3.7×10^{-6}	17,619		<1
Progesterone	4-pregnene-3,20-dione	30	9.5×10^{-10}	4.5	0.75	
17β-Estradiol (E₂)	1,3,5(10)-estratriene-3,17β-diol	2.5 ± 0.8	9.2×10^{-11}	0.4	0.045	
Estrone	3-hydroxy-1,3,5(10)-estratriene-17-one	4.6	1.7×10^{-10}	0.8		

administration of ACTH to castrated animals does significantly increase the growth of sex accessory tissue (5,63,64,69).

Estrogen Production in Men: It is now well established that approximately 75 to 90 per cent of the estrogens in the plasma of young healthy males are derived from the peripheral conversion of androstenedione and testosterone to estrone and estradiol (31,40,56). (See Fig. 3) The synthesis of estrogens in human males have been quantitated by Siiteri and MacDonald (56), who showed that of the total of 7.0 mg of testosterone produced in man each day, 0.35 per cent was converted directly to estradiol, forming 24 µg/day. Of the 2.5 mg of androstenedione produced per day, 1.7 per cent was converted to estrone, producing 42 µg/day. The interconversion of estrone and estradiol yielded a final total peripheral production of approximately 40 µg of estradiol/day. The exact location in the periphery where estrogen production occurs has not been elucidated on a quantitative basis, but it is believed that most of the daily production may involve adipose tissue (40). The small amount of estrogens secreted directly from the testes may originate in part from the Sertoli cells, since in culture, these respond to FSH stimulation by producing small amounts of estradiol. It is also known that Sertoli cell tumors can feminize male dogs and produce large amounts of estrogens (32). The exact location of cellular estrogen synthesis and the balance between Leydig and Sertoli cell synthesis have often been controversial, primarily because of difficulties in assaying the low levels of estrogens.

Men over 50 years of age have an increase in total plasma estradiol levels of approximately 50 per cent, with minimal change (less than 10 per cent) in the free estradiol levels because of increases in binding of the estradiol by elevated testosterone-estrogen-binding globulin (TeBG) levels, which are also age related (66). The result of an age-related decrease in the plasma free testosterone level while the free estradiol level is maintained produces a 40 per cent increase in the value for the ratio of free estradiol/free testosterone (66).

Binding of Steroids To Plasma Proteins: Less than 2 per cent of the total testosterone in human plasma is free or unbound and the remaining 98 per cent is bound to several different types of plasma proteins. The plasma proteins that can bind steroids include human serum albumin, testosterone estrogen-binding protein (denoted TeBG) or SBP, steroid-binding protein, corticosteroid-binding globulin (CBG, also termed transcortin), a progesterone-binding globulin (PBG), and, to a lesser extent, the α-acid glycoprotein (AAG).

11

The total amount of testosterone bound to PBG and AAG is not large and is usually ignored.

The total amount of steroid bound depends on two factors: (1) the affinity of the steroid to bind to the protein, and (2) the capacity, which is the maximal potential binding when all of the protein is saturated with bound steroid; the capacity is governed by the amount of protein in the plasma. Serum albumin has a relatively low affinity for testosterone, but because of its high concentration it can bind appreciable quantities of testosterone. Therefore, albumin is a low affinity, high capacity binding protein. In contrast, a steroid-binding protein (TeBG) that has been isolated from plasma has a high affinity, but the protein is present in relatively low concentration; however, the plasma molarity of each binding protein exceeds the plasma molarity for total testosterone concentration. The majority of the testosterone bound to plasma protein is associated with TeBG protein. For example, Vermeulen has calculated that in the normal human male, 57 per cent of the testosterone in the plasma is bound to TeBG and 40 per cent is bound to human serum albumin. Less than 1 per cent is bound to CBG and only 2 per cent of the total testosterone is free. The normal plasma free testosterone level is therefore 12.2 ± 3.7 ng/100 ml or 4.2×10^{-10}M; this non-protein-bound testosterone is available to diffuse into the prostate and liver cells.

The total plasma levels of TeBG can be altered by hormone therapy. Administration of testosterone decreases TeBG levels in the plasma, while estrogen therapy stimulates TeBG levels (11,65). Estrogen also competes with testosterone for binding to TeBG, but estrogen has only one third the binding affinity of testosterone. Therefore, administration of small amounts of estrogen increases the total concentration of TeBG, and this effectively increases the binding of testosterone and thus lowers the free testosterone plasma concentration. Testosterone-estrogen-binding protein binds dihydro-testosterone and androstanediol more tightly than testosterone, but its association with dehydroepiandrosterone, androstenedione, and conjugated steroids is very weak (11).

Walsh and his colleagues have emphasized that the presence of TeBG in human prostatic tissue can complicate the accurate determination of specific andro-gen-binding proteins unless special precautions are taken in the analytical measurements (43). They point out that if prostatic tissue is contaminated with as little as 4 per cent of serum, then the serum TeBG would contribute approximately 2000 to 3000 femtomoles of high affinity binding.

<u>Castration</u>: Since the testes normally produce approximately 95 per cent of the testosterone in the human male, it is not surprising that bilateral orchiectomy results in a reduction of approximately 93 per cent in the plasma testosterone levels. The value for plasma testosterone following bilateral orchiectomy from six different studies averaged 43 $\pm$ 32 ng/100 ml (13,34,46 49,55,72).

This postcastration level of testosterone in the castrated male is almost identical to the average testosterone level of 45 $\pm$ 16 ng/100 ml for the normal nonpregnant female reported in four studies (8). There is also no significant difference between the low plasma level of testosterone in pre- pubertal boys (6.62 $\pm$ 2.46 ng/100 ml) or girls (6.58 $\pm$ 2.48 ng/100 ml) (18). In summary, the average testosterone levels in the human male are: normal adult, 611 ng/100 ml; castrated adult, 43 ng/100 ml/ prepubertal male, 6.6 ng /100 ml.

<u>Blocking Adrenal Function</u>: The observation that the castrated adult levels of plasma testosterone are over sixfold higher than those in prepubertal boys indicated an extragonadal androgen source. The adrenal glands may be the primary sources of androgen in the castrated male. (See Fig. 3) The adrenal androgens in men have been reviewed by Migeon (44).

Whether or not there is increased adrenal function following castration has not been resolved. In animals there is evidence that castration causes increased levels of ACTH and some degree of adrenal hyperplasia (35). The effects of castration, androgens, estrogens, and hepatic function in regula- ting pituitary-adrenal function are very complex and have not been resolved in detail for man.

Because of the suspected involvement of the adrenal glands in androgen effects on prostatic adenocarcinoma in castrated males, adrenalectomy was performed as a palliative treatment as early as 1945 (51). The current approach to adrenalectomy has been reviewed by Banalaph (6), who did not observe suppression of the plasma testosterone level in castrates after adrenalectomy. Robinson et.al. (47) have also discussed adrenal suppression in treatment of carcinoma of the prostate.

Blocking adrenal steroidogenesis with chemical inhibitors does indeed lower the plasma levels of testosterone in men who have been castrated previously. Spironolactone, a steroidal aldosterone antagoint, is capable of inhibiting the 17,20-1yase enzyme and thus reducing the adrenal synthesis of androgens.

If administration is continued for a month, spironolactone lowers the castrate plasma level of testosterone by over 80 per cent (70).

Aminoglutethimide is capable of suppressing all adrenal steroid synthesis by
producing a reversible inhibition of the enzymatic conversion of cholesterol
to pregnenolone. Aminoglutethimide has been used to treat patients with
prostatic adenocarcinoma who have become refractory to orchiectomy (40).
Glucocorticoid supplement was required when this drug was utilized.

Other pharmacologic approaches to inhibiting steroid synthesis as well as
the regulatory effects of natural factors such as thyroxine and estradiol
have been reviewed in detail by Gaunt et.al. (23).

An additional method of blocking the effects of adrenal steroids is the
administration of antiandrogens, which appear to block adrenal androgen
action directly at the prostate subcellular level through competitive interactions (69).

Gonadotropins: The amount of testosterone produced by Leydig cells in the
testes is controlled in part by the plasma levels of the luteinizing hormone
(LH) released from the anterior pituitary gland. In turn, testosterone is
involved in a negative feedback regulation of the pituitary. When animals
are castrated, thus eliminating the major source of androgens, there is a
dramatic increase in the plasma levels of both LH and FSH. After castration,
specific alterations are observed in the morphology of the pituitary, in
which "castration cells" are observed. The formation of these cells can be
prevented by the administration of exogeneous androgens. Testosterone can
inhibit the synthesis of LH and the release of FSH in castrated male and
female rats, but it is less effective than estrogen.

Testosterone treatment (50 mg) of intact and castrated adult males results
in a marked suppression of pituitary LH release and of plasma LH levels.
With increasing doses of testosterone (100 mg), the FSH plasma level is also
lowered. In contrast, estrogen administered to human males causes a decrease
in both LH and FSH levels. Therefore, testosterone preferentially suppresses
serum LH relative to serum FSH, whereas estradiol produces parallel inhibition of both LH and FSH.

It is now apparent that at least part of the negative feedback by steroids
on the function of the pituitary is mediated by inhibiting the secretion of
the LH-releasing hormone (LRH), which originates as a neuro-humoral factor
in the hypothalamus and is carried to the anterior pituitary via the hypo-

14

physeal portal blood supply. The secretion of these neurohumoral hypotha-
lamic releasing factors is in part under the influence of the central nervous
system (CNS).

Hypophysectomy: Other factors besides testicular androgens have been implicated in prostatic growth; however, they usually have been termed permissive
or synergistic in that either they augment androgenic stimulation or their
absence causes a further involution of an already atrophied gland. Huggins
and Russel (33) reported that hypophysectomy of the dog produced more epithelial atrophy than did castration alone.

The possibility that pituitary factors may contribute to prostatic maintenance in castrated animals raised the possibility that such effects might also
operate in patients with prostatic adenocarcinoma who have relapsed from the
benefits of castration (51,53). At present, hypophysectomy and adrenalectomy
are not routinely performed in patients with disseminated prostatic cancer
because the potential benefits in the control of hormone-insensitive prostatic tumors have not been established.

Prolactin: In hypophysectomized rats, exogenous androgens were not capable
of restoring full prostatic growth unless these animals were given supplements
of exogenous prolactin (27). This observation has now been confirmed in numerous animal experiments, in which prolactin was shown to be synergistic
with androgens on growth (14). Prolactin receptors have been identified in
prostatic tissue (4).

The accumulated evidence that prolactin affects prostatic growth in animals
has led to much speculation about a similar role in humans. Prolactin levels
in human blood are elevated with estrogens, some tranquilizing drugs, and
stress, and can be decreased by L-dopa and ergot derivatives. At present,
with improved assays, the levels are being monitored in patients of advanced
age and in those with benign prostatic hyperplasia, but no clear correlation
of cause and effect is yet apparent (3).

Insulin: Like prolactin, insulin has been reported to have synergistic or
permissive effects on prostatic growth, but these data have been obtained
previously in rodents and often in tissue or organ culture (2,59). There is
little information on the possible role of insulin in the growth of the
human prostate.

Effects at the Cellular Level: Some of the molecular events occurring in the
prostatic cell are depicted in Figure 4. Free testosterone in the plasma

15

FIGURE 4

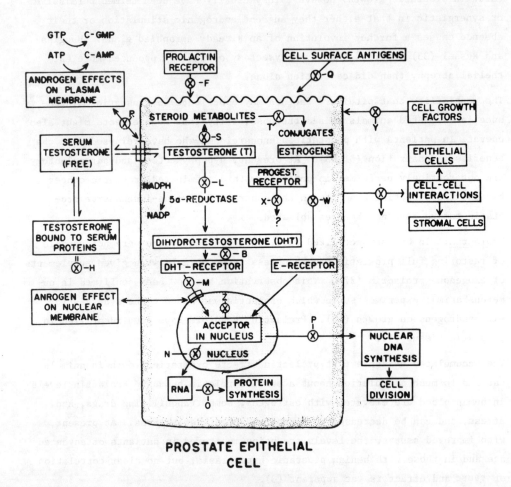

**PROSTATE EPITHELIAL
CELL**

⊗ - TARGET SITE FOR THERAPY

appears to enter the prostate cell by passive diffusion; this conclusion is based on the inability to saturate the uptake and the lack of a marked temperature effect. Steroids such as testosterone also have the potential to interact with plasma membrane components, and through this action many hormones activate membrane adenyl cyclase enzyme complexes, which catalyze the synthesis of the 3':5' nucleotide monophosphate, cyclic AMP (cAMP). Singhal et.al. (58) reported that the administration of cAMP to the castrated rodent caused an increase in prostatic wet weight and the induction of certain glycolytic enzymes. Lesser and Bruchovsky (36) have reported that cAMP administration does not induce cell proliferation, which is an essential element of androgen-induced prostatic growth. Neither did cAMP stimulate RNA polymerase or polyamine levels (41). It therefore appears that cAMP may initiate some effects of testosterone but not other important events related to cellular growth.

Once the free testosterone has entered the prostatic epithelial cell, it is rapidly metabolized to other steroid forms by a series of prostatic enzymes. Over 90 per cent of the testosterone is converted to dihydrotestosterone (DHT) through the action of NADPH and the enzyme 5α-reductase, which reduce the unsaturated bond between the 4 and 5 positions to form the 5α-reduced product of testosterone; the full name for 5α-reductase is Δ^4-3-ketosteroid 5α-oxidoreductase. The 5α-reductase enzyme is located on the endoplasmic reticulum and the nuclear membrane. The formation of DHT, its binding to cytoplasmic receptors, and its subsequent transport into the nucleus have been extensively reviewed (45). Once in the nucleus the DHT-receptor complex interacts with a nuclear acceptor (DNA, chromatin, or nuclear acidic proteins), not fully defined at present, to release genome and DNA template restrictions in an unknown manner. Once the steroid receptor complex binds to the nuclear chromatin a series of orderly and timed events ensue, starting with an increase in (1) a protein initiation factor, (2) messenger RNA and ribosomal RNA synthesis, (3) cellular protein synthesis, and (4) cell replication. The effects of androgens can be blocked in a competitive manner at the cellular level by steroid antagonists (termed antiandrogens), but not by estrogens.

The major effect of estrogens in inhibiting prostate growth appears to take place through the hypothalamic-pituitary-gonadal axis to block testicular synthesis of testosterone and thus lower the plasma testosterone levels. If castrated animals receive injections of both estrogens and androgens, a

17

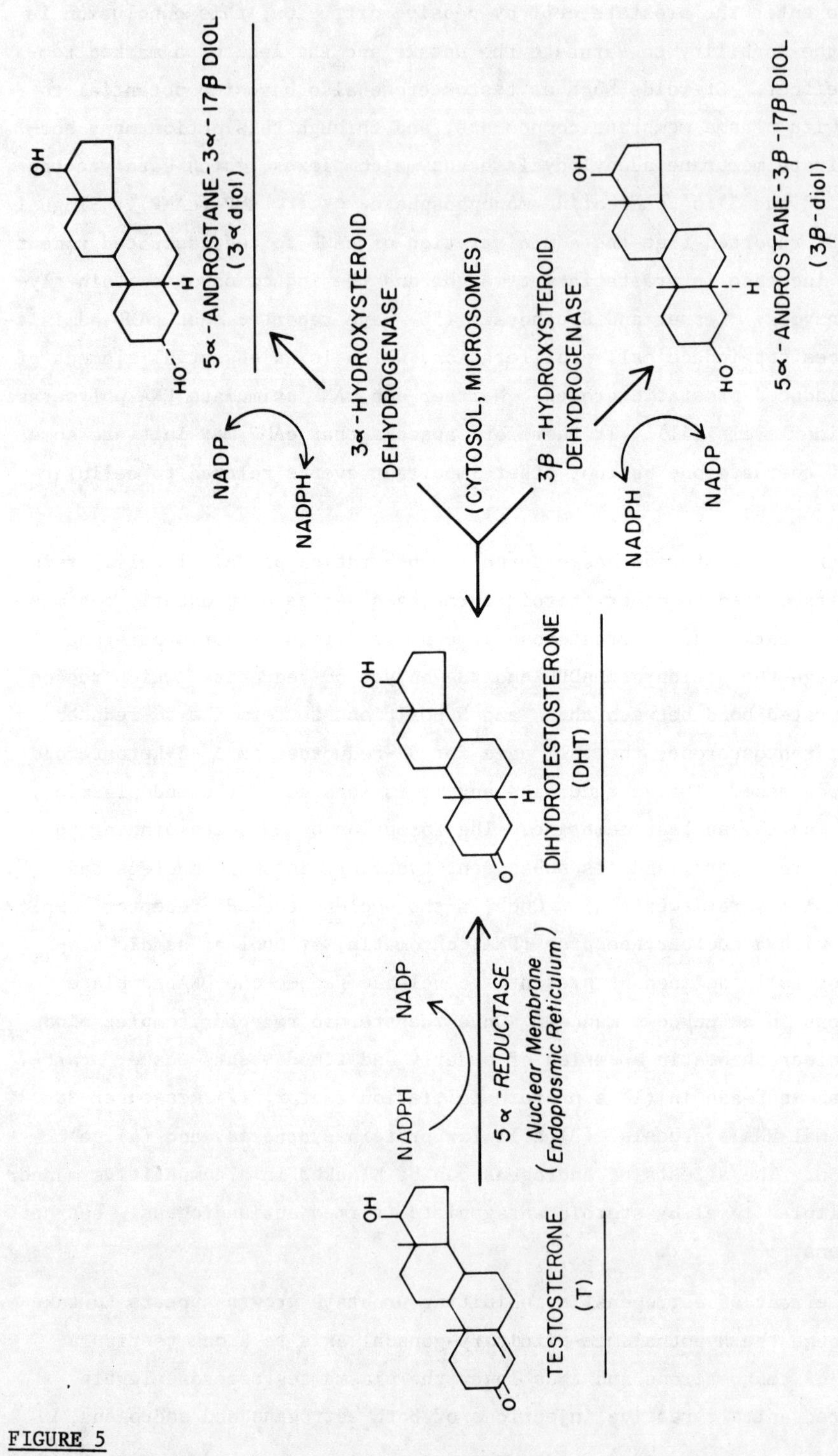
TESTOSTERONE
(T)
NADPH
NADP
5α-REDUCTASE
Nuclear Membrane
(Endoplasmic Reticulum)
DIHYDROTESTOSTERONE
(DHT)
(CYTOSOL, MICROSOMES)
NADPH
NADP
3α-HYDROXYSTEROID
DEHYDROGENASE
5α-ANDROSTANE-3α-17β DIOL
(3α diol)
3β-HYDROXYSTEROID
DEHYDROGENASE
NADPH
NADP
5α-ANDROSTANE-3β-17β DIOL
(3β-diol)

FIGURE 5

full growth of the prostate is realized, indicating the inability of estrogens to block androgen-induced growth at the cellular level. When estrogens do exert a direct effect on the prostate it is usually by stimulation of meta-plastic growth in the cells of the collecting ducts. There may be other unidentified effects of estrogens, particularly since the prostate contains a cytoplasmic receptor for estrogens (30).

Cytoplasmic progesterone receptors have also been observed in human prostatic tissues, and their function is also unknown (42).

Since DHT was established as the active androgen in the prostate nucleus, attention was given to the possible role of this metabolite in abnormal growth of the prostate in both humans and dogs. Wilson and his colleagues esta-blished that prostatic tissue levels of DHT were elevated three- to four-fold in benign prostatic hyperplasia in both dogs and men, but tissue levels of testosterone were not altered (25,57). Walsh and Wilson have induced the first experimental case of benign prostatic hyperplasia in the castrated dog by the administration of exogenous 5α-androstane-3α, 17β diol. This induction was enhanced in the presence of exogenous estrogens. The active 3α-diol meta-bolite is produced from DHT through the reduction of the 3-keto position by 3α-hydroxysteroid dehydrogenase (Fig. 5).

Recent studies by DeKlerk et.al. have also shown that the administration of dihydrotestosterone, particularly in the presence of estrogens, can also induce a marked hyperplastic prostate in young castrate beagles (15).

For more details of the physiological control of the prostate gland, consult the recent review of Coffey (12).

References

1. Anderson, K. M., and Liao, S.: Selective retention of dihydrotestos-terone by prostatic nuclei. Nature, 219: 277-279; 1968.
2. Angervall, L., Hesselsjo, R., Nilsson, S., and Tissel, L. E.: Action of testosterone on ventral prostate, dorsolateral prostate, coagulating glands, and seminal vesicles of castrated alloxandiabetic rats. Diabetologia, 3: 395; 1967.
3. Aragona, C., and Friesen, H. G.: Prolactin and Aging. In Grayhack, J. T., Wilson, J. D., and Scherbenske, M. J. (Eds.): Benign Prostatic Hyperplasia. Proceedings of a workshop sponsored by the Kidney Disease and Urology Program of the National Institute of Arthritis, Metabolism and Digestive Diseases, DHEW Publication No. (NIH) 76-1113.
4. Aragona, C., and Friesen, H. G.: Specific prolactin binding sites in the prostate and testis of rat. Endocrinology, 97: 677; 1975.
5. Arvola, I.: The hormonal control of the amounts of the tissue components of the prostate. Ann. Chir. Gynaecol. Fenn., 50:

Suppl. 102: 1-120; 1961.

6. Banalaph, T., Varkarakis, M. S., and Murphy, C. P.: Current status of bilateral adrenalectomy for advanced prostatic carcinoma. Ann. Surg., 179: 17; 1974.

7. Brandes, D. (Ed.): Male Accessory Sex Organs: Structure and Function in Mammals. New York, Academic Press, 1974.

8. Breuer, H., Hamel, D., and Kruskemper, H. L.: Methods of Hormone Analysis. New York, John Wiley & Sons, 1976.

9. Bruchovsky, N., and Wilson, J. D.: The conversion of testosterone to 5α-androstan-17β-ol-3-one by rat prostate in vivo and in vitro. J. Biol. Chem., 243: 2012-2021, 1968a.

10. Bruchovsky, N., and Wilson, J. D.: The intranuclear binding of testosterone and 5α-androstan-17β-ol-3-one by rat prostate. J. Biol. Chem., 243: 5953-5960, 1968b.

11. Burton, R. M., and Westphal, U: Steroid hormone binding proteins in blood plasma. Metabolism, 21: 253-276, 1972.

12. Coffey, D. S.: The Biochemistry and Physiology of the Prostate and Seminal Vesicles. In Campbell's Urology, 4th ed., Harrison, J. H., Gittes, R. F., Perlmutter, A. D., Stamey, T. A., and Walsh, P. C. (eds.), Volume I, p. 161-201. W. B. Saunders Co., Philadelphia, 1978.

13. Conti, C., Sciarra, F., and Sorcini, G.: Androgen Sources. In Bracci, N., and DiSilverio, F. (Eds.): Hormonal Therapy of Prostatic Cancer. p. 59. Rome, Cofese Publishers, 1975.

14. Danutra, V., Harper, M. E., Boyns, A. K., Cole, E. N., Brownsey, B. G., and Griffith, K.: The effect of certain stilbestrol analogues on plasma prolactin and testosterone in the rat. J. Endocrinol., 57: 207, 1973.

15. DeKlerk, D. P., Coffey, D. S., Ewing, L. L., McDermott, I. R., Reiner, W. G., Robinson, C. H., Scott, W. W., Strandberg, J. D., Talalay, P., Walsh, P. C., Wheaton, L. G., and Zirkin, B. R.: A Comparison of Spontaneous and Experimentally Induced Canine Prostatic Hyperplasia. J. Clin. Invest. (In press), 1979.

16. Doering, C. H., Kraemer, H. C., Brodie, K. H., and Hamburg, D. A.: A cycle of plasma testosterone in the human male. J. Clin. Endocrinol. Metab., 40: 492-500, 1975.

17. Dorfman, R. I.: Methods in Hormone Research. Vol. II. Bioassay. New York, Academic Press, 1962.

18. Forest, M. G., Cathiard, A. M., and Bertrand, J. A.: Total and unbound testosterone levels in the newborn and in normal and hypogonadal children: use of a sensitive radioimmunoassay for testosterone. J. Clin. Endocrinol. Metab., 36: 1132-1142, 1973.

19. Franks, L. M.: Benign prostatic hyperplasia of the prostate. Ann. R. Coll. Surg. Engl., 14: 92, 1954a.

20. Franks, L. M.: Latent carcinoma. Ann. R. Coll. Surg. Engl., 15: 236, 1954b.

21. Franks, L. M.: Latency and progressions in human tumors. Lancet, 2: 1037, 1956.

22. Frieden, E. H.: Chemical Endocrinology. New York, Academic Press, 1976.

23. Gaunt, R., Steinetz, B. G., and Chart, J. J.: Pharmacological alteration of steroid hormone functions. Clin. Pharmacol. Ther., 9: 657, 1968.

24. Gaynor, E. P.: Zur Frage des Prostakrebses. Virchows Arch. Pathol. Anat., 301: 602, 1938.

25. Gloyna, R. E., Siiteri, P. K., and Wilson, J. D.: Dihydrotestosterone in prostatic hypertrophy, II. The formation

and content of dihydrotestosterone in hypertrophic canine prostate and the effect of dihydrotestosterone on prostatic growth in the dog. J. Clin. Invest., 49: 1746-1753, 1970.

26. Goland, M. (Ed.): Normal and Abnormal Growth of the Prostate. Springfield, Illinois, Charles C. Thomas, Publishers, 1975.

27. Grayhack, J. T., Bunce, P. L., Kearns, J. W., and Scott, W. W.: Influence of the pituitary on prostatic response to androgen in the rat. Bull. Johns Hopkins Hosp., 96: 154, 1955.

28. Grayhack, J. T., Wilson, J. D., and Scherbenske, M. J. (Eds.): Benign Prostatic Hyperplasia. Proceedings of a workshop sponsored by the Kidney Disease and Urology Program of the NIAMDD. Washington, D.C., U. S. Gov't. Printing Office, 1976.

29. Harbitz, T. B., and Haugen, O. A.: Histology of the prostate in elderly men. Acta Pathol. Microbiol. Scand., 80: 756-768, 1972.

30. Hawkins, E. F., Nijs, M., Brassinne, C., et al.: Steroid receptors in the human prostate. 1. Estradiol-17β binding in benign prostatic hypertrophy. Steroids, 26: 458-469, 1975.

31. Horton, R. J.: Androgen Hormones and Prehormones in Young and Elderly Men. In Grayhack, J. T., Wilson, J. D., and Scherbenske, M. J. (Eds.): Benign Prostatic Hyperplasia. Proceedings of a workshop sponsored by the Kidney Disease and Urology Program of the NIAMDD, pp. 183-188. Washington, D.C., U. S. Gov't. Printing Office, 1976.

32. Huggins, C., and Moulder, P. V.: Estrogen production by Sertoli cell tumors of the testis. Cancer Res., 5: 510, 1945.

33. Huggins, C. and Russell, P. S.: Quantitative effects of hypophysectomy on testis and prostate of dogs. Endocrinology, 39: 1, 1946.

34. Kent, J. R., Bischoft, A. J., Arduino, L. J., et al.: Estrogen dosage and suppression of testosterone levels in patients with prostatic carcinoma. J. Urol., 109: 858, 1973.

35. Kitay, J. I.: Pituitary-adrenal function in the rat after gonadectomy and gonadal hormone replacement. Endocrinology, 73: 253, 1963.

36. Lesser, B., and Bruchovsky, N.: The effects of testosterone, 5α-dihydrotestosterone and adenosine 3',5'-monophosphate on cell proliferation and differentiation in rat prostate. Biochem. Biophys. Acta, 308: 426-437, 1973.

37. Lipsett, M. B.: Steroid secretion by the human testis. In Rosemberg, E., and Paulsen, C. A. (Eds.): The Human Testis. pp. 407-421. New York, Plenum Press, 1970.

38. Lostroh, A. J.: Effect of testosterone and insulin in vitro on maintenance and repair of the secretory epithelium of the mouse prostate. Endocrinology, 88: 500-503, 1971.

39. Lundberg, S., and Berge, T.: Prostatic carcinoma. An autopsy study. Scand. J. Urol. Nephrol., 4: 93-97, 1970.

40. MacDonald, P. C.: Origin of Estrogen in Men. In Grayhack, J. T., Wilson, J. D., and Scherbenske, M. J. (Eds.): Benign Prostatic Hyperplasia. Proceedings of a workshop sponsored by the Kidney Disease and Urology Program of the NIAMDD, Feb. 20-21, 1975. pp. 191-192. Washington, D.C., U. S. Gov't. Printing Office, 1976.

41. Mangan, F. R., Pegg, A. E., and Mainwaring, W. I. P.: A reappraisal of the effects of adenosine 3':5'-cyclic monophosphate on the function and morphology of the rat prostate gland. Biochem. J., 134: 129-142, 1973.

42. Menon, M., Tananis, C. E., Hicks, L. L., Hawkins, E. F., McLoughlin, M. G., and Walsh, P. C.: Characterization of the

binding of a potent synthetic androgen, methyltrienolone (R1881) to human tissues. J. Clin. Invest., 61: 150-162, 1978.

43. Menon, M., Tananis, C. E., McLoughlin, M. G., and Walsh, P. C.: Androgen receptors in human prostatic tissue: A review. Cancer Treat. Rep., 61: 265, 1977.

44. Migeon, C. J.: Adrenal androgens in man. Am. J. Med., 53: 606, 1972.

45. Moore, R. A., and Wilson, J. D.: Androgen transport and metabolism in the prostate. In Grayhack, J. T., Wilson, J. D., and Scherbenske, M. J. (Eds.): Benign Prostatic Hyperplasia. Proceedings of a workshop sponsored by the Kidney Disease and Urology Program of the NIAMDD, Feb. 20-21, 1975. p. 21-29, Washington, D.C., U. S. Gov't. Printing Office, 1976.

46. Robinson, M. R. G., and Thomas, B. S.: Effect of hormonal therapy on plasma testosterone levels in prostatic carcinoma. Br. Med. J., 4: 391, 1971.

47. Robinson, M. R. G., Shearer, R. J., and Fergusson, J. D.: Adrenal suppression in the treatment of carcinoma of the prostate. Br. J. Urol., 46: 555, 1974.

48. Sanford, E. J., Drago, J. R., Rohner, T. J., Santen, R., and Lipton, A.: Aminoglutethimide medical adrenalectomy for advanced prostatic carcinoma. J. Urol., 115: 170, 1976.

49. Sciarra, F., Sorcini, G., DiSilverio, F., and Gagliardi, V.: Plasma testosterone and androstenedione after orchiectomy in prostatic adenocarcinoma. Clin. Endocrinol., 2: 110, 1973.

50. Scott, W. W.: The lipids of the prostatic fluid, seminal plasma and enlarged prostate gland of man. J. Urol., 53: 712, 1945.

51. Scott, W. W.: Endocrine management of disseminated prostatic cancer, including bilateral adrenalectomy and hypophysectomy. Trans. Am. Assoc. Genitourin. Surg., 44: 101, 1952.

52. Scott, W. W.: Growth and Development of the Human Prostate. In Vollmer, E. P. (Ed.): Biology of the Prostate and Related Tissues. National Cancer Institute Monograph 12. pp. 111-130. Bethesda, Md., National Cancer Institute, 1963.

53. Scott, W. W., and Schirmer, H. K. A.: Hypophysectomy for Disseminated Prostatic Cancer. In Boyland, E., et al.: On Cancer and Hormones. Chicago, University of Chicago Press, 1962.

54. Seidman, H., Silverberg, E., and Holleg, A. I.: Cancer Statistics, 1976. New York, American Cancer Society, 1976.

55. Shearer, R. J., Hendry, W. F., Sommerville, I. F., and Ferguson, J. D.: Plasma testosterone: An accurate monitor of hormone treatment in prostatic cancer. Br. J. Urol., 45: 668, 1973.

56. Siiteri, P. K. and MacDonald, P. C.: Role of Extraglandular Estrogen in Human Endocrinology. In Greep, R.O., and Astwood, E. B. (Eds.): Handbook of Physiology, Section 7. Endocrinology, Vol. II, Chap. 28, pp. 615-629. Baltimore, The Williams & Wilkins Co., 1973.

57. Siiteri, P. K., and Wilson, J. D.: Dihydrotestosterone in Prostatic Hypertrophy, I. The Formation and Content of Dihydrotestosterone in the Hypertrophic Prostate of Man. J. Clin. Invest., 49: 1737-1745, 1970.

58. Singhal, R. L.: Cyclic AMP: Testosterone-like stimulation of prostatic enzymes. Ann. New York Acad. Sci., 185: 181, 1971.

59. Sufrin, G., and Prutkin, L.: Experimental diabetes and the response of the sex accessory organs on the castrate male rat to testosterone propionate. Invest. Urol., 11: 361, 1974.

60. Swyer, G. I. M.: Post-natal growth. Changes in the human prostate. J. Anat., 78: 130, 1944.
61. Tannenbaum, M. (Ed.): Urologic Pathology: The Prostate. Philadelphia, Lea & Febiger, 1977.
62. Tesar, C., and Scott, W. W.: A search for inhibitors of prostatic growth stimulators. Invest. Urol., 1: 482, 1966.
63. Tisell, L. E.: Effect of cortisone on the growth of the ventral prostate, the dorsolateral prostate, the coagulating gland and the seminal adrenalectomized rats. Acta Endocrinol., 64: 637, 1970.
64. Tullner, W. W.: Hormonal Factors in the Adrenal Dependent Growth of the Rat Ventral Prostate. In Vollmer, E. P. (Ed.): Biology of the Prostate and Related Tissues. National Cancer Institute Monograph 12. p. 211. Bethesda, Maryland, National Cancer Institute, 1963.
65. Vermeulen, A.: The Physical State of Testosterone in Plasma. In James, V. H. T., Serio, M., and Martini, L. (Eds.): The Endocrine Function of the Human Testis. Vol. I, pp. 157-170. New York, Academic Press, 1973.
66. Vermeulen, A.: Testicular Hormonal Secretion and Aging in Males. In Grayhack, J. T., Wilson, J. D., and Scherbenske, M. J. (Eds.): Benign Prostatic Hyperplasia. Proceedings of a workshop sponsored by the Kidney Disease and Urology Program of the NIAMDD, Feb. 20-21, 1975, p. 177. Washington, D.C., U. S. Gov't. Printing Office, 1976.
67. Vida, J. A.: Androgens and Anabolic Agents. New York, Academic Press, 1969.
68. Walsh, P. C.: Physiologic basis for hormonal therapy in carcinoma of the prostate. Urol. Clin. North Am., 2 (1): 125, 1975.
69. Walsh, P. C., and Gittes, R. F.: Inhibition of extratesticular stimuli to prostatic growth in the castrate rat by antiandrogens. Endrocrinology, 87: 624, 1970.
70. Walsh, P. C., and Siiteri, P. K.: Suppression of plasma androgens by spironolactone in castrated men with carcinoma of the prostate. J. Urol., 114: 254, 1975.
71. Williams, D. L., and Chisholm, G. D.: Scientific Foundations of Urology, Vol. II. Chicago, Year Book Medical Publishers, 1976.
72. Young, H. H., II, and Kent, J. R.: Plasma testosterone levels in patients with prostatic carcinoma before and after treatment. J. Urol., 99: 788, 1968.

Chapter II.   NEW MORPHOLOGIC FINDINGS RELEVENT TO THE ORIGIN AND
EVOLUTION OF CARCINOMA OF THE PROSTATE AND BPH*

The prostate gland is an organ of complex composition, enclosing within
a single capsule a number of diverse tissues, both glandular and non-
glandular. Historically a concentration of attention on those tissue
components which are of greatest pathologic and physiologic importance
has diverted interest from studying the organ as a whole. Investigation
of anatomic subdivisions has often not been systematic, and conclusions
based on casual observations have led to confusion in terminology and
concepts. Yet proper identification of all components of the prostate
and their anatomic relationships is necessary for a precise definition
of those regions of major interest. In particular, the task of discover-
ing the earliest morphologic and biochemical changes in the evolution of
BPH and carcinoma requires a high degree of anatomic selectivity in choos-
ing tissues for study. Therefore, in order to review the morphologic
evidence for the mode of origin and early evolution of BPH and carcinoma
in the prostate, we should first outline the major anatomic regions of the
gland and relate them to the site of origin of disease.

REGIONAL COMPOSITION OF THE PROSTATE

There are four major anatomic subdivisions in the prostate (8,9). Each
region makes contact with a specific portion of the prostatic urethra,
which can therefore be taken as the primary anatomic landmark for defining
them. The prostatic urethra can be further subdivided at its midpoint
into a proximal or pre-prostatic segment and a distal or prostatic segment
on the basis that all the major ducts of the glandular prostate enter
the urethra in its distal half. The line of division lies at about the
upper end of the verumontanum. Proximal to this point the course of the
urethra is angled abruptly anterior at about 30° to accomodate the ejaculatory ducts, which approach the upper end of the verumontanum along a
nearly vertical course. The regions so identified are as follows:

1.   The anterior fibromuscular stroma comprises up to one third the
total bulk of the prostate and represents almost all of its non-glandular
tissue. It consists of a thick sheet of tissue covering the entire anterior
surface of the organ and hiding the urethra and glandular portions of the
prostate from view anteriorly (Fig. 1). It surrounds the urethra proximally
at its junction with the bladder neck and merges there with the internal

*John E. McNeal

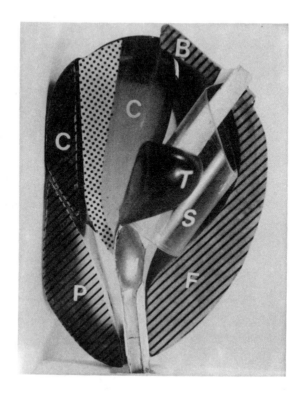

Three dimensional model of prostate anatomy, side view. Sagittal cuts
(lined areas) have removed near side of fibromuscular stroma (F), bladder
neck (B), central zone (C), and peripheral zone (P). Transition zone (T),
sphincter (S), and urethra with verumontanum (V) are seen in full. Periurethral ducts hidden behind transition zone. Ejaculatory ducts (stippled)
traverse center of central zone.

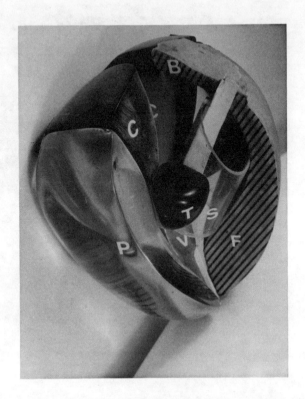

Three dimensional model of prostate anatomy, 3/4 view. Near side of fibro-muscular stroma and bladder neck only removed by sagittal cut. Same symbols as Figure 1.

sphincter and detrusor muscle, from which it originates. It sweeps down-
ward and laterally as an apron of smooth muscle, directly continuous with
that of the bladder wall, and contacts the urethra again at the apex of
the prostate. But near the apex, the smooth muscle is replaced by transverse loops of striated muscle. This proximal extension of the external
sphincter lies behind the smooth muscle apron, forming an incomplete
sphincter along the anterior aspect of the entire distal urethral segment.
Near the verumontanum, both components become increasingly fibrous and
partly blend with each other.

2.   The peripheral zone is the largest anatomic subdivision of the
prostate. It is part of the functioning glandular prostate, and it contains
most of the secretory epithelial tissue of the organ. Its duct orifices
form two rows along the postero-lateral recesses of the urethral wall,
confined to its distal segment between the upper end of the verumontanum
and the prostate apex. The ducts course directly lateral, and the secretory tissue forms a flat disc lateral to the distal urethral segment and
extending a short distance posteriorly. Some duct branches also cup anteriorly at their peripheries to partly surround the striated muscle sphincter.

3.   The central zone is the smaller of the two subdivisions of the
functioning glandular prostate - about 25% of its mass. It contacts the
urethra only at the upper end of the verumontanum, where its duct orifices
open in a tight circle immediately around the ejaculatory duct orifices
and remote from those of the peripheral zone. The central zone ducts
branch proximally, surrounding closely the proximal course of the ejaculatory ducts and fanning out to form a wedge of tissue with its base at the
base of the prostate posterior to the bladder neck. In fanning out laterally, these ducts contact the superior margin of the peripheral zone,
adding a superior quadrant to complete its flat disc of secretory tissue.
Externally, no demarcation can be seen between these two zones.

The separate identity of central and peripheral zones depends primarily
on differences in duct architecture and epithelial appearance; it only
secondarily rests on these distinctions of anatomic location. The peripheral zone ducts are long, narrow, and straight, with short terminal
branches ending in small, simple, round acini. The central zone ducts
are larger, with more complex arborization. They produce large acini of
irregular contour, partly compartmentalized by septa. The peripheral

zone epithelium consists of pale cells in simple columnar arrangement, with basal, small, dark nuclei, and distinct cell borders. The central zone cells have granular, opaque cytoplasm. They are irregularly crowded, so that nuclei lie at different levels. The nuclei tend to be larger and more variable in size.

4.   Finally the pre-prostatic tissue is related to the entire length of the proximal (pre-prostatic) urethral segment. This is the smallest region but the most complex in arrangement of both glandular and non-glandular elements. Its main component is non-glandular - a cylindrical smooth muscle sphincter surrounding the entire course of the urethra above the verumontanum. Closely related to the sphincter are two tiny areas of pre-prostatic glandular tissue, one of these inside the sleeve of sphincteric tissue and the other immediately outside it. The smaller - the periurethral glands - consists of simple, straight ducts of near microscopic size arising from the urethral wall inside the sphincter and coursing for a few millimeters proximally, parallel to the urethra. Their levels of origin and numbers are inconstant, but they tend to be more frequent near the verumontanum than more proximally. They have few branches, few or no acini, and no periductal smooth muscle since their only stroma is that of the urethra itself. Hence they are unlikely to play any significant role in adult prostatic function.

At the lower border of the sphincter, in a very short segment near the upper end of the verumontanum, the lateral urethral wall receives the orifices of the transition zone ducts. These small ducts, of constant origin and location, pass around the distal end of the sphincter and branch proximally toward the bladder neck immediately outside the sphincter. They have a fairly elaborate branch system, which fills the shallow cleft between the peripheral zone and the sphincter but extends for only a short distance proximally toward the bladder neck. The acini in part have their own smooth muscle cuffs, but there is much intermingling of sphincteric stroma with transition zone glandular tissue.

The transition zone epithelium resembles that of the peripheral zone and **is** unlike the central zone epithelium. In fact, both the transition zone ducts and the periurethral ducts represent a continuation proximal to the verumontanum of the lateral line of peripheral zone ducts. All three regions therefore appear to be the product of the same process of embryonic organogenesis. However, the two pre-prostatic components are distinguished by their abortive glandular development and their imperfectly developed stroma, which is partly replaced by non-glandular sphincteric or urethral stroma. The sphincter itself blends proximally with the bladder neck muscle, and so this non-glandular component of the pre-prostatic tissue is related to the fibromuscular region of the prostate, just as its glandular components are related to the peripheral zone. The pre-prostatic tissue therefore is not an entity of unique compostion like the other three regions. It is rather an embryonic transition region between bladder and sphincteric organogenesis proximally and peripheral zone organogenesis distally. In the amalgam of these two inappropriately juxtaposed tissues, it seems likely that the resultant adult function is purely bladder neck and sphincteric rather than prostatic and secretory.

ANATOMY OF PROSTATIC DISEASE

It has recently been found that most BPH develops in the transition zone, especially in that medial portion where there is mingling of glands with sphincteric stroma (9). The periurethral ducts are also involved in BPH origin, though much less prominently. Thus BPH consistently arises in close proximity to the urethra but only along a very short portion of its course through the gland. The total volume of the tissue of origin is very small - perhaps less than 5% of the tissue of the entire glandular portion of the prostate.

Carcinoma has recently been described to arise almost entirely in the peripheral zone (7), and its distribution within that zone was found to be quite uniform between different areas. A very few carcinomas appeared to arise in the central zone, but there was an abrupt decline in frequency exactly at the boundary between the two zones.

These findings are in disagreement with previous studies, which in turn seem to contradict each other. By analysis of specific points of similarity and difference, much of the apparent confusion can be resolved. For example, there is strong agreement in all studies that BPH arises close to the urethra. Franks studied this relationship in detail (2), and his "inner prostate" roughly corresponds to the area of BPH susceptibility identified above (Fig. 2). However, he failed to recognize that BPH origin was limited to a short portion of the urethra. Furthermore, he did not describe the cylindrical sphincter nor the specific duct systems

Figure 2.

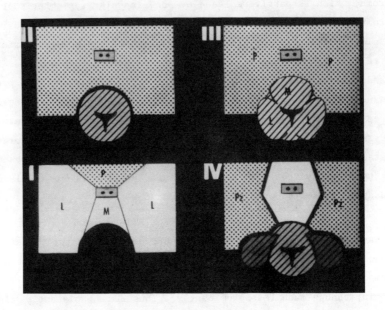

Conflicting concepts of prostate anatomy compared in transverse plane proximal
to verumontanum. There is concensus that origin of BPH (lined area) coincides
with periurethral or inner prostate (I.P.). Divergent views of outer prostate
(O.P.):

    I.   Lowsley - 1912. O.P. is histologically homogeneous but sub-
        divided on embryonic grounds. Carcinoma (stippled) found only
        posterior to ejaculatory ducts. Periurethral (I.P.) region not
        evaluated.

    II. Franks - 1954. O.P. histologically homogeneous with <u>no</u> sub-
        divisions. Carcinoma found everywhere.

    III. Composite (I. & II.). Lowsley's lateral (L) and middle (M) lobe
        terms transferred to I.P. which has BPH nodular deformity. Car-
        cinoma distribution follows Franks, but all O.P. called posterior
        lobe (P).

    IV. McNeal - 1968. O.P. histologically <u>heterogeneous</u>. Central zone
        surrounds ejaculatory ducts, is free of disease. Carcinoma
        diffuse in peripheral zone (Pz). I.P. subdivided by newly
        described transition zone and sphincter.

involved. Such additional, more specific data may hold valuable clues
to pathogenesis of BPH, as well as providing important landmarks for
selecting tissue for study. Franks and others collected data mainly
from transverse sections through the midportion of the prostate near the
verumontanum. The assumption was made that the anatomy of urethra and
prostate both proximal and distal to this plane was the same. Consequently, the sphincter and the transition zone, as well as the central
zone and the relationships of all these structures to disease were probably never visualized in these studies.

Franks reached two other important conclusions. He stated that away from
the periurethral or inner prostate there were no anatomic boundaries in
the gland. He also found that the frequency of carcinoma origin was
uniform throughout the prostate, except for its absence in the inner
gland. These results are actually in perfect agreement with the findings
described here, providing that the only data examined are those which
can be seen on transverse sections taken through the verumontanum. In
this plane, extensively utilized by Franks, the central zone is not
visualized.

The position stated by Franks was intended to refute the findings of
Lowsley, who identified posterior, lateral, and middle lobes in the
prostate away from the periurethral or inner gland (5). Lowsley concluded that carcinoma arose exclusively within the boundaries of the
posterior lobe. This concept had already been challenged previously, and
it is refuted by current data (7) showing most carcinomas to develop
outside the boundaries which Lowsley proposed for the posterior lobe.

Until recently, the prostate has been universally considered to be histologically homogeneous. Lowsley's failure to recognize any heterogeneity
was inevitable since his observations were based on fetal prostates, in
which the distinctive histologic differences have not yet developed.
However, his definitions of the prostate lobes are incompatible with the
current description of central and peripheral zones since the boundary
locations in the two systems conflict. However, the existence of the
posterior lobe has been refuted by LeDuc with injection studies of prostatic ducts in normal adults (4). He demonstrated that all the main
prostatic ducts course laterally; no posteriorly directed ducts, required
to define the posterior lobe, could be identified. Furthermore the exis-

31

tence of Lowsley's lobes is not supported by any anatomic landmarks in the
adult, while the identity of the central and peripheral zones is substantiated both by landmarks and histologic differences.

In recent years, colloquial usage has adapted Lowsley's terminology to a
description of Franks' basic concept. Those nodules of BPH which lie
lateral and posterior to the urethra have been called the "lateral lobes"
and "middle lobe", leaving Franks outer prostate to be misidentified as
"posterior lobe". This compromise view is invalidated by a serious conceptual error. Neither BPH nodules nor their precursors are represented by
any discrete anatomic structures in the normal prostate. It also violates
Lowsley's definition, in which the periurethral tissue was specifically not
included in _any_ of the lobes.

Finally Franks concept of the location of carcinoma origin was later
modified by the idea that within Franks' outer prostate the distribution of
carcinoma was not uniform but rather followed a _gradient_ of susceptibility
such that most cancers developed close beneath the capsule. Studies pur-
porting to show that this is true have been guilty of such anatomic and
geometric inaccuracy that it is doubtful whether their conclusions have any
validity (1).

MODE OF ORIGIN OF BPH

The hallmark of BPH is the nodule. However, discrete nodularity is merely
a secondary change - the result of tissue compression by expansion of an
earlier, pre-nodular lesion. Careful microscopic search of transition zone
tissue shows such tiny prenodular foci, which are the earliest morphologic
manifestation of BPH (9). The main characteristic of these foci is
increased density of small duct branches in a microscopic, circumscribed
area (Fig. 3). Their appearance suggests the creation of new architecture
by repeated budding and branching from pre-existing small ducts. The new
branches often grow inward toward the center of the focus, and sometimes
two or more different ducts may simultaneously engage in branching toward
a common center. So the focus center becomes the architectural organizer
rather than the duct system. As such foci expand by internal branching
and become nodules, they incorporate branches from nearby ducts at the
nodule margin. Passing ducts are often seen to give rise to multiple
branches polarized to the nodule side and simultaneously may show increased
height and volume of epithelial cells limited to the nodule side of the
passing duct. This growth by accretion in later nodules seems to represent

32

Figure 3.

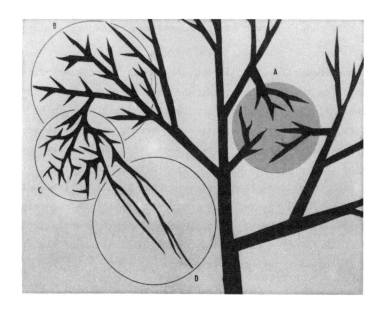

Prostatic duct architecture in BPH (A.) vs premalignant hyperplasia (B.)
superimposed on hypothetical normal pattern. Origin of well differentiated
carcinoma (C.) and moderately differentiated carcinoma (D.) from premalignant
hyperplasia depicted.

the same basic process which initiated the pre-nodular focus. The basic morphologic similarity between nodules of all sizes suggests that the biologic features of nodules do not evolve with time. The focus apparently begins with an abrupt, dichotomous change in tissue characteristics, and all further nodule growth may represent continued expression of that altered character.

The tissue change involved in nodule genesis is probably determined locally, since nodules seem to arise independently of each other. If this is true, then the influence of endocrine alterations in BPH would be relegated to a secondary role. Creation of new organ architecture is generally a feature of embryonic life, and it has been shown that the androgen responsiveness of target tissue becomes qualitatively altered in the adult (10). BPH may represent a focal reawakening of embryonic inductive interactions in which spontaneous, focal reversion to embryonic capacities reinitiates prostatic organogenesis. Furthermore, since nodule growth is polarized toward a center which is not a pre-existing duct, alteration of the stromal component may be the primary pathogenetic event.

MODE OF ORIGIN OF PROSTATIC CARCINOMA

Unlike BPH, the origin of carcinoma in the prostate apparently does not represent a single, dichotomous event but rather one small step in a prolonged evolutionary sequence. Nor is carcinoma origin invariably the first step of the sequence; often a distinct premalignant phase of possibly long duration can also be identified. Though these changes seem to form a continuum, four basic stages can be recognized.

The first stage consists of the persistance of the active histologic appearance of the young adult prostate into old age. Such delayed senescence is quite common and is not necessarily accompanied by any abnormality of histologic appearance (7). Thus in the strict morphologic sense this is not a discrete premalignant change. However it holds a possible clue to the mode of carcinoma origin since both malignancy and premalignant histologic changes are found more often in glands showing persistence of youthful activity. This suggests two hypotheses. First, persistent, high androgen levels may have a carcinogenic effect on the prostate. Second, maintenance of epithelial activity despite declining androgen levels may indicate the emergence of epithelial autonomy.

A second premalignant stage is that of focal adenomatous hyperplasia, most

often seen in prostates which already show a diffusely high level of
epithelial activity (6). In these areas, budding and branching of new,
small ducts creates new architecture in a way reminiscent of the foci of
BPH origin (Fig. 3). In both conditions, newly formed architecture suggests
reversion to embryonic capacities, but morphologic differences between them
suggest different pathogenesis. In BPH growth is strongly polarized toward
the focus center, where new ducts interact with newly formed stroma, as the
old stroma at the margin is pushed aside and compressed. Growth in premalignant hyperplasia is not polarized and often occurs at the focus
periphery, where new branches are in contact with pre-existing stroma.
The new branches probably interact with this stroma, embedding themselves
in it, since there is no evidence of compression of the stroma or any
alteration in its composition. This leads to a hypothesis of pathogenesis
– that BPH represents embryonic induction of a normal epithelium by an
altered stroma, while premalignant hyperplasia arises as a primary embryonic
alteration of epithelium, which becomes autonomous and unresponsive to a
normal stroma.

In a third evolutionary stage, carcinoma appears. Initially it is usually
extremely well differentiated, to the point that its cells cannot be dis-
tinquished from those of normal epithelium. Its duct branches too appear
individually normal. Their appearance suggests that they still retain a
basement membrane, and their relationship to the stroma is not distinctively
different from that in adenomatous hyperplasia. Thus the concept of invasion is difficult to apply properly to this situation. The main morphologic difference from the previous phase is a subtle alteration in architecture. There is now a monotonous uniformity of very small glands, which
may cluster or travel through the stroma in straight lines between muscle
bundles as tubes of uniform diameter and indefinite length.

The evolution of prostatic carcinoma in its second and third stages is
complicated by the existence in perhaps 25% of cases of a totally different
morphologic pattern of progression (6). Rather than creation of new architecture, the second stage consists of progressive alteration of individual
cells contained within pre-existing and unaltered ducts. Several grades of
dysplasia and ultimately carcinoma in situ within ducts are identifiable on
the basis of prominent nuclear atypicalities and intraductal cell proliferation. Transition to the third stage can occur abruptly by the focal
loss of basement membrane and aggressively destructive invasion of the

35

stroma. Though initially very well differentiated, the invasive component retains its distinctive nuclear atypia.

In the fourth and final stage, there is progressive loss of differentiation, which similarly affects both patterns of origin so that they may eventually become morphologically indistinguishable. It has not been proven that all prostatic cancers lose differentiation with time, just as it has not been shown that the previous evolutionary stages are always followed. However, this conclusion is supported by the finding that almost all small prostatic carcinomas are among the best differentiated, and that good differentiation is rare in large tumors except for occasional areas (7,3).

It has also been found that there is a high degree of correlation between degree of differentiation and biologic malignant potential among prostate cancers. This relationship is reliable enough to yield valuable prognostic information in the individual case by quantitating the level of differentiation (3). Only a relatively small percentage of prostatic carcinomas produce metastasis and death; these are almost invariably tumors which show much loss of differentiation. Prostatic carcinoma may be unique among human and animal tumors for the closeness of correlation between morphology and biologic behavior.

In summary, recent morphologic findings have contributed in several ways to the future study of the prostate and its diseases. Morphology has defined and located different areas from which tissues should be selected to study different diseases. It has identified morphologic changes associated with the origins of both BPH and carcinoma which imply a pathogenetic role for reawakened embryonic capabilities. It has described the morphologic and biologic heterogeneity of the entity, prostatic carcinoma, deriving from its uniquely protracted and highly structured evolutionary course. And it has provided a practical method for predicting prognosis in the individual cancer patient.

References

1. Byar, D. P. and Mostofi, F. K.: Carcinoma of the prostate: a prognostic evaluation of certain pathologic features in 208 radical prostatectomies. Cancer, 30, 5-13, 1972.
2. Franks, L. M.: Benign nodular hyperplasia of the prostate: a review. Annals of the Royal College of Surgeons, 14, 92-106, 1954.
3. Gleason, D. F.: Histologic grading and clinical staging of prostatic carcinoma. In Urologic Pathology -- the Prostate. Tannenbaum, M. Ed., p. 171, Philadelphia, Lea & Febiger, 1977.

4. LeDuc, I. E.: The anatomy of the prostate and the pathology of early benign hypertrophy. _Journal of Urology_, _42_, 1217-1241, 1939.

5. Lowsley, O. S.: The development of the human prostate gland with reference to the development of other structures at the neck of the urinary bladder. _American Journal of Anatomy_, _13_, 299-349, 1912.

6. McNeal, J. E.: Morphogenesis of prostatic carcinoma. _Cancer_, _18_, 1659-1666, 1965.

7. McNeal, J. E.: Origin and development of carcinoma in the prostate. _Cancer_, _23_, 24-34, 1969.

8. McNeal, J. E.: The prostate and prostatic urethra: a morphologic synthesis. _Journal of Urology_, _107_, 1008-1016, 1972.

9. McNeal, J. E.: Origin and evolution of benign prostatic enlargement. _Investigative Urology_, _15_, 340-345, 1978.

10. Wilson, J. D.: Recent studies of the mechanism of action of testosterone. _New England Journal of Medicine_, _287_, 1284-1291, 1972.

NEW METHODS FOR THE QUANTITATIVE HISTOPATHOLOGY ANALYSIS OF THE PROSTATE
AT THE LIGHT AND ELECTRON MICROSCOPIC LEVEL: STEREOLOGICAL CORRELATIONS*

CHAPTER III

Introduction

In order to obtain a better understanding of the normal physiological as
well as pathological processes, the quantitative approach to morphology
becomes of obvious importance. The purpose of this chapter is to develop
the possibilities for such quantitative histopathological analysis of the
prostate at the light and electron microscopic level. It should be
stressed, however, that both quantitative morphology and the traditional
descriptive approach must complement each other as much as possible. In
this regard the following points will be discussed:

1. Principles and methods of quantitative morphology.
2. Application of quantitative morphology to the prostate and some
    principal questions which this approach raises:
    -are there advantages when working with stereological methods
     compared with biochemical ones?
    -can the information provided by biochemical work be confirmed,
     supplemented or even extended?
    -what problems arise when working on human biopsy specimens with
     stereological methods?
    -and finally, the most important question: what can be measured and
     when can stereological work not be performed?
3. Experiments results and their correlation to quantitative results on
    human prostatic biopsy specimens.
4. Some preliminary stereological results on the canine prostate under
    different hormonal influences.

Definitions

Quantitative morphology is based on the principles of <u>stereology</u> and
<u>morphometry</u>. Stereology allows the characterization of 3-dimensional
shapes of components by extrapolation from measurements made on
2-dimensional cross sections thereof. Often such interpretations may be
difficult or erroneous when based on a single cross section or profile.
Therefore, it is emphasized that the interpretation obtained by

---

*Hanspeter Rohr, M.D.

 Institute of Pathology, University of Basel,

 Schonbeinstrasse 40, CH-4056 Basel, Switzerland

stereologic methods regarding a 3-dimensional shape of components must be the result of measurements of a sufficient number of strictly randomized cross sections in order for the result to be valid.

In contrast to stereology, which characterizes the shape of a component, morphometry allows one by application of stereological axioms to quantitate the relative volume, the relative surface, and the number of these tissue or cell components. Therefore, tissue or cell components can be analyzed by morphometry in terms of their volume density, surface density or numerical density

Theoretical and experimental basis for quantitative analysis

How can the volume, surface, and numerical densities of cellular components be determined theoretically?

Volume density: For the determination of volume densities, the French geologist Delesse in 1847 demonstrated the equivalence of area and volume fractions, by showing that the area occupied by a mineral component was proportional to its volume in the entire rock (5). Glagoleff (7) and Chalkley (3) extended the Delesse principle and established the basis for the currently applicated so-called pointcounting procedures. In this procedure, a point network is superimposed onto a randomized tissue cross section sample. Each of the test points represents a small unit area. In order to determine the volume density of tissue or cell components, one counts the number of test points on or within the boundaries of the particular component in question (see Figure 1). It can be shown that the fraction of test points contained within the boundaries of the component in question related to the total number of test points is a good estimate of the volume density (V_V) of that component (3). The accuracy of the estimated volume density depends on the number of random samples measured.

Surface density: Tomkeieff (11) demonstrated that surface density (S_V) can be calculated in much the same manner as the volume density. This is based on the fact that the length of all the boundaries formed by a particular component per unit area of a section is proportioned to its surface density. A point counting method to determine surface density can here again be utilized. A lattice as shown in Figure 1 (upper right corner) is superimposed

39

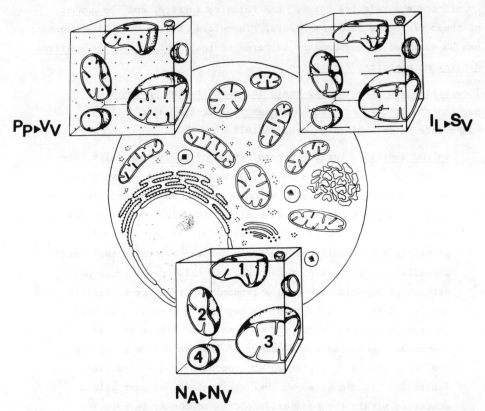

FIG. 1. Measurements of the three main parameters. Volume density (V_V) (*top left*): Fraction of test points (P_P) laying over profiles of a given particle equals volume density (V_V) or $P_P = V_V$. Surface density (S_V) (*top right*): Surface density (S_V) is calculated from the intersection (I_L) of membrane traces with test lines. Numerical density (N_V) (*bottom*): Number of profiles (1 to 4) in the test area (N_A) is converted to N_V by a formula including correction factors for shape and inhomogeneous distribution.

on a randomized tissue cross section. The number of intersections formed by the boundary traces of a particular component (for example mitochondria) with the test line system can be used to calculate the surface density.

Numerical density: The numerical particle density (N_{vi}) is evaluated by counting the number of particle profiles in the test area (see Figure 1 lower half). The value is dependent on the shape and the size distribution of the particle in question. Therefore, correction factors, e.g. for the shape have to be introduced. For spherical particles, such as normal nuclei, the shape factor is usually well definable, whereas for complicated structures, e.g. for distorted mitochondria, the reliability of related calculations is reduced. The values for the numerical densities must be regarded as estimates in most cases.

In summary, stereological analysis is based on counting of points (for V_{vi}), intersection points (for S_{vi}) and particle profiles (for N_{vi}) as illustrated in Figure 1. Detailed information on stereological theory and practice (choice of test lines, point sets and sample size) is given by Weibel et al. (12) and Rohr et al. (9).

Pre-conditions for stereological and morphometrical analysis

The following conditions must be fulfilled if quantitative measurements are to be valid:

(a) The structure to be analyzed must be distributed homogeneously in the reference space.

(b) The study must be done on a representative number of strictly randomized sections or micrographs to perform statistical analysis. As a rule the standard error for a compartment should be less than 10% of the mean, otherwise the sampling volume has to be increased.

(c) For the determination of volume or surface densities the cellular compartments can be simple or complicated structures, discrete or continuous, large or small or variable in size (12). However, for the determination of the numerical density the shape of the cellular component must be geometrically defined.

(d) Standardization of fixation, buffering and embedding procedures should be observed, especially in comparative studies.

Practical considerations for quantitative analysis

In performing a stereological or morphometrical analysis, one must first
establish an appropriate stereological model, a sampling procedure, and
an overall design for stereological analysis. Figure 2 summarizes a
morphometric model for the prostate. This gland can be divided as shown
and each of the components outlined can be quantified (as will be
discussed later).

The different cellular components can not be evaluated at a single stage
of magnification due to the broad differences in shape, size and
frequencies of these components. Therefore, sampling is done at three
magnifications to establish an adequate relationship between the size of
the components and the point or test line sets.

Three magnification levels are used in the determination of the different
parameters listed as follows:

  Level I, primary magnification 1:90 (light microscopy)

  Level II, primary magnification 1:1,300 (electron microscopy)

  Level III, primary magnification 1:4,100 (electron microscopy)

Usually, five animals are studied in a test group which in most cases is
sufficient. However, it is not surprising that under experimental
conditions the individual variability of the tissue and cellular
components increases. Above all, when working on human biopsy specimens
we have to account for this individual variability which results from the
small number of available tissue cubes and the non-homogeneity of the
tissue itself. The tissue preservation must be performed with the
greatest possible care. The problems of random sampling have to be
handled carefully.

What information can be obtained by quantitative analysis which can be helpful to biochemical studies?

One example of such an approach is the question of membrane biogenesis.
One of the best studied models of membrane biogenesis is the response of
the smooth endoplasmic reticulum of hepatocytes to induction by drug
administration or bile duct ligation. Both treatments cause a selective
increase in the amount of the smooth endoplasmic reticulum but result in
different enzymatic patterns of the membranes: after phenobarbital
treatment the rise of the surface density of the smooth endoplasmic
reticulum is paralleled by an increase of the P-450 cytochromes. On the
contrary, the ligation of the bile duct is not followed by raised P-450

Figure 2.

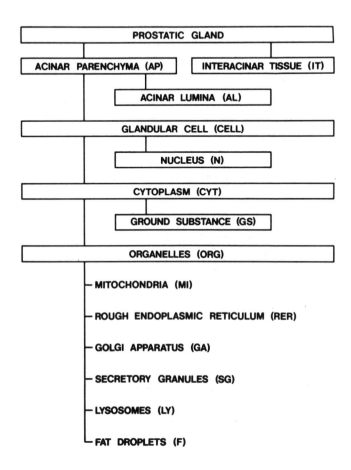

Stereologic model of the prostate gland.

concentrations, resulting in increased center-to-center distances of P-450 on a total ER-membrane basis. Similar model-like calculations of the center-to-center distances of cytochrome molecules in the vitamin E deficient liver revealed nearly double distances (6). The example of smooth endoplasmic proliferation and enzyme induction following drug administration clearly shows the possibilities of interdisciplinary correlation. However, the question of corresponding parameters must be solved carefully.

When working on the prostatic gland it can be shown that in contrast to biochemistry, cellular differentiation is possible by stereological methods. For example, the nuclei of the smooth muscle cell of the prostatic gland cannot be separated by biochemical methods from the glandular ones; however, this distinction is possible with stereological methods.

Weibel's stereological study concerning the distribution of organelles and membranes between hepatocytes and non-hepatocytes in rat liver parenchyma demonstrates to what extent the non-hepatocytic organelles can potentially contaminate subcellular fractions used for biochemical study (12). Special attention must be paid to the interpretation of studies on lysosomes, mitochondria and Golgi apparatus, since an appreciable part of these organelles may be derived from cell types other than hepatocytes. Non-hepatic organelles contaminate subcellular fractions, e.g. non-hepatocytes contribute 55% of the volume of lipid droplets, 43% of the volume of lysosomes and 1.2% of the volume of mitochondria. Non-hepatocytes contain 26.5% of plasma membranes, 32.4% of lysosomal membranes, 15.1% of Golgi apparatus, 6.4% of endoplasmic reticulum and 2.4% of mitochondrial membranes. Therefore, stereological data can supply and even extend biochemical information.

Use of quantitative morphology in the study of the prostate

Several examples will illustrate how quantitative morphology can be applied to the study of prostatic function and disease. The first example deals with an ultrastructural stereological model for the ventral lobe of the rat prostate (Figure 2). This model illustrates how the ventral lobe of prostate can be divided into morphologically well defined compartments. The model has two major divisions, the interacinar tissue (IT) (stromal tissue) and the acinar parenchyma (AP), including the glandular cell and the acinar lumina (AL). The smooth muscle cells were divided into the cytoplasmic compartments as seen in Figure 3. Quantitative morphological

44

Figure 3.

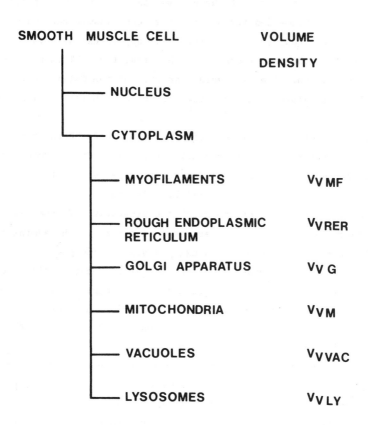

Stereologic model of the prostatic smooth muscle cell.

45

analysis (2) demonstrates that the ventral lobe of the rat prostate consists of 75% acini (AP) and only 25% stromal tissue (IT). Dividing the acini into their two compartments, one finds that the acinar lumina (AL) comprise more than half of the volume (52%) of the whole prostatic gland. The high volume density of the rough endoplasmic reticulum (RER), 31% of the whole cytoplasm, and of the Golgi apparatus (G), 7.5%, demonstrates that the main function of the prostatic cell is protein and

enzyme synthesis. The high volume density of the Golgi apparatus, 7.5%, could be interpreted as an expression of a high rate of membrane synthesis.

Using this approach, the influence of various steroids on the fine structure of the rat glandular prostatic cell was studied in order to get some information about the subcellular reaction pattern of the prostatic glandular cell (2). Two examples will briefly underline these possibilities: The effect of the synthetic progestine 17-ethyl-19-nortestosterone and the synthetic estrogen hexoestrol. The administration of 17-ethyl-19-nortestosterone in a daily dosage of 180 µg per day for three months leads to a reduction of the acinar parenchyma (AP), the glandular cell and its various subcellular compartments. Related to the unit volume of prostatic tissue, there is a significant decrease of the acinar parenchyma, the nucleus, and the cytoplasm as well as of the various subcellular organelles of the glandular cells (Figure 4). Related to the unit volume of cytoplasm, there is a significant decrease of rough endoplasmic reticulum whereas the volume density for the Golgi apparatus, the mitochondria and the lysosomes remains constant. These stereological data demonstrate a persistence of the fine structural integrity of the glandular prostatic cells. Contrary to these findings in the progestine treated rats, the administration of a daily dose of 500 µg hexoestrol for two months leads to an atrophy of the prostatic gland. As seen by the stereological data, there is a significant reduction of the acinar parenchyma, the glandular cell volume, and the various subcellular organelles involved in prostatic fluid synthesis and secretion (Figure 5). Again, the extrapolation of the interpretation of such results to the situation in man can only be made carefully and these interpretations remain difficult and hypothetical.

With certain restrictions, stereological analysis is also possible with needle biopsies. Therefore, an ultrastructural stereological study of the human prostate was performed (1). In the literature there appears

Figure 4.

RAT PROSTATE: PROGESTINE

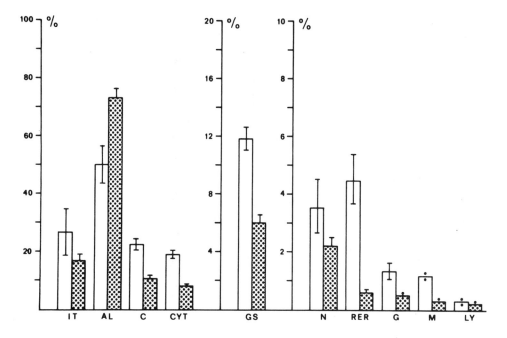

Tissue component and glandular cell components of the ventral prostatic lobe are expressed as a percentage of the total prostatic gland volume. The value of the Progestin-treated animals are shaded. Open bar are for normal controls. Standard errors of the mean are indicated.

Figure 5.

RAT PROSTATE: ESTROGENE

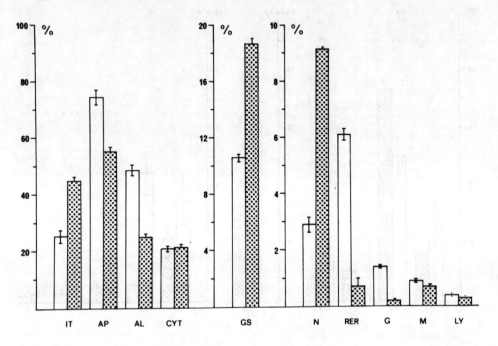

Tissue component and glandular cell components of the ventral prostatic lobe are expressed as a percentage of the total prostatic gland volume. The value of the Estrogen-treated animals are shaded. Open bar are for normal controls. Standard errors of the mean are indicated.

few papers utilizing quantitative morphological analyses on the study of the human prostate. These papers mostly study the prostate of men suffering with benign prostatic hyperplasia, BPH.

Ethical and practical considerations make it difficult to collect material necessary for defining the base-line data from young men for comparative purposes. The stereological analyses were performed, therefore, on prostatic biopsy specimens from healthy young men who underwent vasectomy. The testosterone, 17β-estradiol, LH, FSH and prolactin levels in all volunteers were within the normal range, indicating no pathological lesion in the pituitary-gonadal axis.

A light microscopic stereological analysis (Level I analysis) of these needle biopsies cannot be performed since only few random samples for each needle biopsy specimen are available. This is the most restrictive fact in performing a stereological analysis on needle biopsy specimens. In contrast to needle biopsies on surgical biopsy specimens light and electron microscopic stereological information is available. Some pathological changes, such as e.g. the estrogen induced metaplasia, cannot be quantified by stereological methods.

When comparing the prostatic glandular cell of healthy young men with those of men suffering from BPH, a definite inactivation of the prostatic glandular cell in BPH is observed. There is a decrease of the volume density of the rough endoplasmic reticulum, Golgi apparatus, secretory droplets and lysosomes, thus indicating a strongly diminished secretory activity of the glandular cell in benign prostatic hyperplasia (Figure 6). In order to get some insite into possible epithelial stromal interactions, the fibromuscular tissue of the prostate in man and dog was analyzed by quantitative morphology at the light and electron microscopic level. The results of the stereological analysis of the smooth muscle cell (for stereological subdivisions of smooth muscle cell see Figure 3) of the prostate of healthy young men and of men with BPH were as follows: the volume density of cell organelles (V_{vorg}) such as the rough endoplasmic reticulum, the Golgi apparatus and the mitochondria in BPH is about threefold increased compared with that in young men. Therefore, an activation of the secretory activity - namely synthesis of collagen and mucopolysaccharides - can be assumed (Figure 7). A similar reaction pattern of the smooth muscle cell can be observed in castrated dogs following estrogen administration in a high dosage during a three week period (Figure 8).

Figure 6.

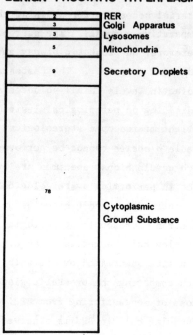

HUMAN PROSTATE:CONTROL

3	RER
5	Golgi Apparatus
4	Mitochondria
42	Secretory Droplets & Lysosomes
46	Cytoplasmic Ground Substance

BENIGN PROSTATIC HYPERPLASIA

2	RER
3	Golgi Apparatus
3	Lysosomes
5	Mitochondria
9	Secretory Droplets
78	Cytoplasmic Ground Substance

Volume of the glandular cell compartments are expressed as a percentage
of the total glandular cell cytoplasm.

Figure 7.

Human smooth muscle cells :
Volume densities per cm^3 cytoplasm

	V_{VGF}		V_{VOrg}	V_{VMF}
Control (n = 75) 5 biopsies	$\overline{m}$ s.e.	0.002 0.001	0.048 0.005	0.950 0.026
B. P. H. (n = 118) 5 biopsies	$\overline{m}$ s.e.	0.013 0.001	0.134 0.006	0.853 0.032

Volume density of cellular Golgi apparatus alone = V_{VGF}

Volume density of cellular myofilaments = V_{VMF}

Volume density of total cell organelles (RER, Golgi apparatus, mitochondria, etc.) = V_{VORG}

Figure 8.

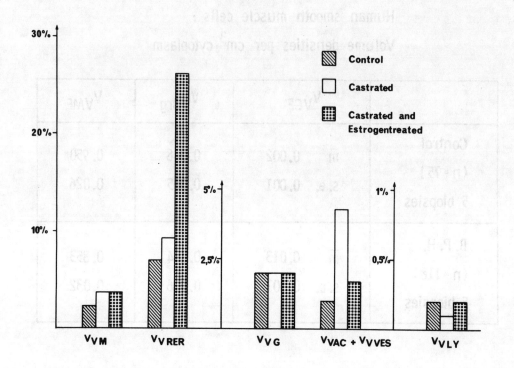

Effects of Castration and Estrogen treatment on prostatic smooth muscle cell component.

V_{VM} = volume density of mitochondria

V_{VRER} = volume density rough endoplasmic reticulum

V_{VG} = volume density Golgi apparatus

$V_{VAC} + V_{VVES}$ = volume density of vaculoes and vesicles

V_{VLY} = volume density of lysosomes

Most probably, the activation of smooth muscle cells is one of the important keys in the morphogenesis of the BPH. In previous papers an activation of the smooth muscle cell has been reported for the uterus of the prepubetal rat following injection of 17-β-estradiol (10). It could be demonstrated that these activated smooth muscle cells can participate in the synthesis of the ground substance of connective tissue (8). Remembering the high volume density of the fibromuscular tissue (60% of the whole adenoma) and the activation of the smooth muscle cells in BPH, special attention should be paid to the smooth muscle of the prostate regarding the etiology of this disease. However, the mechanism of the smooth muscle cell activation is rather complex and most probably not exclusively mediated by estrogens.

Such an assumption can also be supported by the preliminary stereological results which were obtained on the canine prostate in a joint study with the Johns Hopkins School of Medicine.

Some of these results will be presented shortly. Further details will be given by Dr. Coffey.

The experimental design was as follows: Intact dog prostates (I) and so-called "large intact dog prostates" (LI) as well as prostates of dogs with spontaneous BPH served as "controls" (see Figure 9 first column). Groups of 10 dogs each, intact (I) and castrated (Ca) were treated with androgens such as testosterone, DHT or 5α-androstane-3α-17β-diol by the protocol reported by De Klerk et al. (4). Half of these groups were treated moreover with estrogens (E2). Finally, a group of five intact and five castrated dogs was treated with estrogen alone. The quantitative morphological results can be briefly summarized as follows (Figure 9): The stereologically elaborated reaction pattern of the dog prostate following androgen and/or estrogen treatment and that of spontaneous BPH is mostly dominated by a relative and/or absolute increase of the glandular parts (AP), shown as the top portion of each bar. The bottom portion represents the stromal components (IT). The total height of the bar represents the total prostate weight in grams. It should be stressed that in all groups the androgen metabolites DHT and 5α-androstan-3α-17β-diol are more effective in inducing an increase of the prostate than testosterone. It is striking that the growth inducing activity of these androgenic metabolites can be increased by estrogens in both the intact and the castrated groups. Highest stromal induction is observed in groups treated with androgen metabolites and estrogens.

Figure 9.

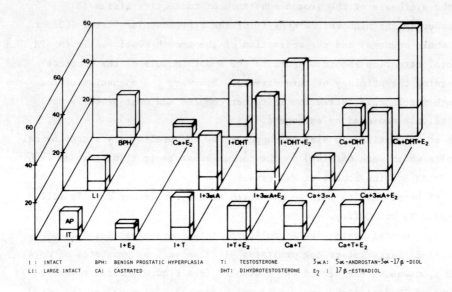

| I : | INTACT | BPH: | BENIGN PROSTATIC HYPERPLASIA | T: | TESTOSTERONE | 3αA: | 5α-ANDROSTAN-3α-17β-DIOL |
| LI: | LARGE INTACT | CA: | CASTRATED | DHT: | DIHYDROTESTOSTERONE | E₂ : | 17β-ESTRADIOL |

However, it must be stressed that an extrapolation of these data to BPH in man is only possible with greatest caution, since in man the histopathology in BPH is mostly dominated by stromal changes.

References

1. Bartsch, J.: Stereology, a new quantitative morphological approach to study prostatic function and disease. Eur. Urol., 3: 85-91, 1977.
2. Bartsch, G.; Fischer, E.; Rohr, H. P.: Ultrastructural morphometric analysis of the rat prostate (ventral lobe). Urol. Res., 3: 1-11, 1975.
3. Chalkley, H. W.: Method for the quantitative morphological analysis of tissues. J. natn. Cancer Inst., 4: 47-53, 1943.
4. DeKlerk, D. P.; Coffey, D. S.; Ewing, L. L.; McDermott, I. R.; Reiner, W. G.; Robinson, C. H.; Scott, W. W.; Strandberg, J. D.; Talalay, P.; Walsh, P. C.; Wheaton, L. G., and Zirkin, B. R.: A comparison of spontaneous and experimentally induced canine prostatic hyperplasia. J. Clin. Invest. (In press), 1979.
5. Delesse, M. A.: Procede mecanique pour determiner la composition des roches. C.r. Acad. Sci., Paris, 25: 544-545, 1947.
6. Frigg, M.; Rohr, H. P.: Morphometry of liver mitochondria in vitamin E deficiency. Expl molec. Path., Submitted 1975.
7. Glagoleff, A. A.: On the geometrical methods of quantitative mineralogic analysis of rocks. Trans. Inst. Econ. Mineral., Moscow, 59, 1933.
8. Rohr, H. P.; Jurukova, Z.: Beitrage zur Bildung bindegewebiger Matrix in glatten Muskelzellen. Path. Eur., 3: 571-592, 1968.
9. Rohr, H. P.; Oberholzer, M.; Bartsch, G.; Keller, M.: Morphometry in experimental pathology (methods, baseline data and applications). Int. Rev. exp. Path., 54: 233-325, 1976.
10. Ross, R.; Klebanoff, J. S.: Fine structural changes in uterine smooth muscle and fibroblasts in response to estrogen. J. Cell Biol., 32: 155-167, 1967.
11. Tomkeieff, S. I.: Linear intercepts, areas and volumes. Nature, 155: 107-110, 1945.
12. Weibel, E. R.; Kistler, G. S.; Scherle, W. F.: Practical stereological methods for morphometic cytology. J. Cell Biol., 30: 23-38, 1966.

It would have been too good to be true had epidemiologic risk data from three separate prostatic cancer populations (K-P, VA, NW) turned out to be similar, with trends and results parallel for all studied variables, at least at first glance. It isn't true, although some of the sexual attributes, events and practices characterizing patients and controls appear consistent in direction. Some of these results will be summarized in this paper, along with background information designed to develop the general area of risk variables possibly associated with oncogenic transformation of prostatic epithelium and initiation of carcinomatous foci.

The discovery of risk variables which condition the proportions of male populations destined to be found with prostatic cancer, and those individual men for whom such an outcome can be predicted, subserves the additional objective of structuring a rationale for carcinogenesis in the prostate. No such fund of information existed until recently, no clues, no understanding of the origins and development of what may be the key carcinoma in searching for generalizations possibly covering most solid cancers.

It appears now that first transformations may take place very early in life as a consequence of diverse physiologic and secretory patterns associated with puberty; and also that these events may differ in time and extent for different populations, by race and by sociocultural levels.

MORBIDITY AND MORTALITY

Information related to the distribution and risk of prostatic cancer which appears to hold up in worldwide populations is derived mostly from studies in the United States, where proportions by race, age, and sociocultural levels are available for comparison, Figure 1; and also from certain Oriental popu-

*I. D. Rotkin. This work was supported by Public Health Service grant CA-16925 from the National Prostatic Cancer Project of the National Cancer Institute, National Institutes of Health, U.S. Department of Health, Education and Welfare. Sampling described in this report was obtained through the cooperation of the following institutions, hospitals and urologists: 1) Kaiser-Permanente Medical Center (K-P), Los Angeles, Dr. J. F. Cooper, Chief of Urology; 2) University of Illinois/West Side Veterans Administration Hospital (VA), Chicago, Dr. S. S. Clark, Head, Department of Urology; and 3) Northwestern University (NW), Chicago, Dr. John T. Grayhack, Chairman, Department of Urology.

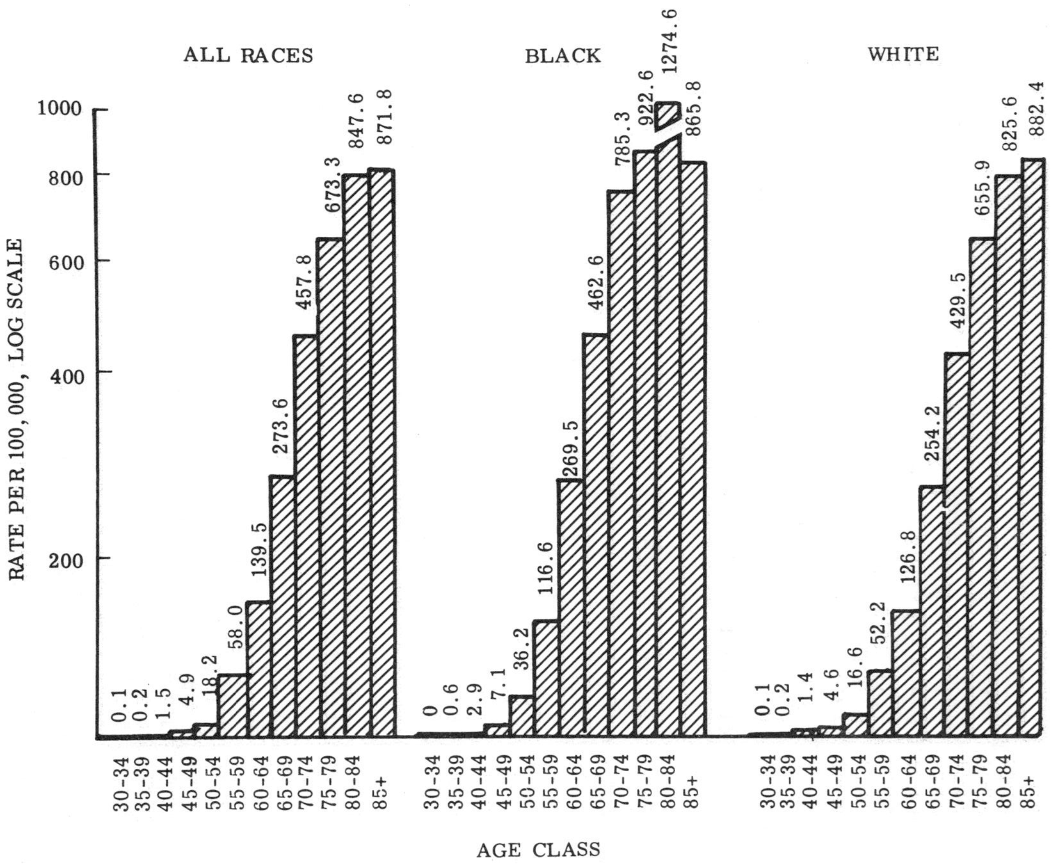

FIGURE 1. Average annual U.S. age-specific incidence rates for prostatic cancer per 100,000 males, 1969-1971. Derived from the Third National Cancer Survey, National Cancer Institute, USDHEW.

lations elsewhere in the world (32). These observations are:

1. Highest incidence rates are found among black men. In the United States
more prostatic cancer is diagnosed in blacks than in their combined cancers of
the lung, bronchus, and trachea (7,19). The impression that incidence in
black African populations is much lower than in the United States (19,38) may
be misleading. Separate populations from Africa show incidence rates ranging
from 9.4 to 19.2 per 100,000 (32), fairly substantial frequencies in themselves, yet life expectancies cannot be overlooked in estimating incidence for
age-related cancers where rates rise steeply in older age classes. Few prostatic cancers are diagnosed anywhere in men under age 50, and mean life
duration in many African black populations does not extend much past age 40,
providing a minimal pool of men at risk. Jackson, et al. (19) reported 67 of
1000 prostates from autopsies with carcinomas in Nigerian black men with a
median age of 50 years. It is difficult to know how many of these lesions
would have become clinically manifest, or how many of the normal prostates in
the series might have contained oncogenically transformed but not ascertain-
able cells which might have progressed after the age of 50, since mean age of
clinical discovery is near 70 years of age. Comparisons of worldwide populations, Figure 2, might lead to the conclusion that black men are at high
risk in Africa as well as in the United States, but there is no question other
than that studies are needed among blacks everywhere in the world, particularly
in East Africa and among island populations of the Pacific.

2. For some unknown reason, perhaps related to lifelong sexual patterns, the
Japanese and probably all Orientals seldom die from prostatic cancer despite
incidences of latent lesions which are as high as those found in other races.
This single ethnic comparison is the most important available demographic
clue to which specific biologic risk variables may be fitted. Life expectancy
in Japan is parallel to that in Germany, Scandinavia, Britain and the United
States. Levels of diagnostic and pathologic education and ability also are
similar. Sociologic and medical reporting are as advanced as any elsewhere,
and we must be convinced that the extremely low prostatic cancer death rates
are real. Studies from Japan (23,24) report 13 to 18 percent of prostates
with latent lesions in serial unselected autopsy cases, ages 45-90 at death in
one series (23). Distribution of the lesions covered the posterior, lateral
and anterolateral regions of the prostate; some were diffusely infiltrated
throughout the organ, and several showed multiple foci. Yet, none at any age
had penetrated the musculofibrous capsule. This suggests some type of re-

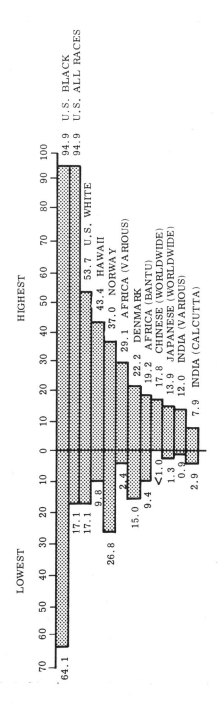

FIGURE 2. Worldwide prostatic cancer incidence rates per 100,000, all ages: range of estimates. Derived from various sources.

straint or failure of development to which the concept of cocarcinogenesis may perhaps be fitted. It would be tempting to consider an exogenous modifier in resolving this racial difference, yet Bean et al. (2) have revealed no relation between radiation in Hiroshima and Nagasaki Japanese taken at autopsy, and rates, histologic type or degree of activity of prostatic cancer. From worldwide mortality rates, and from autopsy series, it would seem that unless some attribute or event, perhaps an interaction of endogenous, environmental and genetic variables, forces the development of the latent lesion, it will not become invasive.

3. Unless it is kept clearly in mind that worldwide data, as taken from reports to the World Health Organization, probably do not reflect reality, over- and underestimates may be taken too seriously. For example, I visited Peru in 1976 and found no concern over mortality from prostatic cancer, especially since exceptionally high rates of stomach and cervix cancer overshadowed an appraisal. Yet, I found that mortality from prostate cancer is substantial in Peru, where only 10 percent of males survive after age 50 (4). Collectors of information, such as WHO, must depend upon reliability at the sources, and they can only report what is being conveyed to them. The situation further is complicated by the following:

4. A large proportion of prostatic carcinomas in any population remain stationary, yet morbidity and mortality differ worldwide, perhaps as a consequence of genetic endowment (attributes), or of differential exposures and practices (events). This may be true also of other adenocarcinomas, particularly of the breast; and perhaps other solid carcinomas. Comparisons of latent lesions with diagnosed invasive cancers often are presented as ratios, ranging from 3 to 8 latent for each diagnosed lesion (9,32). Taking these ratios as upper and lower limits, it has been estimated that 1 white man in every 25 to 57 in the United States will harbor a prostatic cancer, latent or manifest. For black men in the United States the outlook is more severe, 1 in 17 to 39. These estimates cover most age classes at risk, 50 and older (32). Since the proportion of latent lesions which will progress cannot be forecast, accurate estimates of total prostatic carcinomas in any population can only be derived from autopsy series, yet these cannot be applied to national rates unless each series is a representative sample of the entire nation. Oota and colleagues (23,24) have shown that virtually all carcinomas appearing in Japanese men are nonprogressive, with occasional exceptions contributing to a small death rate. It is possible that a much larger proportion of latent

lesions in blacks, and also in whites, progress into invasive pathologic
stages. Henschke et al. (15) list as reasons for the "rapid" increase of
certain cancers in the black U.S. population such variables as underreporting
in death certificates, errors in census enumeration, changes in racial age
distributions, genetic differences, cure rates and environmental factors,
and they settle upon environmental carcinogens as most likely, but this
can only be considered as a speculation. As I will show in this paper there
is reason to consider a hormonal rationale, although modification by exogenous
cocarcinogens is possible.

Worldwide mortality rates reflect the several foregoing observations.
Table 1 lists death rates from prostatic cancer for 45 countries, with
corresponding life expectancies. Rates generally are correlated with life-
spans, as would be expected. However, certain key departures are interesting.
At the bottom of the list, where low rates are fitted to low expectancies,
Japan appears with a male life expectancy of 72 years against a rate of only
2 prostate cancers per 100,000. This, and other such exceptions which are
diagnostic, are summarized in Figure 3, showing the correlation of mortality
with average life expectancy. Table 1 and Figure 3 both are derived from
material assembled from a number of sources, principally the World Health
Statistics Annual, 1970-1971, and presented in a recent review of prostate
cancer epidemiology (32). Whereas most countries cluster as would be expected
around the correlation axis, Figure 3, exceptions exist in Singapore, with
a generally Oriental population and a fairly long life expectancy, and in
Japan with a very long life expectancy, both with extremely low death rates
from prostatic cancer. On the other end of the comparison is South Africa,
with a largely black population, a short life expectancy for the black segment, and a high death rate from prostate cancer, although not as high as in
U.S. blacks whose life expectancy is longer. White men in the United States,
on the other hand with a life expectancy equivalent to other European white
populations, show a higher death rate than any of the European countries.

RISK INFORMATION

Other than geographic and racial differences in morbidity and mortality
rates, which by themselves are indicators of risk levels, demographic studies
have provided no useful information. No differences by incidence or age
distribution were found between urban and rural populations in Iowa (13)
or in California (17,20). Relationships to risk of prostate cancer have
failed to surface in case control studies for marital status, social class,

61

TABLE 1: Comparison of worldwide mortality rates per
100,000 population with life expectancies (32).

COUNTRY	LIFE EXPECTANCY	MORTALITY RATE
Sweden	74	18.3
Switzerland	74	18.3
Norway	74	18.1
Barbados	68	16.5
New Zealand	70	15.5
Australia	68	15.3
Belgium	69	14.7
Netherlands	74	14.6
Hungary	70	14.6
France	72	14.5
Canada	72	14.3
Germany, F.R.	71	14.1
United States	70	13.9
Austria	70	13.5
Finland	72	13.5
Portugal	64	13.0
Northern Ireland	70	12.8
Denmark	73	12.8
Ireland	70	12.7
Luxembourg	67	12.5
Spain	70	12.4
England and Wales	72	11.5
Italy	70	10.5
Scotland	72	10.3
Venezuela	66	10.3
Czechoslovakia	71	09.7
Panama	61	08.6
Israel	72	08.5
Peru	53	08.5
Poland	69	08.3
Romania	68	08.0
Malta	69	07.4
Yugoslavia	65	06.9
Bulgaria	70	06.5
Costa Rica	65	06.5
Greece	69	05.8
Mexico	60	05.6
Mauritius	59	03.1
Singapore	62	02.2
Japan	72	01.9
Hong Kong	--	01.8
Egypt	53	01.4
El Salvador	58	00.9
Philippines	58	00.9
Thailand	56	00.2

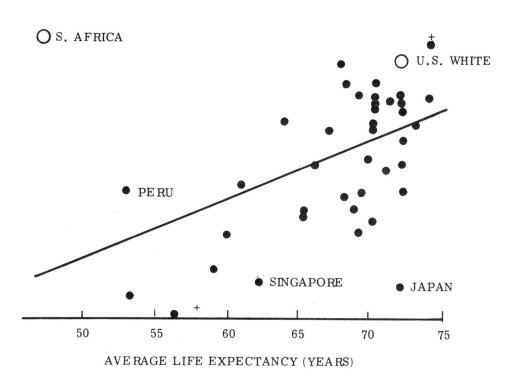

religion, place of birth and educational levels (17,20,38). The effect of
migration upon mortality from prostatic cancer for Japanese is subject to
assessment (14). Rising rates in migrant populations reaching Hawaii and
the United States, and in first generation Japanese, appears to have taken
place. However, the emergence of latent endogenous variables, possibly
conditioned in continuing generations by a genetic mix from new mating patterns, could influence such an effect, as also could admittedly, the presence
of a mysterious cocarcinogenic variable that appears to protect Orientals
with latent lesions, but not as many blacks or whites. Orientals also in
other parts of the world are at low mortality risk from prostate cancer,
and mortality rates from prostatic cancer in Nissei and farther removed Japanese remain lower than those of other races in Hawaii and the United States.

King et al. (21) has summarized levels of risk by occupation and socioeconomic
status for British, Netherlands and United States men, but without well designed case control studies such comparisons are risky since so much arbitrary
judgment enters into assignment of status by both occupation and economic
level. Until recently, attempts to relate diet, physical characteristics,
circumcision, tobacco and alcohol, ABO blood groups, prostatitis, fertility,
and medical history all have failed to reveal differences between prostatic
cancer patients and the general male population (10,21,32,38).

It is reasonable to assume that risk research of a prevalent hormone-dependent
cancer would be heavily weighted with investigations of endocrine malfunction
or differences, yet the deficit of literature is as extreme as it is for
other risk variables. From his negative results comparing pituitary characteristics of prostatic cancer patients with the general population, Liavag
et al. (22) concluded that no useful hormonal information has been uncovered
regarding endocrine imbalance as a risk factor. Possibly this is because
studies were conducted only with old rather than also with very young populations. Franks (10) agrees that a hormonal effect has not yet been demonstrated.

Although Wynder et al. (38) regarded information on sexual activity as
"notoriously difficult to obtain" one would assume that the entire range
of sexual variables hardly could be overlooked in epidemiologic studies of
a hormone-dependent adenocarcinoma of the reproductive system. Several investigators have ventured into this area of inquiry (34, 38) with limited
surveys, as have we with full exploratory studies in 3 different hospitals
of 2 major metropolitan areas, Chicago and Los Angeles (30,32,33). Sequellae

of sexual activity can relate to 2 major risk areas: an exogenous rationale
based upon venereal transmission of an oncogenic agent, and the endogenous
effect of sexuality upon the production, balance and/or accumulation of
androgens and other products in relation to risk.

Some information exists regarding venereal disease in relation to risk (16,34)
but no populations of celibates have been sampled to discover an effect of
abstinence upon risk. Urologists serving Catholic populations appear to
diagnose prostatic cancers quite regularly in priests. Nor have there been
until recently any structured studies of lifetime diet patterns in comparing
prostatic cancer patients with the population matrices from which they are
derived, or in which they live. Wynder et al. (38) has speculated upon the
effect of cholesterol from the ingestion of fats, presumably upon the synthesis of androgenic steroids, but they presented no evidence for this.

Other variables under study include circumcision of nonJewish patients and
controls (38), with no resolution, air pollution in a search for the effect
of cadmium oxide upon risk, for which results were negative in the age class
60-69 (36); and also a range of chronic conditions ascribing relationship
to prostatic cancer with cirrhosis of the liver, hypertension, diabetes
mellitus, stroke, and coronary heart disease. All are diseases of old age
and it is not surprising that correlations exist, but that any of these
conditions increase risk of prostatic cancer hardly can yet be held secure
for prevalent entities occuring together at the same time in life.

A purportedly high increase in risk of prostatic cancer for men with an
antecedent benign prostatic hypertrophy has been reported (1,11) but the
information cannot be held secure for reasons which are discussed elsewhere
(5,17,27,29,32). Still, we were influenced sufficiently by this claimed
association to undertake exclusion of clinically detectable BPH control
candidates from our studies, an extremely difficult and time consuming procedure.

Three familiar investigations for genetic contribution to risk (20,34,37)
reported excesses of prostatic cancers in the families of patients compared
to those of controls. An endogenous theory for carcinogenesis calls for
a heritable contribution to risk, expressing as differences in hormonal
levels and components, in susceptibility of target cells, in receptor molecules, or in defense systems.

It should be evident from the foregoing that the epidemiologic literature

65

for prostate cancer hardly parallels those of several other cancers. Very few exploratory studies have been undertaken and reported, nor until recently have solid hypotheses been advanced which lend themselves to testing. It is possible now to propose a theoretical construct which is derived from our multivariate studies, together with a summary of evidence which has been submitted for publication (33) and more of which will be detailed in the future.

A MODEL FOR CARCINOGENESIS IN THE HUMAN PROSTATE

In making reference to my rationale for the origin and development of prostatic carcinoma, Figure 4, certain assumptions, reservations and questions must be outlined. These are:

1. A hormonal etiology is assumed, with a pubertal excess of androgen. This is derived from interpretation of our case-control epidemiologic studies comparing diagnosed patients with clinically BPH-free controls matched by age and race. Assumed also are genetic and external modifiers which operate not only upon initiation of the cancer but also upon development of the lesion.

2. No claim is made that the information from which this model is structured comprises hard data or that the interpretations are secure.

3. Keeping in mind the extreme race and population diversity of morbidity and mortality rates, it is necessary to assume that certain attributes and events will condition risk more than others, with oncogenic transformation of perhaps genetically selected cells which may or may not thereafter continue to develop into carcinomatous foci according to a timetable, depending upon the presence of modifying events.

4. In defense of what may appear to be premature model-making, the effort assigned to such a pursuit can be justified by the possibility of utilization. Figure 4 is an attempt to provide early data-based hypotheses where none exist. It is legitimate with multivariate exploratory studies also to analyze data and to reach conclusions. Utility for Figure 4 also is found in merging epidemiologic interpretations with the classical model for carcinogenesis, and further to extend such conjecture to stages of tumor development.

5. It is not possible to profile the candidate at increased risk until other variables have been sorted out, and their relative contribution to variance has been determined.

66

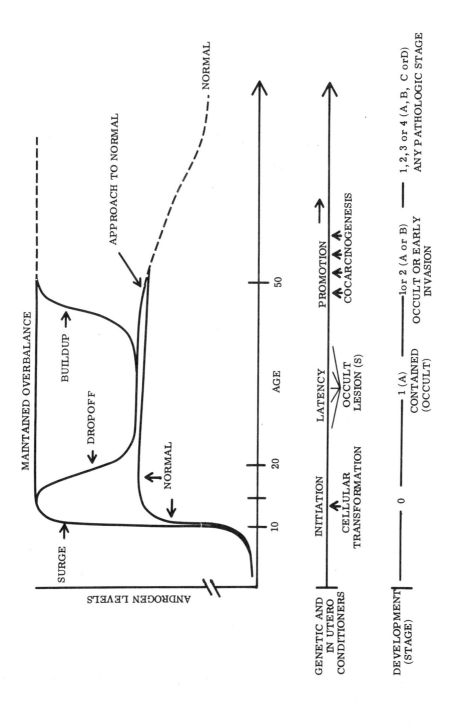

FIGURE 4. Model for carcinogenesis in the human prostate, including events paralleling the animal model, and conformance of the model to staging of the lesion. See text for explanation.

Explanation of the model. Evidence at sampled institutions focused upon
early adolescence when differences between prostatic cancer patients and
controls emerged. Age classes varied for each variable and for each hospital,
as would be expected for populations which differed in composition ethnically
and by sociocultural level, but all such primary differences are within ages
10 to 17, the pubertal, prepubertal and postpubertal ranges. Generally
described, these variables are the secondary sexual characteristics, those
concerned with sexual drive and development, early gynecomastias and pubertal
obesity. Results for some of these variables are stronger than others,
and for some are only suggestive, but with some exceptions they trend in the
same directions: more patients developed secondary sexual characteristics
at specific pubertal ages than corresponding groups of controls, and also
more were excessively driven sexually during these periods. Further, despite
their strong libidos, a proportion of patients appear to have been repressed
sexually throughout life. Also, fewer patients developed gynecomastias and
obesity early in life than expected by comparison with controls, suggestive
of a strong overbalance of androgenic components even when excessive estrogenic secretion could be expected to produce feminizing characteristics in
a certain number of young males.

Referring to Figure 4, the model shows an excessive androgenic rise during
puberty. This may be considered as a temporary surge with a consequent
dropoff to almost normal, or as a maintained abnormal overbalance which
persists through life. In either case, the assumption is that a high level
of unbound androgens is available to operate upon active pubertal and postpubertal prostatic tissue.

The curves in Figure 4 compare the high levels of androgen against normal.
No scale is provided for the Y axis, since the trend is what is being established. The development of carcinogenesis, underneath the curves, indicates
cellular transformation leading to initiation of the carcinoma with potential
for further neoplastic development. Data from the individual and combined
samples appear to suggest that although patients are characterized by a
stronger sexual drive than the general male population, also as a consequence
of excessive androgenic secretion, their sexual capacity is underutilized,
indicating sexual repression for unknown reasons.

If an overbalance is maintained during life it would continue throughout
the latent period into the later years. A surge would drop back, approaching
normal later in life. Since onset of the cancer is presumed to begin at

68

puberty and the mean age at diagnosis is about age 65, the average latent
period following initiation is very long, as predicted by Whitmore (35),
perhaps 50 or more years, after which a reinforcing event is required to
promote the lesion into malignancy. This is the well known cocarcinogenic
modification following the animal model of Berenblum (3) and all others
who have demonstrated classical carcinogenesis with laboratory animals.
A human model paralleling the animal model has been proposed for cervix
cancer (25,26) based upon strongly convincing research results, but without
resolution of cocarcinogenesis. An approach to this may, however, be made
for prostate cancer.

Latency is variable in duration. Early carcinomatous foci are expected to
develop during this period, probably toward the end since few such foci have
been found in autopsy material from young men. Appearance of the lesion
in earliest detectable stages may not take place until the sixth decade or
even later, depending upon rate of development and also possibly maintained
hormonal levels or the presence of other unknown factors. From our data
which suggest a repression of sexuality by patients throughout life, a
constant accumulation of prostatic residues may take place which would have
no effect until the latent lesion was sufficiently developed for progression
into advanced stages. If the approach to actuality in the model is a surge
of androgen with a later dropoff, we can assume that there is a buildup
again of hormonal and other residues at age levels when carcinomas begin to
be diagnosed, failing an adequate sexual outlet. If this does not take place,
the lesion remains latent without progressing. In the case of a maintained
overbalance, if tenable as a hypothesis, the high level of androgens would
remain so until the focus of cells is sufficiently advanced to progress later
in life as programmed. The cocarcinogenic event may affect the latent lesion
at any time after it matures sufficiently, with an increasing probability
that this will take place as the candidate becomes older, which is why morbidity rates rise with age.

Relationship of the model to any specific hormonal precursor, metabolite or
enzyme is not proposed, nor are other substances or influences possibly
operating upon initiation or promotion identified. The objectives are to
show an effect at puberty and to relate epidemiologic findings to carcinogenesis.

Other speculations are possible for promotion of the lesion after latency:
external cocarcinogens, failure of inhibitors or immunologic defenses to

69

protect against invasion, or even a genetic timetable which can operate within the modified cell in later years. The evidence so far seems to indicate continuing secretory production for which an adequate sexual program might bring relief from risk.

There is no intent to overlook possible epidemiologic alternatives to a hormonal hypothesis, nor to the possibility that external modifiers can operate upon a key endogenous variable. These domains include migratory patterns to search for environmental influence, sociocultural patterns, occupational exposures, diet, physical and psychologic stress, use of tobacco and alcohol, and interaction with other disease processes.

From the model, a theory of a subsiding surge followed by a later buildup of prostatic secretion which may or may not occur depending upon sexual behavioral patterns, would explain the large number of latent lesions which never develop, and also those that do. This may serve additionally to explain the lazy carcinoma which does not remain stationary but develops very slowly past promotion. The concept of a maintained high level of androgen might be useful in explaining the aggressive cancer.

Detailed comparisons of sexual and hormonal-related variables are being reported (33) and also will be published in later papers. Results from studies of other investigated areas in the research will be presented. Evidential support and interpretations for the model are provided in the following summary.

Percentage frequencies of sexual variables covering totals for all samples are shown in Table 2. Where only three years are shown the age class represents the specific time of life when trends or excesses developed; where more than three years are shown, the age ranges include separate classes for each sampled hospital.

Trends show excesses of patients with pubertal onset of masturbation, after which a reversal takes place favoring controls. Fewer patients failed to practice masturbation during life. Since masturbatory activity does not require a partner, the conclusion is that a high level of hormonally mediated eroticism took place during puberty, followed by repression. That patients were highly driven sexually also is suggested by frequencies showing fewer who failed to masturbate during life. Attempts at seduction (referred to as necking and petting in detailed reports) continue the trend of excessive libidinous output by patients, yet for some reason there seems to have been

70

TABLE 2:   SEXUAL DRIVE AND DEVELOPMENT:
SUMMARY OF SEXUAL VARIABLES.*

VARIABLES	N Pairs	Patients %	Controls %	Trend or Excess	P Values
Onset Masturbation:					
Ages 12-14	413	33.4	25.2	Patients	<.005
Ages 14-17	413	26.7	36.3	Controls	<.002
Never Masturbation	413	20.1	29.0	Controls	<.001
Heavy Seduction:					
Ages 11-14	413	17.9	10.0	Patients	<.0005
Ages 15-19	413	34.6	31.0	Patients	NS
Ages 20-39	413	22.5	21.8	Patients	NS
Unfulfilled Erections					
Ages 11-14	413	14.5	11.6	Patients	NS
Ages 15-19	413	52.8	50.1	Patients	NS
Ages 20=39	413	44.3	44.1	=	NS
Heavy Nocturnal Emissions					
Ages 11-14	413	25.2	19.6	Patients	<.03
Ages 15-19	413	57.2	51.1	Patients	<.05
Ages 20-39	413	45.3	42.1	Patients	NS
$\bar{X}$ Coital Acts Per Year	413	63.7	72.3	Controls	--
$\bar{X}$ Age, Greatest Coital	Pat. 395				
Activity	Cont. 387	30.75	32.34	Controls	--

*Condensed from detailed data presented at the XIIth Int'l Cancer Congress, Buenos Aires, October 1978, to be published in a forthcoming report.

an underdevelopment of actual sexual encounters, shown by mean coital acts per year. Trends for unfulfilled erections and heavy nocturnal emissions, both involuntary indicators of sexual drive and least inhibited by availability of sexual opportunity, both were shown in other publications (30,31,33) with excesses of patients during adolescence, and with a diminution of frequencies approaching those of controls later in life.

Hormonal-related variables, Table 3, are those usually accepted as indicators of endocrine activity. Trends for these are similar at each hospital for all 4 variables: ages voice change, onset hirsutism, growth acceleration and genitalia development, settling upon puberty as the time when differences developed between patients and controls. Although not shown, these trends reverse or disappear at all sampled hospitals after the pubertal age periods where they were found, indicating that they are substantial enough to consider in support of the model.

Additionally, fewer patients developed early gynecomastias and obesity compared to controls. These findings are strong in the Los Anglese samples, but considerably weaker in the Chicago samples, although the trends are observable in accumulated frequencies. Again, different populations are not directly comparable, yet totals reveal the trend. If true, and repeatable in other populations, failure to develop effeminate characteristics early in life by an expected proportion of the male population can be viewed as an estrogenic deficit, or of so preponderant an androgenic component that an excess of estrogen is masked.

The domain of voluntary coital sexuality is indirect in measuring erotic drive since all variables calling for participating partners are conditioned by cultural background, proximity, opportunity and approach. That these sociologic modifiers contribute to the biologic sexual process undoubtedly provides some explanation for the diversity we have found in coital patterns for the 3 hospital populations, by age,class and trend.

A more direct variable is the nocturnal emission, an involuntary sexual episode that reflects background but requires no partner. Figure 5 demonstrates excessive sexual drive by patients at one hospital (Los Angeles) throughout the early years, with reversal in the late twenties. The Chicago hospitals are similar in trend, although both show a departure from the excess characterizing the Los Angeles patients at about age 20. These show early and late excesses of patient sexual drive, but with similarity at age

TABLE 3: HORMONE-RELATED VARIABLES: SUMMARY*

| VARIABLES | N | | Patients % | Controls % | Trend or Excess | P Values |
	Patients	Controls				
Voice Change Ages 10-17	284	269	50.7	36.8	Patients	<.0005
Onset Hirsutism Ages 12-17	337	347	43.0	33.1	Patients	<.004
Accelerated Growth, Ages 10-14	193	165	40.4	32.7	Patients	<.07
Genitalia Develmt, Ages 12-15	308	312	39.9	31.4	Patients	<.02
Gynecomastias, Ages 12-13	413	413	1.6	2.6	Controls	NS
Pubertal Obesity Ages 17	413	413	5.8	8.2	Controls	<.09

*Condensed from detailed data presented at the XIIth Int'l Cancer Congress, Buenos Aires, October 1978, to be published in a forthcoming report.

20. All samples indicate strong drive following adolescence. However, Figure 6 demonstrates a uniform deficit of coital activity extending into the later years by patients at all sampled hospitals, and into old age at 2 hospitals.

A separate sexual variable, unfulfilled erections, Figure 7, measures drive but also describes the well known experience following attempts at seduction, closeness to the arousing partner or sexual reveries, although our question specifically designated the outcome of encounters. Excesses of patients at 2 hospitals were found with these experiences peaking during late adolescence. The trend at the third hospital generally is similar, losing the effect at late adolescence but confirming it in the early and middle years. The repeated unfulfilled erection can be considered a source of trauma to the urogenital system, often with extremely painful sequellae following engorgement. Whether it is an adequate or adjunct event for initiation of neoplasia is open to speculation; our interest in this variable was in relation to sexual drive.

DISCUSSION AND MORE SPECULATION

That sexuality has emerged as a suggested component contributing to risk is not surprising. Ismail et al. (18) demonstrated that during abstention of coitus by young men a cyclic pattern of urinary testosterone production was observed, with peaks of excretion at about eight-day intervals. Episodes of sexual intercourse resulted in a rise of testosterone excretion, indicating that androgens were being removed as a result of coitus. Further, Gupta (12) in studying prepubertal boys from 8 to 11 years of age, found a correlation between urinary testosterone and skeletal maturity, larger boys excreting more hormone. Hormone levels of girls did not correlate with bone maturity. Of the three other papers investigating epidemiologic associations with prostate cancer, only two developed sexual material. Steele et al. (34) found a gradient of "sustained sexual interest" and sexual drive which was greatest by prostatic cancer patients, less by BPH patients, and least by controls. Measurement of sexual drive was by multiple premarital and extramarital partners, and by an interest in "more coitus." Krain (20) discovered more prostatic cancer patients with a history of multiple coital acts per week than controls, and also more coital partners before marriage. Both studies are characterized by problems with which we are sympathetic: small samples, a very sensitive subject in communicating with older men, and choice of indicators to measure sexual drive.

SEXUAL DRIVE AND DEVELOPMENT: HEAVY NOCTURNAL EMISSIONS

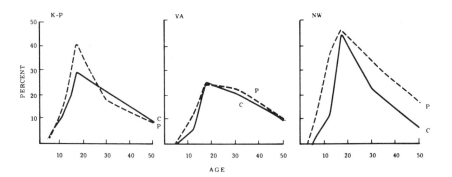

SEXUAL DRIVE AND DEVELOPMENT: COITAL ACTS PER YEAR

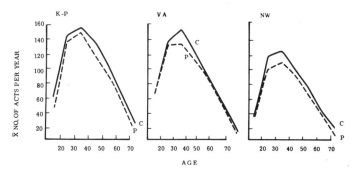

SEXUAL DRIVE AND DEVELOPMENT: UNFULFILLED ERECTIONS

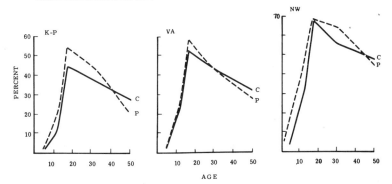

FIGURE 5.   Sexual drive and development in 3 hospital populations: heavy nocturnal emissions. (Upper)

FIGURE 6.   Sexual drive and development in 3 hospital populations: coital acts per year. (Middle)

FIGURE 7.   Sexual drive and development in 3 hospital populations: unfulfilled erections. (Lower)

75

From our experience, it would be hazardous to predict that a single key variable will arise for prostatic cancer as it has in lung cancer (and the subject has not been exhausted for lung cancer) other than a possible contribution to risk of some degree by sexual patterns and their influence upon cellular oncogenic transformation through physiologic process, probably endocrinologic, with the cell as target for secretory imbalances or excesses of some sort. The possibility cannot be overlooked that an oncogen or carcinogen can be venereally transmitted, although our studies so far have not provided convincing evidence to support such an outcome of sexuality.

Is there a necessary virus? Research into the possible role of viruses in association with human prostatic tumors has not been as aggressively pursued as in cancers of the cervix and breast, leukemias and lymphomas. Although not strictly an epidemiologic pursuit, the merging of virologic and epidemiologic disciplines occurs in seroepidemiologic studies where antibody response to identified agents is measured in cases and controls. So far, it is doubtful that any human neoplastic condition has been convincingly associated with the presence of a virus either as an initiating agent or a promoter, yet the opportunity for viral nucleotides to interfere with normal cellular function is attractive as a hypothesis for oncogenesis, and it is well demonstrated that certain neoplastic diseases of fowl, mice, rabbits and frogs are virally induced. Two currents exist in studies of prostatic cancer: investigations of relationships with oncornaviruses, particularly type C; and also herpesvirus simplex type 2. Dmochowski and Horoszewicz (8) found virus-like particles in samples of poorly differentiated prostatic adenocarcinomas, and also in undifferentiated cancers. These particles, resembling type C viruses, were found in 10 of 35 prostatic cancers and in 1 of 8 BPH prostates. Centifanto et al. (6) suggested that the human prostate is the reservoir for type 2 herpesviruses which then are available for transmission to the female at risk of cervix cancer. However, the case for HSV2 as a venereal oncogenic agent initiating cervix cancer still is unresolved (28).

There are difficulties with human virologic investigations: individual viruses are selected for study and other possible agents are not excluded, the evidence necessarily must be circumstantial since human subjects may not be experimentally inoculated and human cancers require long periods for development, and selected viruses so far have been found to be relatively ubiquitous. The use of tumor tissue in viral investigations is open to

procedural question since any relationship is then not with the initiation
or promotion of the cancer but with the cancer after it already has developed.   This latter has been a problem with hybridization experiments incorporating portions of viral nucleic acids into the genome of tumor cells, where
the relationship would better be made with normal cells at risk, if they
could be identified.   To date, researchers in prostatic cancer have made
little headway on the question, but if such a viral relationship does exist,
a venereal mode is likely.   There is the possiblity of an interaction of
hormones with viruses, especially if a vertically transmitted particle is
postulated which can be switched on by specific androgenic components.

Outlook for new research.   The usual demurrer that much more work will need
to be done before the situation clarifies must be introduced here since
little work has been done.   Our research is only a beginning and has been
featured because there is very little other epidemiologic effort to cite.
I have presented some background in this paper, and also limited results
of selected variables, sexual and hormonally related.   From these I have
proposed a model for the initiation and development of prostatic cancer,
not as an end result but in an effort to organize continuing epidemiologic
interest into directional patterns.

From results so far, continuing research could focus upon testing limited
selections of variables as our interpretations proceed.   More work upon the
true nature of a relationship between benign prostatic hyperplasia and prostatic cancer should be attempted, if only defensively to eliminate or to
maintain the hypothesis, studies so far having been inconclusive.

The effect of prostatitis upon initiation of prostatic cancer often has
been proposed, yet such a hypothesis calls for prospective designs requiring
30 or more years for resolution.   Prostatic infections do not normally arise
until early adulthood, in contradiction to our theory of adolescent initiation.   An important suggestion for new research would be to begin investigations of pubertal boys, with ages perhaps ranging from 10 to 17, and with
focus upon the age class 12-14, for those individuals who are found with
significant departures of hormonal assay, and with extended followup to
determine continuing trends of abnormal levels, or possible dropoffs toward
the end of adolescence.   Although circumstantial, this would provide a basis
for establishing puberty as the time when cellular transformation can take
place.

It might be useful for urologic clinicians to routinely obtain information
from male patients at age 40 and over about continuing sexuality to
distinguish those who are active against those who are not, and for
correlation with eventual diagnoses of both BPH and prostatic cancer. If
our speculations hold promise, repression of sexuality might be another
indicator for detection of prostatic cancer.

REFERENCES

1. Armenian, H. K., Lilienfeld, A. M., Diamond, E. L. and Brose, I. D.
    J.: Relation between benign prostatic hyperplasia and cancer of the
    prostate. Lancet, II: 115, 1974.
2. Bean, M. A., Yatani, R., Lin, P. I., Fukazawa, K., Ashley, F. W. and
    Fujida, S.: Prostatic carcinoma at autopsy in Hiroshima and Nagasaki
    Japanese. Cancer, 32: 498, 1973.
3. Berenblum, I.: The mechanism of carcinogenesis. A study of the
    significance of cocarcinogenic action and related phenomena. Cancer
    Research, 1: 807, 1941.
4. Brandon, J. G.: Un programa de registro de incidencia de cancer su
    Lima metropolitana. Instituto Nacional de Enfermedades Neoplasicas,
    Ministerio de Salud, Lima, Peru, 1973.
5. Byar, D. P.: Benign prostatic hyperplasia and cancer of the prostate.
    Lancet, I: 866, 1975.
6. Centifanto, Y. M., Drylie, D. M., Deardourff, S. L., and Kaufman, H.
    E.: Herpesvirus type 2 in the male genitourinary tract. Science,
    178: 318, 1972.
7. Cutler, S. J. and Young, J. L.: Third National Cancer Survey:
    Incidence Data. USDHEW Publ. No. (NIH) 75-787, PHS, NIH, NCI.
    National Cancer Monograph 41, Bethesda, Maryland, 1975.
8. Dmochowski, L. and Horoszewica, J. S.: Viral oncology of prostatic
    cancer. Seminars in Oncology, 3: 141, 1976.
9. Franks, L. M.: Latent carcinoma of the prostate. Journal of
    Pathology and Bacteriology, 68: 603, 1954.
10. Franks, L. M.: The incidence of carcinoma of prostate: an
    epidemiological survey. In: Recent Results in Cancer Research,
    Vol. 39, Eds: E. Grundmann and H. Tulinius, Springer-Verlag, Berlin,
    1972.
11. Greenwald, P., Kirmss, V., Polan, A. K., and Dick, V. S.: Cancer of
    the prostate among men with BPH. Journal of the National Cancer
    Institute, 33: 335, 1974.
12. Gupta, D.: Separation and estimation of testosterone and
    epitestosterone in the urine of pre-pubertal children. Steroids, 10:
    475, 1967.
13. Haenszel, W. M., Marcus, S. C. and Zimmerer, E. G.: Cancer morbidity
    in urban and rural Iowa. PHS Monograph 37, USDHEW, Bethesda, Md.,
    1957.
14. Haenszel, W., and Kurihara, M.: Studies of Japanese migrants.
    1. Mortality from cancer and other diseases among Japanese in the
    United States. Journal of the National Cancer Institute, 40: 43,
    1968.
15. Henschke, U. K., Leffall, L. D., Jr., Mason, C. H., Reinhold, A. W.,
    Schneider, R. L. and White, J. E.: Alarming increase of the cancer
    mortality in the U.S. black population (1950-1967). Cancer, 31:
    763, 1973.

16. Heshmat, M. Y., Herson, J., Kovi, J., and Niles, R.: An epidemiologic study of gonorrhea and cancer of the prostate gland. Medical Annals of the District of Columbia, 42: 378, 1973.
17. Hutchison, G. B.: Epidemiology of prostatic cancer. Seminars in Oncology, 3: 151, 1976.
18. Ismail, A. A. A. and Harkness, R. A.: Urinary testosterone excretion in men in normal and pathological conditions. Acta Endocrinologica, 56: 469, 1967.
19. Jackson, M. A., Ahluwalia, B. S., Attah, E. B., Connolly, C. A., Herson, J., Heshmat, M. Y., Jackson, A. G., Jones, G. W., Kapoor, S. K., Kennedy, J., Kovi, J., Lucas, A. O., Nkposong, E. O., Olisa, E. and Williams, A. O.: Characterization of prostatic carcinoma among blacks. A preliminary report. Cancer Chemotherapy Reports, 59: 3, 1975.
20. Krain, L. S.: Epidemiologic variables in prostatic cancer. Geriatrics, 2: 93, 1973.
21. King, H. K., Diamond, E., and Lilienfeld, A. M.: Some epidemiological aspects of cancer of the prostate. Journal of Chronic Diseases, 16: 117, 1963.
22. Liavag, I., Harbitz, T. B., and Haugen, O. A.: Latent carcinoma of the prostate. In: Recent Results in Cancer Research, Vol. 39, Eds: E. Grundmann and H. Tulinius, Springer-Verlag, Berlin, 1972.
23. Oota, K. and Misu, Y.: A study on latent carcinoma of the prostate in Japanese. GANN (Japanese Journal of Cancer Research), 49: 283, 1958.
24. Oota, K.: Latent carcinoma of the prostate among the Japanese. Acta Union Internationale Cancra, 17: 952, 1961.
25. Rotkin, I. D.: Adolescent coitus and cervical cancer: associations of related events with increased risk. Cancer Research, 27: 603 1967.
26. Rotkin, I. D.: Cervical carcinogenesis: an epidemiologic model adaptable to control programs. In: Recent Results in Cancer Research, Vol. 39, Eds: E. Grundmann and H. Tulinius, Berlin, Springer-Verlag, 1972.
27. Rotkin, I. D.: Benign prostatic hyperplasia, prostatic cancer and carcinogenesis. Lancet, II: 359, 1975.
28. Rotkin, I. D.: Another view of Herpes simplex virus type 2. Journal of the American Medical Association, 235: 2188, 1976.
29. Rotkin, I. D.: Epidemiology of benign prostatic hypertrophy: review and speculations. In: Benign Prostatic Hyperplasia, NIAMDD Workshop Proceedings, 1975. Eds: John Grayhack and Gene D. Wilson. DHEW Publ. No. (NIH) 76-1113, USDHEW, PHS, NIH. Gov't Printing Office, Washington, D. C., pp. 105, 1976.
30. Rotkin, I. D.: Studies in the epidemiology of prostatic cancer: expanded sampling. Cancer Treatment Reports, 61: 173, 1977.
31. Rotkin, I. D.: Risk variables associated with prostatic cancer. In: Cancer Prevention and Detection (Proceedings of the Third Int'l. Symposium on the Detection and Prevention of Cancer). Ed. H. E. Nieburgs. Marcel Dekker, Inc., New York, 1978.
32. Rotkin, I. D.: Epidemiology of prostatic cancer. In: Cancer Epidemiology in the United States and the Soviet Union. Ed: D. L. Levin. Monograph, NCI, NIH, Bethesda, Md. In press.
33. Rotkin, I. D., Cooper, J. F., Benjamin, J. A., Osburn, W. C., Moses, V. K. and Kaushal, D.: Effect of sexual events and attributes upon risk of prostatic cancer: Los Angeles samples. Submitted for publication.

34. Steele, R., Lees, R.E. M., Kraus, A. S. and Rao, C.: Sexual factors in the epidemiology of cancer of the prostate. Journal of Chronic Diseases, 24: 29, 1971.
35. Whitmore, W. F.: The natural history of prostatic cancer. Cancer, 32: 1104, 1973.
36. Winkelstein, W. and Kantor, S.: Prostatic Cancer: relationship to suspended particulate air pollution. American Journal of Public Health, 59: 1134, 1969.
37. Woolf, C. M.: An investigation of the familial aspects of carcinoma of the prostate. Journal of Chronic Diseases, 24: 29, 1971.
38. Wynder, E. L., Mabuchi, K., and Whitmore, W. F., Jr.: Epidemiology of cancer of the prostate. Cancer, 28: 344, 1971.

In view of the postulated hormone dependency of benign prostatic hyperplasia (BPH) and prostatic carcinoma (PCA), it is of importance to have an exact knowledge of the hormonal environment in which these tumors develop and to investigate whether in patients with either BPH or prostatic cancer, plasma sex hormone levels are different from those in controls.

This raises however some difficult problems. First, we really do not know when BPH or carcinoma really begins. Many urologists believe that a small periurethral nodule requires 15-25 years before it is transformed into clinical BPH (2,10). If BPH does not occur when castration is performed before puberty, but does occur if castration is performed between age 20 and 30, then it may be a valid working hypothesis that BPH begins early in adulthood. Second, if prepubertal castrates do not develop BPH even when treated with androgens, then it may be assumed that besides testosterone (T), the testes contribute (an) other factor(s), important in the development of BPH.

Hence, it appears that in evaluating the hormonal environment in which BPH develops, we should:

1. study sex hormone secretion not only in elderly males but also in young individuals.

2. not only look at testosterone but also at other testicular hormones.

3. not only make cross-sectional studies, but also make longitudinal studies over 30-40 years.

It is unrealistic however to hope that such data will be available in the next few years; hence, we are bound for many more years to rely upon cross-sectional studies. Finally, in view of the high incidence of BPH and PCA in elderly males, the rationale for comparing hormonal levels in patients with clinical prostatic neoplasia to levels in elderly males may be questioned.

---

*A. Vermeulen[1], A. Van Camp[2], J. Mattelaer[3], and W. De Sy[4]
[1]Dept. of Endocrinology & Metabolic Diseases, Academic Hospital, State University Ghent.
[2]Dept. of Urology, University of Antwerp.
[3]Dept. of Urology, Onze Lieve Vrouw Clinic Kortrijk.
[4]Dept. of Urology, Academic Hospital, State University Ghent (Belgium)

I. Sex hormone levels in normal males

1. After puberty <u>plasma T</u> levels reach a plateau with individual values
    between 280 and 1000 ng/dl, and a mean of about 600 ng/dl. The mean
    metabolic clearance rate (MCR) is about 1000 liters/24 hrs and the
    blood production rate (BPR) varies between 4 and 10 mg/24 hrs.

    This testosterone is largely bound to plasma proteins: about 50-60%
    is bound to a high affinity, low capacity specific binding globulin,
    variously called testosterone-estradiol binding globulin (TeBG) or
    sex hormone binding globulin (SHBG); approximately 40% is loosely
    bound to albumin and 2% is free. Only the non specifically bound
    testosterone is biologically active. The albumin bound fraction is
    linearly related to the free fraction, the proportionality factor
    being determined only by the albumin concentration in plasma.

    From the sixth decade of life on, there occurs a gradual decrease in
    plasma T levels, with however broad interindividual variations, and
    in the ninth decade of life the mean plasma T level is $\pm$ 250 ng/dl
    with individual levels as high as 600 or as low as 50 ng/dl.

    Due to the progressive increase with age of the TeBG concentration,
    the free testosterone concentration starts to decrease already in
    the 5th decade of life and the combined effect of a decrease of the
    total T levels and of the increase in TeBG results in a steeper
    decline with age of free testosterone.

2. Total and/or free <u>dihydrotestosterone</u> (DHT) levels also decrease with
    age (21), but the decrease is by far less important than for testos-
    terone (31,6,15).

3. Similarly, <u>5α-androstane-3α,17β-diol</u> levels decrease from a mean of
    17ng/dl in normal young males to a value of approximately 8ng/dl in
    elderly males.

4. Plasma <u>androstenedione</u> (A) has a mixed adrenal and testicular origin
    (31). Although Pirke et al (21) observed a moderate decrease with age
    of A levels, the relative levels of A are independent of age.

5. 17-hydroxy Progesterone (17-OHP) has essentially a testicular origin.
    Hence it is not surprising that an age dependent decrease of 17-OHP
    levels is observed.

6. <u>Progesterone</u> levels are age independent.

7. Along the $\Delta 5$ pathway, the immediate precursor of testosterone is
    androst-5-en-3β,17β-diol ($\Delta 5$-diol) (see chapter 2). Pirke et al (21)
    as well as we ourselves observed an age dependent decrease of plasma
    levels of $\Delta 5$-diol.

8. The immediate biosynthetic precursor of $\Delta 5$-diol is DHEA, plasma levels
    of which originate largely from the adrenal cortex. Considering its
    adrenal origin, plasma levels of DHEA as well as of DHEA-sulfate sur-
    prisingly decrease rapidly in elderly males (and women). In view of
    the fact that cortisol secretion does not decrease significantly in
    old age, this observation suggests a specific shift in the bio-
    synthetic pathways in aging adrenals. Indeed, the decrease in plasma
    levels is not a consequence of a change in metabolism, as the MCR
    is certainly not increased in elderly persons.

9. Plasma 17-hydroxypregnenolone has a mixed adrenal-testicular origin
    with about equal contribution from both glands.

    Again in elderly males the plasma levels are significantly lower than
    in young males; the same applies to pregnenolone levels.

From these results we may conclude that in aging males secretion of T and its
precursors is decreased and that moreover there occur important changes in
adrenal steroid biosynthesis, resulting in a dramatic decrease in DHEA and
DHEA-sulfate levels.

What is the biological origin of this decrease in androgen secretion? Several
morphological studies have shown that the biochemical evidence for an age
dependent impairment of testicular function finds its anatomical equivalent
in a decrease in testicular volume, progressive thickening of basal membranes,
interstitial fibrosis, decreased spermatogenesis and a decrease in the number
of Leydig cells. It has been shown that the distribution pattern of the
testicular lesions is closely related to testicular blood flow, being more
pronounced in the testicular segments at the periphery of arterial supply.

This raises the question whether testicular senescence has a primary testicular
or a secondary hypothalamo-pituitary origin.

It is well known that, whereas in postmenopausal females there occurs a large
increase in gonadotropin secretion, not nearly as great an increase is
observed in elderly men.

Nevertheless, most authors studying plasma gonadotropin levels observed a

significant increase in both LH and FSH levels in old age, pointing towards
a primary testicular origin of the decreased testicular function (27,23,8,13,
26).

Nevertheless there appears to exist an adequate Leydig cell secretory reserve
since upon human chorionic gonadotropin stimulation plasma T levels increase,
although the absolute and possibly also the relative increase is less than
in younger subjects (23). On the other hand the pituitary gonadotrophs react
to gonadotropin releasing hormone (GnRH) stimulation with increased LH and
FSH output, although again the response may be somewhat weaker than in young
individuals (23,8,9). Therefore, subtle age related alterations in the hypothalamo-pituitary function may exist with the resultant lowering of the feedback set point.

However, other explanations may be advanced. It is well known that in males
estradiol (E2) levels do not decrease as a function of age and several authors
observed an increase in E2 levels in elderly males (21,23). Moreover, due
to the increase in TeBG and the lower affinity of TeBG for E2 than for T,
the free E2 fraction decreases less than the free T fractions in elderly
males. As a consequence there occurs an age related increase in the ratio
of the concentration of available free estradiol to available free testosterone
(AFE2C/AFTC). Hence it is possible that this increased E2 level might suppress LH secretion which normally would be stimulated in response to the age
related decrease in T levels.

II. Sex hormone levels in BPH and prostatic carcinoma

The question may be raised whether subjects with BPH or prostatic carcinoma have a different hormonal spectrum. Schematically aging is characterized by a decline in androgen secretion and at least a relative increase
in estrogen secretion.

In view of the fact that androgens and perhaps estrogens are necessary
for BPH to develop, one may wonder in subjects that develop BPH, whether
higher androgen and/or estrogen levels are found. The difficulty however
resides in the fact:

1. that BPH becomes only clinically manifest after a silent evolution
   of at least 20 yrs.

2. that clinical symptomatology is only poorly related to the volume
   of the prostate.

3. that at the time of clinical symptomatology, the critical period
   for growth stimulation may be over.

As no prospective studies are available and as subjects that <u>will</u> develop
BPH or prostatic carcinoma cannot be distinguished early in life, the <u>only</u>
<u>data available concern patients in an advanced stage of the disease</u>. There
is some evidence for distinct differences in hormonal plasma levels between
patients with clinically evident BPH and "normal controls".

1. In comparison to normal controls, BPH patients appear to have higher
   mean plasma T (fig. 1) and DHT levels (11,12,29,30); the differences
   being greatest within patients 70-80 yrs old. The individual values
   overlap, however, the whole normal range. In PCA the mean T level,
   although higher, was not significantly increased in comparison to
   control.

2. Whereas in young males, 75% of plasma DHT originates by peripheral
   conversion of T, in elderly males (with BPH?) over 50% of DHT is
   secreted as such either by the testes or the prostate.

   It is possible that the hypertrophied prostate secretes DHT. Mahoudeau et al. (17) found the mean DHT levels in prostatic venous
   plasma to be 69 vs 41 ng/dl in peripheral plasma, although the
   difference was not statistically significant. However, if we estimate
   the prostatic blood flow at about 20 ml/min, the secretion of the
   hyperplastic prostate would be $\pm$ 10 μg/24 hrs or relatively negligible.

   After prostatectomy neither Mahoudeau et al. (17) nor Vermeulen &
   De Sy (30) found any decrease in DHT levels, suggesting again that
   prostatic DHT secretion does not contribute significantly to the
   total DHT blood production rate (300-600 μg/24 hrs).

3. Mean plasma estradiol levels, (3.0 $\pm$ 0.2 ng/dl) appear to be slightly
   higher in BPH patients than in controls (2.2 $\pm$ 0.2 ng/dl), however
   with individual values overlapping again the whole normal range.(Fig.2)
   This confirms the data of Sköldefors et al. (24) which demonstrated
   an increase in urinary excretion of estrogens in BPH. In this
   connection it is interesting to recall that Lloyd et al. (16) reported
   that in dogs with BPH, E2 and E1 plasma and prostatic tissue levels
   were significantly increased.

   Bayard et al. (1) on the other hand found similar T and E2 blood

Figure 1.

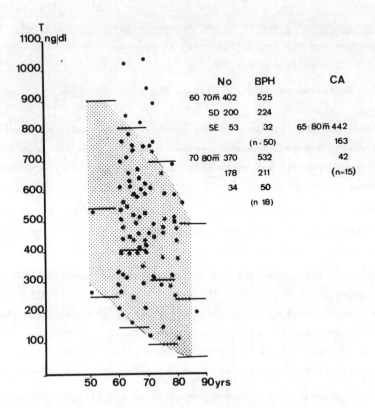

T levels in function of age, in normal subjects (No) and in patients with prostatic neoplasm. • = BPH * = PCA

Figure 2.

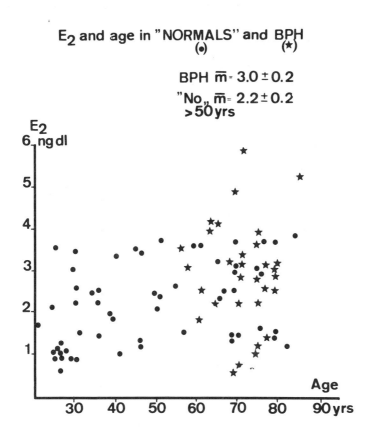

Estradiol levels in aging males with and without BPH.

production rates in 6 patients with BPH and in sex age matched controls.

4. As shown in fig. 3 there is an evident increase of the E2/T ratio with age but in patients with clinical BPH, this ratio is not higher than in "normal" controls.

5. In patients with either BPH or prostatic carcinoma, LH but not FSH levels appear to be lower than in controls (7), as is the increase upon GnRH stimulation (4,7).

6. As far as prolactin is concerned, data in the literature are divergent as Harper et al. observed increased levels in patients with BPH, whereas Hammond et al. (7) did not observe any difference with normal controls.

In summary, data from literature as well as from our laboratory suggest that in patients with clinical BPH and possibly also with prostatic carcinoma, both mean androgen and estrogen levels, are slightly higher than in normal controls. Moreover there is evidence for at least relatively increased secretion of DHT, but available data so far do not indicate that the prostate is a major source of the extra DHT. In the individual patient with BPH however, low, normal or increased androgen and/or estrogen levels may be observed. As to the significance of these findings with respect to pathogenesis of either BPH or prostatic carcinoma, one can only speculate. Androgens do stimulate prostatic growth and there is suggestive evidence that the combined action of androgens and estrogens might be synergistic. On the other hand increased plasma levels may be the consequence rather than the cause of prostatic neoplasia. For example, in BPH tissue the conversion of DHT to Adiol could be impaired (5,20); this might block further uptake of DHT, and although rather unlikely, increase indirectly plasma DHT levels. Malathi & Gurpide (18) in superfusion experiments found that at least under in vitro conditions release of DHT to cell medium is a main route of disposition of DHT, whereas most of Adiol and T are metabolized to other products. Wilson et al. (33) were unable to produce BPH with injection of either T or DHT in castrated dogs, although the intracellular DHT concentration was as high as in the control hypertrophic group. Androstane-3α,17β-diol, alone or in combination with estrogens on the other hand did induce BPH in castrated dogs (32) and, in distinction with other authors Shida et al. (25) observed an increased Adiol formation in hypertrophic in comparison to normal prostates (14). On the

Figure 3.

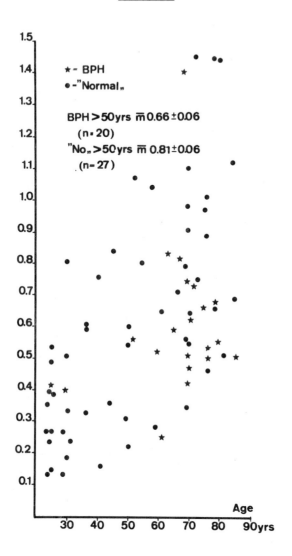

E2/T in males with and without BPH.

other hand, in the view of the low Adiol concentration in plasma, its decrease in old age and its high affinity binding to TeBG, it appears however difficult to conceive how plasma Adiol would play a major role in the pathogenesis of BPH.

One should finally bear in mind that all the data concerning hormone levels in prostatic neoplasia are obtained at the time when BPH or PCA are well developed, and that their developments took 10-20 yrs. We do not know whether patients in whom increased hormone levels are observed have had increased hormone levels for the whole period while they developed prostatic neoplasia. Prospective longitudinal studies in young subjects with elevated sex hormone levels should furnish data to decide whether increased sex hormone levels play a causal role in the pathogenesis of prostatic neoplasia.

References

1. Bayard, F., Louvet, J. P., Thyssens J. L., Thouvenot, J. P., & Boulard, C. L. Taux de production de la testosterone et de l'oestradiol 17 chez le sujet proteur d'une hypertrophie prostatique. Annales d'Endocrin., 34: 563-571 (Paris), 1974.
2. Brendler H.: Benign prostatic hyperplasia. Natural history. In: "Benign prostatic hyperplasia" p. 101-103, NIAMDD workshop Proceedings, 1975.
3. Demisch, K., Magnet, W., Lenbauer, W., & Schoffling, K.: Studies about unconjugated androstenediol in human peripheral plasma. J. Clin. Endocrinol. Metab., 37: 129-134, 1973.
4. Geller, J., Baron, A., & Kleinman, S.: Pituitary luteinizing hormone reserve in elderly men with prostatic disease. J. of Endocrinol., 48: 289-290, 1970.
5. Geller, J., Albert, J., Lopez, D., Geller, S., & Niwayama, G.: Comparison of androgen metabolites in benign prostatic hypertrophy (BPH) and normal prostate. J. Clin. Endocrinol. Metab., 45: 686-688, 1976.
6. Hallberg, M. C., Wieland, R. G., Zorn, E. M., Firrst, B. H., & Wieland, J. M.: Impaired Leydig cell reserve and altered serum androgen binding in the aging male. Fert. & Steril., 27: 812-814, 1976.
7. Hammond, G. L., Konturri, M., Maatala, P., Puukka, M., & Vihko, R.: Serum FSH, LH and prolactin in normal males and patients with prostatic diseases. Clin. Endocrinol., 7: 129-135, 1977.
8. Hashimoto, T., Miyai, K., Izumir, K., & Kumahasa, Y.: Gonadotropin response to synthetic LHRH in normal subjects: correlation between LH and FSH. J. Clin. Endocrinol. & Metab., 37: 910-926, 1973.
9. Haug, E., Aakvaag, E., Sand, T., & Torgesen, I. A.: The gonadotrophin response to synthetic gonadotropin releasing hormone in males in relation to age, dose and basal serum levels of testosterone, oestradiol,-17β and gonadotrophins. Acta Endocrinol., 77: 625-635, 1974.
10. Hirst, A. E., Jr., Bergman, R. T.: Carcinoma of the prostate in men 80 or more years old. Cancer, 7: 136-141, 1954.

11. Horton, R., Hsich, P., Barberia, J., Pages, L., & Cosgrove, M.: Altered blood androgens in elderly men with prostate hyperplasia. <u>J. Clin. Endocrinol.</u>, <u>41</u>: 793-796, 1975.

12. Ishimari T., Pages L., & Horton R.: Altered metabolism of androgens in elderly men with benign prostatic hyperplasia. <u>J. Clin. Endocrinol. & Metab.</u>, <u>45</u>: 695-701, 1977.

13. Isurugi K., Fukutani K., Takayasu H., Wakabayashi K., & Tamaoki B. I.: Age related changes in serum luteinizing hormone (LH) and follicle stimulating hormone (FSH) levels in normal men. <u>J. Clin. Endocrinol. & Metab.</u>, <u>39</u>: 955-957, 1974.

14. Jacobi, G. H. & Wilson, J. D.: Formation of 5α-androstane-3α,17β-diol by normal and hypertrophic human prostate. <u>J. Clin. Endocrinol. & Metab.</u>, <u>44</u>: 107-115, 1977.

15. Lewis, J., Ghanadian B., & Chisholm, G. D.: Serum 5α-dihydrotestosterone and testosterone changes with age in man. <u>Acta Endocrinol.</u>, <u>82</u>: 444-448, 1976.

16. Lloyd, J. W., Thomas, J. A., & Mawhinney, M. G.: Androgens and estrogens in the plasma and prostatic tissue of normal dogs and dogs with benign prostatic hypertrophy. <u>Investigative Urology</u>, <u>13</u>: 220-222, 1975.

17. Mahoudeau, J. A., Delassalle, A., & Bricaire, H.: Secretion of dihydrotestosterone by human prostate in benign prostatic hypertrophy. <u>Acta Endocrinol.</u>, <u>77</u>: 401, 1974.

18. Malathi, K., & Gurpide, E.: Metabolism of 5α-dihydrotestosterone in human benign hyperplastic prostate. <u>J. Ster. Biochem.</u>, <u>8</u>: 141-145, 1977.

19. Mobbs, B. G., Johnson, T. E., & Connolly, S. G.: Hormonal responsiveness of prostatic carcinoma: In vitro technique for prediction. <u>Urology</u>, <u>3</u>: 105-106, 1974.

20. Morfin, R. F., Di Stefano, S., Bercovici, J. P., & Floch, H. H.: Comparison of testosterone, 5α-dihydrotestosterone and 5α-androstane, 3β,17β-diol metabolisms in human normal and hyperplastic prostates. <u>J. Ster. Biochem.</u>, <u>9</u>: 245-252, 1978.

21. Pirke, K. M., & Doerr, P.: Age related changes in free plasma testosterone, dihydrotestosterone and oestradiol. <u>Acta Endocrinol.</u>, <u>89</u>: 171-178, 1975.

22. Rosenfield, R. L., & Otto, P.: Androstenediol levels in human peripheral plasma. <u>J. Clin. Endocrinol. & Metab.</u>, <u>35</u>: 818, 1972.

23. Rubens, R., Dhont, M. & Vermeulen, A.: Further studies on Leydig cell function in old age. <u>J. Clin. Endocrinol. & Metab.</u>, <u>39</u>: 40-45, 1974.

24. Skoldefors, H., Carlstrom, K., & Furuhjebm.: Urinary hormone excretion in benign prostatic hyperplasia. <u>J. Ster. Biochem.</u>, <u>7</u>: 447-480, 1976.

25. Shida, K., Shimazaki, J., Ito, Y., Yamanaka, H., & Nagai-Yuasa, H.: 3α-reduction of dihydrotestosterone in human normal and hypertrophic prostate tissues. <u>Invest. Urol.</u>, <u>13</u>: 241, 1975.

26. Snyder, P. J.: Effect of age on the serum LH and FSH response to gonadotropin releasing hormone. In: "Benign Prostatic Hyperplasia" p. 161, NIAMDD Workshop Proceedings, 1965.

27. Stearns, E. L., MacDonnell, S. A., Kaufman, B. J., Padua, R., Lucman, T. S., Winter, J. S. D., & Faiman, C.: Declining testicular function with age. Hormonal and clinical correlates. <u>Amer. J. of Med.</u>, <u>57</u>: 761-766, 1974.

28. Stenis, P., Horming, D., Lindenmeyer, D., & Theile, L.: Biological and radioimmunological determinations of pituitary hormones, especially of prolactin in patients with prostatic carcinoma

(Abstract). <u>Acta Endocrinol.</u> (Kbh)., 1975, suppl. <u>193</u>, 68.

29. Szymanorski, J., Baranowska, B., Migdalska, B., & Kozlowicz, I.: Etude sur l'interdependance de l'hypertrophie prostatique et les troubles de bilan hormonal. Rapport preliminaire. I. Etude de la testosterone serique. <u>J. d'Urologie et de nephrologie</u>, 10: 827-836, 1976.

30. Vermeulen, A., & De Sy, W.: Androgens in patients with benign prostatic hyperplasia before and after prostatectomy. <u>J. Clin. Endocrinol. & Metab.</u>, <u>43</u>: 1250, 1976.

31. Vermeulen, A. & Verdonck, L.: Radioimmunoassay of 17β-hydroxy-5α-androstan-3 one, 4-androstene-3,17-dione, dehydroepiandrosterone, 17-hydroxyprogesterone and progesterone and its application to human male plasma. <u>J. Ster. Biochem.</u>, <u>7</u>: 1-10, 1976.

32. Walsh, P. C., & Wilson, J. D.: The induction of prostatic hypertrophy in the dog with androstanediol. <u>J. Clin. Invest.</u>, <u>57</u>: 1093, 1976.

33. Wilson, J. D., Gloyna, R. E., & Siiteri, P. K.: Androgen metabolism in the hypertrophic prostate. <u>J. Ster. Biochem.</u>, <u>6</u>: 443-445, 1975.

A COMPARATIVE STUDY OF BINDING, METABOLISM AND ENDOGENOUS LEVELS OF
ANDROGENS IN NORMAL, HYPERPLASTIC AND CARCINOMATOUS HUMAN PROSTATE*
CHAPTER VI

INTRODUCTION

Possible differences between human normal prostate (NPR), prostatic
carcinoma (PCA) and benign prostatic hyperplasia (BPH) concerning their
"androgen status" at the cellular level could lead to further ideas about
the as yet completely unknown role which androgens may play with respect
to the pathogenesis and hormone responsiveness of prostatic tumours. We
have therefore compared androgen binding, in vitro metabolism and
endogenous tissue concentration of androgens in PCA, BPH and NPR. The
data found indicate that the NPR seems to be protected against excessive
accumulation of testosterone (T) and 5α-dihydrotestosterone (DHT) due to
the shift of androgen metabolism to the 5α-androstanediols[x], while in
BPH and especially in PCA the androgen metabolism is shifted to T and/or
DHT, both of which display a high affinity for the cytosolic androgen
receptor.

MATERIAL AND METHODS

Chemicals: All chemicals used were purchased from companies mentioned in
earlier publications (39,40).

Tissue: The origin and handling of the PCA as well as BPH tissue have
been described in detail earlier (39,40). The number of investigated
aliquots may be depicted from the "RESULTS" section. The 7 NPR were
obtained from the Institute of Forensic Medicine. The men were in the
age range 19-43 years (mean: 33), and the time span between death of the
men and tissue processing lasted up to 6 h. The absence of any
pathological alteration was proven by histological examination.

Binding studies: Qualitative and quantitative studies were performed as
described recently (39,40), using agargel electrophoresis according to

---

[x] The following abbreviations and terms were used: 5α-androstanediols
(DIOL) = 5α-androstane-3α, 17β-diol + 5α-androstane-3β, 17β-diol.
$NADPH_2$ = reduced form of nicotinamide-adenine dinucleotide phosphate.
5α-reductase = 3-oxo-5α-steroid $\triangle^4$-dehydrogenase. 5α-reduction = amount
of DHT plus 5α-androstanediols found after DHT incubation. 3α(β) -
reduction = amount of 5α-androstanediols found after DHT incubation.

*Chapter by M. Krieg, W. Bartsch, W. Janssen[+], and K. D. Voigt,
Department of Clinical Chemistry, 2nd Medical Clinic, and Institute of
Forensic Medicine[+], University of Hamburg, D-2000 Hamburg 20, F.R.G.
This paper is a copy of an article, originally published by Pergamon
Press, Oxford, in "The Journal of Steroid Biochemistry", Vol. 10, 1979.

Wagner (70). The homogenate of the BPH and NPR were incubated in exactly
the same way, as described earlier for the BPH (39). The incubation of
the PCA tissue was slightly modified due to the lack of sufficient material,
and to the standardization of the procedure according to the European Group
of Prostatic Cancer Research. Details have been described elsewhere (40).
Sex hormone-binding globulin (SHBG) binding capacity in plasma was
measured by the method of Dennis et al. (18).

Metabolic studies: Metabolic studies were performed for the PCA, BPH and
NPR in exactly the same way, as described for the PCA and BPH in an
earlier publication (40). For clarity some experimental details were
outlined in the "RESULTS" section.

Determination of endogenous androgen tissue levels: The tissue concentrations
were measured by radioimmunoassay after thorough steroid extraction.
Details for measuring T, DHT and 5α-androstane-3α, 17β-diol (3α-diol)
were reported elsewhere (39,41). The handling was exactly the same for
PCA, BPH and NPR.

Miscellaneous: Further details for measuring enzyme and heat sensitivity
of the binding proteins, cytosolic protein concentration, and radioactivity
were published earlier (39). The statistical significance of the difference
of the means were checked with the Wilcoxon-Mann-Whitney-test ("U-test"),
the correlation of the plasmatic and cytosolic SHBG concentration with
the Spearman rank correlation coefficient.

RESULTS

Binding studies: In Fig. 1 typical DHT-binding patterns in human organ
cytosols are shown as obtained by agargel electrophoresis. Concerning
PCA (left panel), three charcoal resistant binding peaks were regularly
found, in addition to small amounts of unbound radioactivity in slice
nos. 18-28, in the 14 analyzed cytosols. While peak 2 and 3 decreased in
the presence of an excess of unlabelled DHT (shaded areas), peak 1
remained unaffected. From a series of binding studies (39,40) we know
that peak 2 represents the cytosolic androgen receptor and peak 3 the
plasmatic SHBG. In 12 out of 14 BPH cytosols (middle panel) a
qualitatively identical binding profile as found in PCA cytosols could
be demonstrated. In two cytosols peak 2 was absent. In the seven
analyzed cytosols of NPR (right panel), only peak 1 and 3 were regularly
assayable, while receptor bound DHT (peak 2) could not be detected. If
calculating the assayable cytosolic receptor (peak 2) and SHBG (peak 3)

94

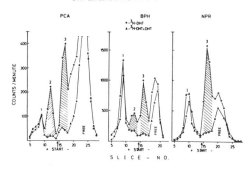

DHT-BINDING IN HUMAN ORGAN CYTOSOLS

Fig. 1 In vitro binding of tritiated DHT in the 100,000 x g cytosol of
human prostatic carcinoma (PCA), benign prostatic hyperplasia (BPH) and
normal prostate (NPR). Organ homogentates or cytosols were incubated with
tritiated DHT alone (•) or in the presence of an excess of unlabelled DHT
(△). Before binding was analyzed by agargel electrophoresis, the cytosol
was treated with charcoal to remove the excess of unbound steroids.
Cytosol (40 μl) was applied between slice Nos. 14 and 15. Anodic pool left,
cathodic pool right from the start. Electrophoresis: 90 min at 10 V/cm.
Temperature within the gel <5°C. Radioactivity was measured in CPM/slice,
each slice being 3 mm wide. The shaded area of peak 2 indicated the
amount of specifically bound DHT to the receptor protein, of peak 3 to
the sex hormone-binding globulin.

concentration in PCA and BPH by the amount of displaced tritiated DHT

through an excess of unlabelled DHT, as indicated by the shaded areas of

Fig. 1, it was found (Table 1) that in PCA cytosol a significantly (P<0.04)

higher receptor and SHBG concentration was assayable than in BPH. Furthermore

(Fig. 2), if the PCA group is divided in a group consisting exclusively of

adenocarcinomas and a group consisting predominantly of a cribriform and/or

low differentiated tumour type, the latter group has a significantly

(P<0,05) higher mean assayable receptor concentration. Concerning SHBG,

this significant difference within the PCA group could not be demonstrated.

In Fig. 3 the statistically significant Spearman rank correlations between

cytosolic and respective plasmatic SHBG concentration are shown, that is

to say the higher the cytosolic assayable concentration of SHBG the higher

is also the respective plasmatic SHBG concentration.

Metabolic studies: In Table 2 the main metabolites found after incubation

of the PCA, BPH and NPR homogenate with either tritiated T, DHT or 3α-diol

are summarized. Four points seem remarkable: 1. In PCA significantly

more of the added T remained unmetabolized than in BPH and NPR, accompanied

by an approximately 15% lower amount of formed DHT plus 5α-androstanediols.

However, the amount of formed DHT was as high as in the BPH and NPR

respectively. 2. In PCA significantly more of the added DHT remained

95

Table 1

Receptor and sex hormone-binding gloubulin (SHBG) concentration in the 100.000 x g cytosol of human prostatic carcinoma (PCA), benign prostatic hyperplasia (BPH) and normal prostate (NPR)

		Receptor conc.	Cytosolic assayable (fmol/mg protein)	SHBG conc.	
	n	mean	range	mean	range
PCA	14	30.9[1]	6.0 - 93.5	93.2[2]	35.7 - 225
BPH	14	12.3	0 - 37.8	39.9	18.1 - 84.7
NPR	7	not assayable		not determined	

Significantly different to BPH: [1] = P<0.04, [2] = P<0.01

Table 2

Main metabolites (mean + SD) obtained by thin layer chromatography in the homogenate of human prostatic carcinoma (PCA), benign prostatic hyperplasia (BPH), and normal prostate (NPR), found after incubation of the 1:2 with buffer diluted homogenate with tritiated testosterone (TESTO), 5α-dihydrotestosterone (DHT), and 5α-androstane-3α, 17β-diol (3α-DIOL) for 30 min at 37°C in the presence of $NADPH_2$ (for TESTO and DHT) or NADP (for 3α-DIOL).

	Metabolites found (pmol)	Tritiated steroids added per g homogenate		
		TESTO (15.4+2.4 pmol)	DHT (16.8+2.5 pmol)	3α-DIOL (23.2+1.6 pmol)
PCA	TESTO	5.1+2.8[1] (10)	<0.5 (5)	<0.5 (4)
	DHT	6.6+3.2 (10)	13+2.5 (5)	1.8+0.2 (4)
	DIOL	3.3+2.4[2] (10)	3.9+2.1[2] (5)	20+0.6 (4)
BPH	TESTO	0.8+0.5 (16)	<0.5 (16)	<0.5 (6)
	DHT	5.5+1.7 (16)	6.8+1.9 (16)	1.2+0.4 (6)
	DIOL	6.2+2.7 (16)	7.3+3.0 (16)	21+1.3 (6)
NPR	TESTO	1.2+0.8 (7)	<0.5 (7)	<0.5 (2)
	DHT	4.3+1.7 (7)	5.5+2.7 (7)	<0.5 (2)
	DIOL	7.3+2.5 (7)	10.5+3.6 (7)	22.6+1.8 (2)

DIOL = 5α-androstane-3α, 17β-diol + 5α-androstane-3β, 17β-diol
Significantly different to BPH and NPR: [1] = P<0.01, [2] = P<0.05

CYTOSOLIC ASSAYABLE RECEPTOR CONC.
(f mol / mg PROTEIN)

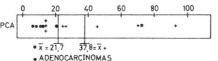

• ADENOCARCINOMAS

+ CRIBRIFORM AND/OR LOW DIFFERENTIATED TUMOR

Fig. 2   Cytosolic assayable receptor concentration found in the 100,000 x g cytosol of 14 prostatic (PCA). The PCA was divided in two groups: • group consisting exclusively of adenocarcinoma; + group showing predominantly a cribriform or cribriform and low differentiated tumour pattern. The means were statistically significantly different with P<0.05.

Fig. 3   Spearman rank correlation between assayable sex hormone-binding globulin(SHBG) concentration in plasma and the respective prostatic carcinoma (PCA) or benign prostatic hyperplasia (BPH).

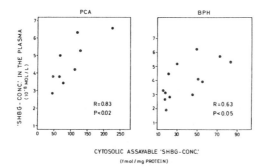

unmetabolized than in BPH and NPR, accompanied by a significantly lower
amount of formed 5α-androstanediols. 3. If 3α-diol was added, in all
three organs very little was converted to DHT. 4. Comparing BPH and NPR,
the latter converted much more of added DHT to 5α-androstanediols,
although the difference is slightly above the 5% confidence limits.
Fig. 4 shows a further difference between BPH and NPR: In the absence of
NADPH$_2$ in the incubation medium a significant amount of T is converted to
DHT plus 5α-androstanediols in BPH, while in NPR this conversion stops
dramatically, the shaded bars being significantly different between BPH
and NPR. On the contrary, after DHT incubation of the homogenates, the
conversion of DHT to the 5α-androstanediols stops nearly completely and
identically in both homogenates, if NADPH$_2$ supplementation has been
omitted. In Table 3 the metabolic data are compiled according to relative
metabolic activities. Besides the significantly higher ratios in the PCA
compared to BPH and NPR, which confirm the significant differences in
metabolism mentioned above, it seems remarkable that the ratio 5α-reduction
to 3$\alpha(\beta)$-reduction is significantly lower in NPR than in BPH.
Endogenous androgen tissue levels: Table 4 summarizes the endogenous
androgen concentrations found in the PCA, BPH and NPR homogenates. Three
differences being statistically significant: 1. The high T concentration
in PCA compared to BPH and NPR. 2. The low DHT concentration in NPR
compared to PCA and BPH. 3. The low 3α-diol concentration in BPH
compared to PCA and NPR.

DISCUSSION
This comparative study clearly demonstrates statistically significant
quantitative differences between human PCA, BPH and NPR with respect to
their androgen binding, in vitro metabolism and endogenous androgen
concentrations.
Concerning androgen binding in BPH four points should be discussed:
1. We have characterized and quantified the binding of tritiated DHT to
the cytosolic androgen receptor in BPH very carefully (39) and could find
no qualitative differences to respective studies in rat prostate (42).
The same similarities were found by others (5,10,17,27,45,52,58,69) and,
compiling the literature (5,10,17,27,28,33,35,38,43,45,48,52,58,59,61,65,
67,69,64), DHT-binding data in BPH display generally identical
characteristics to those found in accessory sexual glands of experimental
animals. However, as also emphasized very recently by Wagner (71), some
doubts still exist as to whether in all reports, in which gel column

98

Fig. 4 NADPH$_2$- dependency of the in vitro metabolism of testosterone (TESTO) and 5α-dihydrotestosterone (DHT) in human benign prostatic hyperplasia (BPH) and normal prostate (NPR) analyzed by thin layer chromatography. 1:2 with buffer diluted homogenates were incubated for 30 min at 37°C with tritiated TESTO (15.4+2.4 pmol/g homogenate) or DHT (16.8+2.5 pmol/g homogenate) in the presence (●) or absence (Θ) of 30 μmol/g homogenate NADPH$_2$. The conversion of TESTO to DHT + DIOL (DIOL = 5α-androstane-3α, 17β-diol plus 5α-androstane-3β, 17β-diol) was without adding NADPH$_2$ significantly higher in BPH than in NPR.

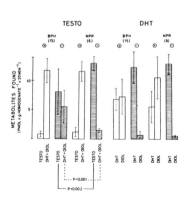

Table 3

Relative metabolic activities found in human prostatic carcinoma (PCA), benign prostatic hyperplasia (BPH), and normal prostate (NPR) after incubation of the organ homogenates with tritiated testosterone (TESTO) or 5α-dihydrotestosterone (DHT) for 30 min at 37°C in the presence of 30 μmol/g homogenate NADPH$_2$

	TESTO 5α-Reduction	5α-Reduction 3α(β)-Reduction	DHT DIOL
PCA	0.62+0.42[1] (10)	3.1+1.8 (5)	4.3+2.4[2] (5)
BPH	0.07+0.04 (16)	2.0+1.4 (16)	1.4+1.4 (16)
NPR	0.10+0.08 (7)	1.2+0.4[3] (7)	0.7+0.5 (7)

DIOL = 5α-androstane-3α, 17β-diol + 5α-androstane-3β,17β-diol

5α-Reduction = DHT + DIOL found after TESTO-incubation

3α(β)-Reduction = DIOL found after DHT-incubation

DHT/DIOL = DHT and DIOL found after DHT-incubation

[1] = significantly different to BPH and NPR, P<0.01

[2] = significantly different to BPH and NPR, P<0.02

[3] = significantly different to BPH and PCA, P<0.05

Table 4

Endogenous levels of testosterone (TESTO), 5α-dihydrotestosterone (DHT)
and 5α-androstane-3α, 17β-diol (3α-DIOL) in the homogenate of human
prostatic carcinoma (PCA), benign prostatic hyperplasia (BPH) and normal
prostate (NPR), measured by radioimmunoassay

| | Endogenous androgen level (ng/g tissue) | | |
	PCA	BPH	NPR
TESTO	1.2 ± 0.8^{1} (7)	0.3 ± 0.1 (11)	0.2 ± 0.1 (7)
DHT	3.9 ± 0.3 (3)	4.5 ± 1.4 (14)	$1.6^{2} \pm 1.0$ (6)
3α-DIOL	1.6 ± 0.8^{3} (7)	0.6 ± 0.7 (14)	1.7 ± 0.3^{3} (3)

[1] = significantly different to BPH and NPR, $P < 0.002$
[2] = significantly different to PCA and BPH, $P < 0.05$
[3] = significantly different to BPH, $P < 0.05$

chromatography, density gradient ultracentrifugation or charcoal
absorption technique were applied to characterize in crude BPH cytosols
the androgen binding, a precise discrimination between DHT-binding to the
cytosolic receptor and the cytosol contaminating plasmatic SHBG was
really possible. Using the ultracentrifugation technique we were unable
to discriminate in crude cytosol between the SHBG and cytosolic receptor
in BPH (66), and Mobbs et al. (50) in an earlier paper demonstrated, by
using a charcoal absorption technique, that the DHT-binding in the crude
human tissue cytosols is probably more related to the SHBG than to an
androgen receptor protein. Various authors (10,48,64,65,59,20,4,28)
circumvented this problem using tritiated methyltrienolone (R 1881) as
binding marker, which is not bound to the SHBG (11). However, it has
become recognized (48,59,20,4,16) that R 1881 binds with high affinity
to a binding protein in BPH cytosol, which resembles the progestin
receptor of the uterus, and very recently Gustafsson et al. (31) using
a new synthetic progestin (R 5020) actually characterized such a
progestin receptor in BPH and PCA cytosols. One approach might overcome
this problem of interference between androgen and progestin binding sites,
namely the saturation of the progestin binding component with unlabelled

R 5020, in order to prevent tritiated R 1881 interacting with such sites.
By this procedure Sirett et al. (64) found only very small amounts of
unoccupied androgen receptor sites (about 4 fmol/mg cytosol protein).
On the other side, the measurement of occupied specific androgen receptor
sites, which are present in a five-to ten-fold higher amount than the
unoccupied, seems possible using tritiated R 1881 (10,28,59), probably
due to heat denaturation of the interfering progestin component in the
course of the exchange procedure. We believe that the use of tritiated
DHT in combination with agargel electrophoresis, which discriminates
precisely between receptor protein and SHBG allows a reliable comparative
quantitative assay of the cytosolic androgen receptor protein in various
human prostates, knowing furthermore that the progesterone receptor has
only a very faint affinity to DHT, as shown by competition studies in
calf mammary gland (71).

2. So far, compiling the published cytosolic androgen receptor concentration
in BPH (39,10,48,64,61,59,71,73,28,38,65), great variation within a
series as well as great differences of the mean concentration between the
various authors can be stated, the latter at least partly due to quite
different methodological approaches. On the contrary, the great variation
of the values within one series is mainly due to the individual
biological status of the patients. In this respect, the endogenous
androgen concentrations and the tissue composition must be carefully
regarded. Concerning endogenous androgen concentration we could
demonstrate (39) that there is a significant negative correlation between
the androgen concentration in the tissue and the amount of assayable
receptor sites, that is to say the higher the tissular androgen
concentration the lower the assayable cytosolic androgen receptor
concentration. Concerning the variation of the tissue composition it is
well known that the BPH consists of a mixture of epithelial and stromal
elements, and Cowan et al. could demonstrate striking differences in
R 1881-binding (16) and DHT-metabolism (15) between these two elements.

3. Our incubation procedure (0°C, 2 - 24 h, high excess of tritiated DHT)
does not allow to discriminate between occupied and unoccupied binding sites,
therefore we used the term "assayable". Whether this parameter has any
biological significance in terms of hormone responsiveness of the tissue,
remains as yet unclear. However, the same holds true if the cytosolic
binding sites are divided into occupied and unoccupied amounts, especially
as the ratio occupied to unoccupied was in a series of 15 analyses, with

two exceptions, rather constant (28). At the moment concerning the biological significance of the cytosolic androgen receptor in BPH, it may only be tentatively concluded that its role is similar to the known action of the androgen receptor of the rat prostate (44), i.e. the BPH cytosol displays a receptor apparatus, which allows the translocation of DHT into the nucleus. This conclusion is substantiated by the very recent findings of various authors (17,43,48,64,67) who have described for the BPH specific nuclear binding sites with similar characteristics as found for the respective sites in the rat prostate nuclei.

4. Finally, concerning the hormones which might be involved in the development of the BPH oestrogens must also be regarded in addition to the aforementioned androgens as well as progestins. We could demonstrate a significant competition between tritiated DHT and unlabelled oestradiol for the receptor sites (39), and furthermore using tritiated oestradiol various authors have described a specific binding (34,73,72,7), which seems to be able to translocate the oestradiol into the BPH nuclei (7). Compared to binding studies in BPH, up to now less data have been published with respect to the PCA, mainly due to the difficulty in getting sufficient histologically proven carcinomatous tissue for biochemical analysis. We have stressed this point in a recent paper (40). The characterization of the cytosolic androgen binding therefore remains fragmentary, although as far as investigated the androgen receptor seems to be qualitatively identical to respective findings in BPH and rat prostate. The receptor quantitation performed by us (40) and others (52,65,71,73) revealed a wide range of values. This is also known for the oestrogen receptor in mammary breast cancer and as discussed there (47) cellular heterogeneity and endogenous steroid levels might be the main factors for this great variation. As discussed for the BPH, it is too early to make, on the basis of quantitation of cytosolic androgen receptor sites, predictions with respect to hormone responsiveness of this malignant tumour, although Mobbs et al. (52) and Wagner (71) have made some suggestions in this respect. However, it seems remarkable that we found in the PCA group statistically higher assayable cytosolic receptor concentrations than in the BPH, a finding which might be important since Lieskovsky and Bruchovsky (43) found more nuclear binding sites in PCA than in BPH and NPR. Furthermore, the higher cytosolic receptor concentration in cribriform and/or low differentiated prostatic tumours is evident and has been confirmed by Snochowsky et al. (65) in so far

that in their series of 8 BPH and 3 PCA specimens the highest receptor concentration was found in a punch biopsy of a cancer with low degree of differentiation. Further investigations at the cellular level will give an answer as to whether this difference in cytosolic androgen receptor concentration between high and low differentiated carcinomas is reflected by the same difference in the nuclei. Finally, besides androgens, oestrogens and progestins must also be regarded as steroid hormones influencing the growth and hormone responsiveness of the carcinomas. Using tritiated oestradiol, we (40) and others (71,73,8) found significant amounts bound to a cytosolic protein with low binding capacity. We could find this oestradiol-binding in each of 7 analyzed cytosols, the amount of bound oestradiol being, however, significantly lower than parallely analyzed DHT-binding. Wagner (71) on the other side found specimens, which bind either both steroids or which bind only DHT or oestradiol. This may indicate that two different receptor proteins are involved. Concerning progestin-binding, Gustafsson et al. (31) have reported very recently about a specific binding of tritiated R 5020 in three cytosols of human prostatic carcinomas. On the other hand, we have incubated aliquots of 4 carcinomas parallely with tritiated DHT and tritiated R 1881, and although the affinity of R 1881 to the progesterone receptor is evident as discussed above, displacement of tritiated R 1881 with either R 1881 or DHT revealed identical amounts of limited binding sites which are furthermore identical to the amount of binding sites found parallely with tritiated DHT. Thus, in our specimens a progestin binding component seems to be absent.

Our negative results in unequivocally demonstrating cytosolic androgen receptors in 7 NPR must be discussed primarily in the light of the time span between death of the young men and tissue processing, which lasted up to 6 h. Simulating this time span using rats, the amount of assayable binding sites decreases dramatically in castrated and uncastrated animals (unpublished own data), thus in humans the very labile cytosolic receptor protein will probably extensively be denaturated during this time span so that the receptor becomes undetectable. In contrast to this assumption is the finding of Davies and Griffiths (17) who demonstrated a cytosolic androgen binding by sucrose gradient ultracentrifugation in one normal prostate specimen removed from a cadaver within 12 h of death, and the finding of Mobbs et al. (51) who assayed very little of a cyproterone-acetate-inhibitable-androgen-binding in three NPR from cadavers of subjects who had died within 6-24 h of analysis. Further cytosolic binding studies were performed in NPR specimens obtained by needle biopsy or during the course of an open operation (61,71). Both groups demonstrated androgen binding sites in varying amount, although the data by Shimazaki et al. (61) seem to be overestimated due to the interference of DHT-binding to SHBG. Therefore, compiling these data, in NPR cytosol an androgen receptor, which does not show as far as investigated striking differences to findings in human BPH, PCA and rat prostate, can tentatively be assumed. Probably this receptor is translocated into the nucleus, as Lieskovsky and Bruchovsky (43) demonstrated significant amounts of androgen receptor molecules in NPR nuclei, the amount being, however, statistically lower than the respective quantities found in BPH and PCA nuclei. Further quantitative binding studies in NPR, PCA and BPH are needed to confirm the above mentioned differences in receptor content. Besides androgen receptor studies, androgen metabolism in human BPH, PCA and NPR has gained much interest since 1963, when Farnsworth and Brown (22) first described the formation of DHT as the main metabolite after incubation of human BPH tissue slices with tritiated T. This finding was later confirmed by in vivo studies of Becker et al. (9) and by Pike et al. (56). The first report concerning quantitative differences in the conversion of T to DHT between BPH, PCA and NPR was published by Shimazaki et al. (62), who found a ranking of metabolic activity as NPR> BPH >PCA. Thereafter numerous publications dealt with the in vitro metabolism of T in BPH, PCA and NPR (5,15,13,14,49,29,63,60,36,46,54,55, 57,19) as well as the extent to which it can be influenced by oestrogens, progestins and antiandrogens (62,14,30,6,53,24,68,37,2,3,21). Without going into detail, only the decreased androgen metabolism in carcinomatous tissue was unequivocally found. However, the number of investigated specimens were often very low and thus a statistical evaluation of differences in the androgen metabolism between BPH, PCA and NPR not possible. Therefore, our comparative study can only be compared with a few in part similar studies recently done by others (13,60,36,54,19,55,51). Concerning the PCA irrespective of the kind of differentiation of the PCA, a statistically lower 5α-reductase activity than in BPH and NPR may be assumed. This is in accordance with findings of others (5,13,57,19), while Morfin et al. (55) as well as Jenkins and McCaffery (37) could find only in poorly differentiated carcinomatous tissue a decreased formation of 5α-reduced metabolites. For the first time we described furthermore a statistically lower $3\alpha(\beta)$-hydroxysteroid dehydrogenase activity in PCA compared to BPH and NPR. This drastically decreased conversion of DHT to 5α-androstanediols leads to a relatively higher 5α-reductase than $3\alpha(\beta)$-hydroxysteroid dehydrogenase activity in the PCA, thus shifting the androgen metabolites to T as well as DHT. Concerning the comparison of androgen metabolism between BPH and NPR, Bruchovsky and Lieskovsky (13) demonstrated a statistically higher 5α-reductase and lower $3\alpha(\beta)$-hydroxysteroid dehydrogenase activity in BPH compared to NPR. This is in contrast to the findings of Jacobi and Wilson (36), who found just the opposite concerning the $3\alpha(\beta)$-hydroxysteroid dehydrogenase activity, namely significantly higher activity in BPH than NPR. When considering the absolute amounts of formed metabolites after incubation of BPH and NPR with T, DHT or 3α-diol, we could not demonstrate statistically significant differences, although the tendency of higher 5α-reductase and lower $3\alpha(\beta)$-hydroxysteroid dehydrogenase activity in BPH compared to NPR was evident. The same may be depicted from the data of Djoseland et al. (19). However, other groups (60,37) could not find any difference in this respect.

When considering the ratio of 5α-reductase to $3\alpha(\beta)$-hydroxysteroid dehydrogenase activity, it was in our series, as in the series of Bruchovsky and Lieskovsky (13), statistically higher in BPH compared to NPR, indicating that the T metabolism is shifted in BPH towards DHT while in NPR towards 5α-androstanediols. A further proof of a higher 5α-reductase activity in BPH compared to NPR is given by the significantly different $NADPH_2$ dependency of the T conversion to DHT. While in BPH without cofactor supplementation of the incubates a significant 5α-reduction of T occurs, in NPR this reduction is nearly completely stopped. If it is assumed that the metabolism in organ homogenates without cofactor supplementation is a better reflection of the actual in vivo condition, this finding might indicate that in BPH the 5α-reductase is better supplied with reduced cofactors than in NPR. Bearing in mind the longer time span up to the final tissue processing of NPR compared to BPH, one might argue that this is the reason for the differences. However, Morfin et al. (54) could demonstrate the same difference, although the NPR and BPH specimens were both processed immediately. Furthermore, we could not find such differences between BPH and NPR with respect to the $3\alpha(\beta)$-hydroxysteroid dehydrogenase activity.

If it is assumed that the in vitro metabolism at the cellular level of the human prostate regulates at least partly the endogenous androgen concentrations in these tissues, then from our metabolic data the following predictions can be made: In PCA relatively high levels of T and DHT and low levels of 3α-diol, in BPH relatively high levels of DHT and low levels of T and 3α-diol, and finally in NPR relatively high levels of 3α-diol and low levels of T and DHT should be found. Concerning the T concentration, actually in PCA statistically higher levels were found than in BPH and NPR. This findings has been excellently confirmed by Habib et al. (32) and with less statistical significance, by Farnsworth and Brown (23), while Albert et al. (1) found a higher mean T level in BPH than PCA. The equally low concentration in BPH and NPR has also been reported by Siiteri and Wilson (63). With respect to the DHT tissue concentrations, it has been known since 1970 (63) that the BPH has significantly higher levels than the NPR, a finding confirmed later by us (74) and Geller et al. (25). On the contrary, the significantly higher DHT level in PCA compared to NPR was reported only very recently by Geller et al. (26). Conflicting results were published when considering comparatively the DHT values between BPH and PCA. While Geller et al. (26) and Habib et al. (32) found significantly lower DHT levels in PCA than in BPH, a finding confirmed at the nuclear level by Bruchovsky et al. (12), Farnsworth and Brown (23) reported just the opposite. We could not find significant differences in this respect between PCA and BPH, reflecting well our metabolic findings. Concerning the 3α-diol concentrations, our findings of significantly higher levels in NPR than in BPH was in accordance with a report of Geller et al. (25). The unexpectedly high 3α-diol levels found in PCA by us, and in even higher concentrations by Albert et al. (1) and Farnsworth and Brown (23), cannot, at the moment, be explained by our metabolic studies.

With only one exception our predictions of endogenous tissue concentrations due to the metabolic data in vitro were fulfilled completely, thus indicating that the in vitro metabolism might reflect the in vivo situation. Finally, taking together these comparative data on androgen binding, in vitro metabolism and androgen concentrations at the cellular level of the BPH, PCA and NPR the following may be stated:

1. The NPR seems to be protected against excessive accumulation of T and DHT due to the shift of androgen metabolism to the 5α-androstanediols, which are, in general, not bound with high affinity to the cytosolic

androgen receptor.

2. Compared to NPR, in PCA and BPH the androgen metabolism is shifted significantly to T and DHT, both of which have a high affinity for the cytosolic androgen receptor.

3. It is attractive to speculate that this acquired error in androgen metabolism could play an important role in the development and hormone responsiveness of BPH and PCA.

4. Further studies on androgen binding and metabolism must be correlated to the histological type of the tumour as well as extended to the nuclear level of these tissues. Then predictions with respect to hormone responsiveness of the individual tumours might be possible in the future.

ACKNOWLEDGEMENT

This work was supported by the DFG, Sonderforschungsbereich 34 "Endokrinologie".

References

1. Albert J., Geller J., Geller, S. and Lopez, D.: Prostate concentrations of endogenous androgens by radioimmunoassay. J. Steroid Biochem. 7: 301-307, 1976.
2. Altwein, J. E., Orestano, F. and Hohenfellner, R.: Testosterone turnover in cancer of the prostate. Suppression by gestagens in vitro. Invest. Urol. 12: 157-161, 1974.
3. Altwein, J. E., Rubin, A., Klose, K., Knapstein, P. and Orestano, F.: Kinetik der 5-alpha-Reduktase im Prostataadenom in Gengenwart von Oestradiol, Diäthylstilböstrol, Progesteron und Gestonoron-Capronat (Depostat). Urologe A13: 41-46, 1974.
4. Asselin, J., Labrie, F., Gourdeau, Y., Bonne, C. and Raynaud, J.-P.: Binding of (^{3}H)-methyltrienolone (R1881) in rat prostate and human benign prostatic hypertrophy (BPH). Steroids 28: 449-459, 1976.
5. Attramadal, A., Tveter, K. J., Weddington, S. C., Djoseland, O., Naess, O., Hansson, V. and Torgersen, O.: Androgen binding and metabolism in the human prostate. Vitamins Horm. 33: 247-264, 1975.
6. Bard, D. R. and Lasnitzki, I.: The influence of oestradiol on the metabolism of androgens by human prostatic tissue. J. Endocr. 74: 1-9, 1977.
7. Bashirelahi, N., O'Toole, J. H. and Young, J. D.: A specific 17β-estradiol receptor in human benign hypertrophic prostate. Biochem. Med. 15: 254-261, 1976.
8. Bashirelahi, N. and Young, J. D.: Specific binding protein for 17β-estradiol in prostate with adenocarcinoma. Urology 8: 553-558, 1976.
9. Becker, H., Kaufmann, J., Klosterhalfen, H. and Voigt, K. D.: In vivo uptake and metabolism of ^{3}H-testosterone and ^{3}H-5α-dihydrotestosterone by human benign prostatic hypertrophy. Acta endocr. 71: 589-599, 1972.
10. Bonne, C. and Raynaud, J.-P.: Assay of androgen binding sites by exchange with methyltrienolone (R1881). Steroids 27: 497-507, 1976.

11. Bonne, C. and Raynaud, J.-P.: Methyltrienolone a specific ligand for cellular androgen receptors. Steroids 26: 227-232, 1975.

12. Bruchovsky, N., Callaway, T., Lieskovsky, G. and Rennie, P. S.: Markers of androgen action in human prostate: Potential use in the clinical assessment of prostatic carcinoma. Proc. Conf. Clin. Biochem. in Med. (in press).

13. Bruchovsky, N. and Lieskovsky, G.: Increased ratio of 5α-reductase: 3α-hydroxysteroid dehydrogenase activities in hyperplastic human prostate. J. Endocr. (in press).

14. Chung, L. W. K. and Coffey, D. S.: Androgen Glucuronide. II. Differences in its formation by human normal and benign hyperplastic prostates. Invest. Urol. 15: 385-388, 1978.

15. Cowan, R. A., Cowan, S. K., Grant, J. K. and Elder, H. Y.: Biochemical investigations of separated epithelium and stroma from benign hyperplastic prostatic tissue. J. Endocr. 74: 111-120, 1977.

16. Cowan, R. A., Cowan, S. K. and Grant, J. K.: Binding of methyltrienolone (R1881) to a progesterone receptor-like component of human prostatic cytosol. J. Endocr. 74: 281-289, 1977.

17. Davies, P. and Griffiths, K.: Similarities between 5α-dihydrotestosterone-receptor complexes from human and rat prostatic tissue: Effects on RNA polymerase activity. Mol. Cell. Endocr. 3: 143-164, 1975.

18. Dennis, M., Horst, H.-J., Krieg, M. and Voigt, K. D.: Plasma sex hormone-binding globulin capacity in benign prostatic hypertrophy and prostatic carcinoma: Comparison with age dependent rise in normal human males. Acta endocr. (Kbh.) 84: 207-214, 1977.

19. Djoseland, O., Tveter, K. J., Attramadal, A., Hansson, V., Haugen, H. N. and Mathisen, W.: Metabolism of testosterone in the human prostate and seminal vesicles. Scand. J. Urol. Nephrol. 11: 1-6, 1977.

20. Dubé, J. Y., Chapdelaine, P., Tremblay, R. R., Bonne, C. and Raynaud, J.-P.: Comparative binding specificity of methyltrienolone in human and rat prostate. Hormone Res. 7: 341-347, 1976.

21. Farnsworth, W. E.: A direct effect of estrogens on prostatic metabolism of testosterone. Invest. Urol. 6: 423-427, 1969.

22. Farnsworth, W. E. and Brown, J. R.: Metabolism of testosterone by the human prostate. JAMA 183: 436-439, 1963.

23. Farnsworth, W. E. and Brown, J. R.: Androgen of the human prostate, Endocr. Res. Comm. 3: 105-117, 1976.

24. Geller, J., Albert, J., Geller, S., Lopez, D., Cantor, T. and Yen S.: Effect of megestrol acetate (Megace) on steroid metabolism and steroid-protein binding in the human prostate. J. Clin. Endocr. Metab. 43: 1000-1008, 1976.

25. Geller, J., Albert, J., Lopez, D., Geller, S. and Niwayama, G.: Comparison of androgen metabolites in benign prostatic hypertrophy (BPH) and normal prostate. J. Clin. Endocr. Metab. 43: 686-688, 1976.

26. Geller, J., Albert, J., Lopez, D., Geller, S., Stoeltzing, W. and Vega, D. dela: DHT concentrations in human prostate cancer tissue. J. Clin. Endocr. Metab. 46: 440-444, 1978.

27. Geller, J., Cantor, T. and Albert, J.: Evidence for a specific dihydrotestosterone-binding cytosol receptor in the human prostate. J. Clin. Endocr. Metab. 41: 854-862, 1975.

28. Ghanadian, R., Auf, G., Chaloner, P. J. and Chisholm, G. D.: The use of methyltrienolone in the measurement of the free and bound

cytoplasmic receptors for dihydrotestosterone in benign hypertrophied human prostate. J. Steroid Biochem. 9: 325-330, 1978.

29. Giorgi, E. P., Stewart, J. C., Grant, J. K. and Scott, R.: Androgen dynamics in vitro in the normal and hyperplastic human prostate gland. Biochem. J. 123: 41-55, 1971.

30. Giorgi, E. P., Stewart, J. C., Grant, J. K. and Shirley, I. M.: Androgen dynamics in vitro in the human prostate gland. Effect of oestradiol-17β. Biochem. J. 126: 107-121, 1972.

31. Gustafsson, J.-A., Ekman, P., Pousette A., Snochowski, M. and Högberg, B.: Demonstration of a progestin receptor in human benign prostatic hyperplasia and prostatic carcinoma. Invest. Urol. 15: 361-366, 1978.

32. Habib, F. K., Lee, I. R., Stitch, S. R. and Smith, P. H.: Androgen levels in the plasma and prostatic tissues of patients with benign hypertrophy and carcinoma of the prostate. J. Endocr. 71: 99-107, 1976.

33. Hansson, V., Tveter, K. J., Attramadal, A. and Torgersen, O.: Androgen receptors in human benign nodular prostatic hyperplasia. Acta endocr. (Kbh.) 68: 79-88, 1971.

34. Hawkins, E. F., Nijs, M. and Brassinne, C.: Steroid receptors in the human prostate. 2. Some properties of the estrophilic molecule of benign prostatic hypertrophy. Biochem. Biophys. Res. Comm. 70: 854-861, 1976.

35. Hsu, R. S., Middleton, R. G. and Fang, S.: Androgen receptors in human prostates. In: "Normal and Abnormal Growth of the Prostate." (Edited by M. Coland) C. C. Thomas, Springfield, Illinois. 663-675, 1975.

36. Jacobi, G. H. and Wilson, J. D.: Formation of 5α-androstane-3α, 17β-diol by normal and hypertrophic human prostate. J. Clin. Endocr. Metab. 44: 107-115, 1977.

37. Jenkins, J. S. and McCaffery, V. M.: Effect of oestradiol-17β and progesterone on the metabolism of testosterone by human prostatic tissue. J. Endocr. 63: 517-526, 1974.

38. Kodama, T., Honda, S. and Shimazaki, J.: Androphilic proteins in cytosols of human benign prostatic hypertrophy. Endocrinol. Japon. 24: 565-573, 1977.

39. Krieg, M., Bartsch, W., Herzer, S., Becker, H. and Voigt, K. D.: Quantification of androgen binding, androgen tissue levels, and sex hormone-binding globulin in prostate, muscle and plasma of patients with benign prostatic hypertrophy. Acta endocr. (Kbh.) 86: 200-215, 1977.

40. Krieg, M., Grobe I., Voigt, K. D., Altenähr, E. and Klosterhalfen, H.: Human prostatic carcinoma: Significant differences in its androgen binding and metabolism compared to the human benign prostatic hypertrophy. Acta endocr. (Kbh.) 88: 397-407, 1978.

41. Krieg, M., Smith, K. and Bartsch, W.: Demonstration of a specific androgen receptor in rat heart muscle: Relationship between binding, metabolism, and tissue levels of androgens. Endocrinology 103: 1686-1695, 1978.

42. Krieg, M. and Voigt, K. D.: Biochemical substrate of androgenic actions at a cellular level in prostate, bulbocavernosus/levator ani and in skeletal muscle. Acta endocr. Suppl. 214: 43-89, 1977.

43. Lieskovsky, G. and Bruchovsky, N.: Measurement of androgen receptors in human prostate. J. Urol. (in press).

44. Mainwaring, W. I. P.: The Mechanism of Action of Androgens, Springer, Verlag, Heidelberg, 1977.

45. Mainwaring, W. I. P. and Milroy, E. J. G.: Characterization of the specific androgen receptors in the human prostate gland. J. Endocr. 57: 371-384, 1973.
46. Malathi, K. and Gurpide, E.: Metabolism of 5α-dihydrotestosterone in human benign hyperplastic prostate. J. Steroid Biochem. 8: 141-145, 1977.
47. McGuire, W. L., Zava, D. T., Horwitz, K. B. and Chamness, G. C.: Steroid receptors in breast tumors-current status. In: "Current Topics in Experimental Endocrinology." (Edited by L. Martini and V. H. T. James), Academic Press, New York, Vol. III: 93, 98-99, 1978.
48. Menon, M., Tananis, C. E., Hicks, L. L., Hawkins, E. F., McLoughlin, M. G. and Walsh, P. C.: Characterization of the binding of a potent synthetic androgen, methyltrienolone, to human tissues. J. Clin. Invest. 61: 150-162, 1978.
49. Mercier-Bodard, C., Marchut, M., Perrot, M., Picard, M.-T., Baulieu, E.-E. and Robel, P.: Influence of purified plasma proteins on testosterone uptake and metabolism by normal and hyperplastic human prostate in "constant-flow organ culture". J. Clin. Endocr. Metab. 43: 374-386, 1976.
50. Mobbs, B. G., Johnson, I. E. and Conolly, J. G.: In vitro assay of androgen binding to human prostate. J. Steroid Biochem. 6: 453-458, 1975.
51. Mobbs, B. G., Johnson, I. E., Conolly, J. G. and Clark, A. F.: Evaluation of the use of cyproterone acetate competition to distinguish between high-affinity binding of (^{3}H)-dihydrotestosterone to human prostate cytosol receptors and to sex hormone-binding globulin. J. Steroid Biochem. 8: 943-949, 1977.
52. Mobbs, B. G., Johnson, I. E., Conolly, J. G. and Clark, A. F.: Androgen receptor assay in human benign and malignant prostatic tumour cytosol using protamine sulphate precipitation. J. Steroid Biochem. 9: 289-301, 1978.
53. Morfin, R. F., Bercovici, J.-P., Charles, J.-F. and Floch, H. H.: Testosterone and progesterone metabolism and their interaction in the human hyperplastic prostate. J. Steroid Biochem. 6: 1447-1352, 1975.
54. Morfin, R. F., Di Stefano, S., Bercovici, J.-P. and Floch, H. H.: Comparison of testosterone, 5α-dihydrotestosterone and 5α-androstane-3β, 17β-diol metabolism in human normal and hyperplastic prostates. J. Steroid Biochem. 9: 245-252, 1978.
55. Morfin, R. F., Leav, I., Charles, J.-F., Cavazos, L. F., Ofner, P. and Floch, H. H.: Correlative study of the morphology and C19-steroid metabolism of benign and cancerous human prostatic tissue. Cancer 39: 1517-1534, 1977.
56. Pike, A., Peeling, W. B., Harper, M. E., Pierrepoint, C. G. and Griffiths, K.: Testosterone metabolism in vivo by human prostatic tissue. Biochem. J. 120: 443-445, 1970.
57. Prout, G. R., Kliman, B., Daly, J. J., MacLaughlin, R. A. and Griffin, P. P.: In vitro uptake of ^{3}H-testosterone and its conversion to dihydrotestosterone by prostatic carcinoma and other tissues. J. Urol. 116: 603-610, 1976.
58. Rosen, V., Jung, I., Baulieu, E. E. and Robel, P.: Androgen-binding proteins in human benign prostatic hypertrophy. J. Clin. Endocr. Metab. 41: 761-770, 1975.
59. Shain, S. A., Boesel, R. W., Lamm, D. L. and Radwin, H. M.: Characterization of unoccupied (R) and occupied (RA) androgen binding components of the hyperplastic human prostate. Steroids

<u>31</u>: 541-556, 1978.

60. Shida, K., Shimazaki, J., Ito, Y., Yamanaka, H. and Nagai-Yuasa, H.: 3α-Reduction of dihydrotestosterone in human normal and hypertrophic prostatic tissues. <u>Invest. Urol.</u> <u>13</u>: 241-245, 1975.

61. Shimazaki, J., Kodama, T., Wakisaka, M. and Katayama, T.: Dihydrotestosterone-binding protein in cytosols of normal and hypertrophic human prostates, and influence of estrogens and antiandrogens on the binding. <u>Endocrinol. Japon.</u> <u>24</u>: 9-14, 1977.

62. Shimazaki, J., Kurihara, H., Ito, Y. and Shida, K.: Testosterone metabolism in prostate; Formation of androstan-17β-ol-3-one and androst-4-ene-3, 17-dione and inhibitory effect of natural and synthetic estrogens. <u>Gunma J. Med. Sci.</u> <u>14</u>: 313-325, 1965.

63. Siiteri, P. K. and Wilson, J. D.: Dihydrotestosterone in prostatic hypertrophy. 1. The formation and content of dihydrotestosterone in the hypertrophic prostate of man. <u>J. Clin. Invest.</u> <u>49</u>: 1737-1745, 1970.

64. Sirett, D. A. N. and Grant, J. K.: Androgen binding in cytosols and nuclei of human benign hyperplastic prostatic tissue. <u>J. Endocr.</u> <u>77</u>: 101-110, 1978.

65. Snochowski, M., Pousette, A., Akman, P., Bression D., Andersson, L., Högberg, B. and Gustafsson, J.-A.: Characterization and measurement of the androgen receptor in human benign prostatic hyperplasia and prostatic carcinoma. <u>J. Clin. Endocr. Metab.</u> <u>45</u>: 920-930, 1977.

66. Steins, P., Krieg, M., Hollmann, H. J. and Voigt, K. D.: In vitro studies of testosterone and 5α-dihydrotestosterone binding in benign prostatic hypertrophy. <u>Acta endocr. (Kbh.)</u> <u>75</u>: 773-784, 1974.

67. Symes, E. K., Milroy, E. J. G. and Mainwaring, W. I. P.: The nuclear uptake of androgen by human benign prostate in vitro: Action of antiandrogens. <u>J. Urol.</u> <u>120</u>: 180-183, 1978.

68. Tan, S. Y., Antonipillai, I. and Murphy, B. E. P.: Inhibition of testosterone metabolism in the human prostate. <u>J. Clin. Endocr. Metab.</u> <u>39</u>: 936-941, 1974.

69. Tveter, K. J., Unjhem, O., Attramadal, A., Aakvaag, A. and Hansson, V.: Androgenic receptors in rat and human prostate. <u>Adv. Biosci.</u> <u>7</u>: 193-207, 1971.

70. Wagner, R. K.: Characterization and assay of steroid hormone receptors and steroid-binding serum proteins by agargel electrophoresis at low temperature. <u>Hoppe-Seyler's Z. Physiol. Chem.</u> 253: 1235-1245, 1972.

71. Wagner, R. K.: Extracellular and intracellular steroid binding proteins. Properties, discrimination, assay and clinical applications. <u>Acta endocr. (Kbh.)</u> Suppl. 218: 1-73, 1978.

72. Wagner, R. K., Schulze, K. H. and Jungblut, P. W.: Estrogen and androgen receptor in human prostate and prostatic tumor tissue. <u>Acta endocr. (Kbh.)</u> Suppl. 193: 52, 1975.

73. Voogt, H. J. de and Dingjan, P.: Steroid receptors in human prostatic cancer. A preliminary evaluation. <u>Urolog. Res.</u> <u>6</u>: 151-158, 1978.

74. Voigt, K. D. and Krieg, M.: Biochemical endocrinology of prostatic tumors. In: "Current Topics in Experimental Endocrinology." (Edited by L. Martini and V. H. T. James). Academic Press, New York, Vol. III, 173, 177-184, 1978.

ANDROGENIC CONTROL OF PROSTATIC GROWTH:

REGULATION OF STEROID LEVELS*

CHAPTER VII

INTRODUCTION

The relationship between androgens and the development of prostatic cancer is at present unclear. Adenocarcinoma of the human prostate does not develop, however, in the absence of functioning testes. This conclusion is based on the early work of R. A. Moore who found upon microscopic examination of the prostates of eunuch, eunuchoids, or of individuals with pituitary infantilism, who lost their secondary sexual characteristics before the age of 40, no incidence of prostatic neoplasia (21). This work remains the best evidence that prostatic cancer has endocrine dependent determinants. Prostatic cancer is also age dependent. This form of cancer is rarely seen in males under the age of 40. Aging is also associated with changes in the levels of circulating androgens in the blood. Studies by several groups have shown that while the total circulating levels of androgen decrease only slightly in the aging male, the concentration of free non-protein bound androgen does decline significantly with age (31). This reduction of free androgen coupled to a slight rise in free estrogen levels results in a significant decrease in the ratio of free androgen to free estrogen in the aging male. Therefore, alteration in the sex hormonal environment may be causally related to prostatic cancer. Attempts to induce prostatic cancer experimentally in animals by sex hormonal manipulation have proven, however, to be remarkably difficult. Only one report in the vast literature has reported limited success. Noble reports that following a complex schedule of sex hormonal manipulations, induction of prostatic adenocarcinoma of the dorsal prostate of the Nb rat was achieved (24). In direct contrast to the difficulty in producing experimental prostatic cancer, the experimental production of another type of prostatic neoplasia, benign prostatic hyperplasia (BPH), has been achieved rather easily. Dogs have been induced to develop BPH by the simple injection of various androgen metabolites alone or in combination with estrogens (6, 32). It is thus clear that an understanding of how sex hormones control the normal growth and function of the

*John T. Isaacs and Donald S. Coffey, James Buchanan Brady Institute, Department of Urology, The Johns Hopkins University School of Medicine, Baltimore, Maryland 21205. This work was supported by Grant No. CA15416, awarded by the National Cancer Institute, DHEW.

prostate is critical to the understanding of how these hormones could possibly induce prostatic neoplasia.

Along these lines, it is pertinent to recall that the prostate of a mature individual is chronically dependent on a continuous supply of androgen to maintain the normal cell content and functional activity of the gland. Normally this androgen induced stimulation of the prostate results in a delicate balance between cell loss and cell renewal (maintenance growth) such that a continuous proliferative overgrowth of the prostate does not occur. Some type of constraint mechanism(s) exists to prevent the over-stimulation of the prostate by continuous chronic exposure to androgen while still allowing maintenance growth to occur. The net result is an androgen-dependent cellular homeostatis of the normal prostate. In prostatic cancer, these constraint mechanisms are either completely lacking or deficient and massive malignant overgrowth of the gland may result. Understanding of the normal constraint mechanism for the androgen-dependent growth of the prostate is extremely complicated. Attempts to define and study possible mechanisms are just beginning.

Can Constraint Mechanisms on Prostatic Overgrowth be Experimentally Demonstrated?

Using the rat as a model, the existence of constraint mechanisms on prostatic overgrowth is clearly documented by the following experiment. If intact adult male rats are injected daily for three weeks with 10 mg/day of cyproterone acetate, a known antiandrogen, involution of the ventral prostate results, Table 1. Cyproterone acetate's mechanism of action has

Table 1.　　Reversibility of Cyproterone Acetate Induced Atrophy
of the Rat Ventral Prostate of Intact Animals

	Ventral Prostate	
	Total Weight (mg/100 g B.W.)	Total DNA (µg/100 g B.W.)
Treatment None (Intact Control)	120 ± 20	200 ± 35
Intact-injected daily with Cyproterone Acetate (10 mg/d) for three weeks	30 ± 15	55 ± 8
Intact-injected daily with Cyproterone Acetate (10 mg/d) for three weeks-then not in-jected for 1 month	100 ± 15	185 ± 19

B. W. = Body Weight

113

been shown to be via competition in the prostate for the androgen receptor thereby preventing the nuclear uptake and retention of androgens (29). The cyproterone acetate injections have no effect upon either the serum testosterone levels nor the weight of the testes in the rat (29). If after three weeks, the cyproterone acetate injections are stopped, the complete restoration of the involuted prostate by endogenous androgen occurs over the following month, Table 1. However, while endogenous androgen is able to stimulate the regrowth of the involuted prostate once the normal weight and DNA content is reached, no further proliferative overgrowth occurs even if several additional months are allowed. Clearly this demonstrates that endogenous androgen levels are completely able to induce proliferative restoration of the involuted prostate but eventually some type of constraint mechanism intervenes in this growth response when normal size of the adult prostate is restored. Also since the serum levels of androgen are not changed at all by any of these treatments, the constraint mechanisms on prostatic overgrowth appears to be intrinsic to the prostate itself and not dependent upon changes in serum androgen levels.

Can The Natural Constraint Mechanism on Prostatic Growth Be Overcome In The Normal Intact Adult Male?

Experimentally it is rather easy to overcome the constraint mechanism on prostatic growth. For example, the prostates of intact adult male rats are capable of being stimulated into a proliferative overgrowth response by simply injecting these animals with exogenous dihydrotestosterone (DHT). DHT, the 5α-reduced product of testosterone, has been shown in a series of classical papers to be the active androgenic growth factor in the prostate (1, 4) and injection of 2 mg/day (pharmacological dose) of this steroid dramatically increases the ventral prostatic wet weight of the rat, Figure 1. This growth response lasts about 1-3 weeks and is a truly proliferative overgrowth as documented by the concomitant increase in total cell content of the prostate. A similar proliferative overgrowth of the prostate can be induced in the intact adult dog by DHT injections. When intact adult beagles were injected with DHT at a dose of 25 mg three times a week for four months, the prostates increased in wet weight to a volume approximately 290% of that for the intact noninjected control dogs. The total DNA content (cellular content) likewise increased 220% indicating that the response was truly proliferative (6). Clearly, the constraint mechanism on proliferative overgrowth of the prostate of an intact adult animal can be overcome by

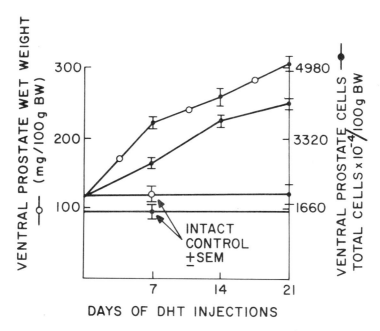

<u>Figure 1.</u>　　　Effects of daily DHT injections (2 mg/day) on the ventral
　　prostatic wet weight and cell content. All starting animals were
　　intact, adult male rats. —O— = total wet weight, —●— = total cells.

high levels of androgen. It must be pointed out, however, that the proliferative overgrowth response of both the rat and dog stimulated by high
levels of androgen is not unlimited. Eventually, even with continuous high
levels of exogenous androgen, proliferative overgrowth of the prostate
ceases (after 3-4 weeks in the rat and after 4 months in the dog). Therefore,
it is apparent that there may be several types of constraint mechanisms
responsible for the normally tightly regulated androgen-dependent cellular
homeostatis of the prostate.

<u>Is There a Difference Between the Dose of Androgen Needed to Overcome the</u>
<u>Constraint Mechanisms on Proliferative Growth and the Dose Required to</u>
<u>Maintain the Prostate?</u>

There is a difference between the doses of exogenous androgen needed to
induce these two separate growth responses. This is illustrated by the
following experiment: male adult rats are castrated and immediately begun
on daily injections of various doses of DHT. After 7 days the animals are
killed and the ventral prostatic wet weight RNA, and DNA content determined.

115

This treatment results in involution, maintenance, and indeed, overgrowth of the ventral prostate depending upon the dose of DHT injected, Figure 2.

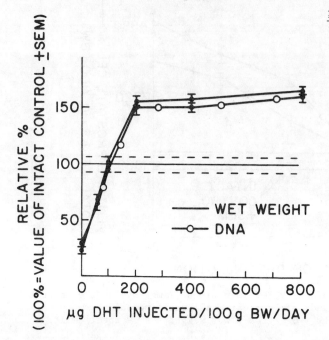

Figure 2. Ability of various dosages of daily DHT injections to maintain or stimulate the wet weight and DNA content of the ventral prostate in adult male rats castrated and immediately begun on steroid injection schedule (total period of injection = 7 days).

At a dose of 100 µg DHT/100 g body weight/day, neither the wet weight nor DNA and RNA changes following castration. The cell morphology of the secretory epithelial cells is maintained in the normal tall columnar manner. Therefore, a dose of 100 µg DHT/100 g body weight/day is sufficient to induce complete maintenance growth of the prostate. Indeed, in other experiments, it has been found that this dose of DHT is capable of completely maintaining the prostate on a long term basis (months). At doses less than 100 µg DHT/100 g body weight/day, maintenance growth is not sufficient and involution of the ventral prostate results. The epithelial cells are no longer tall columnar but instead are cuboidal. If doses larger than 100 µg DHT/100 g body weight/day are injected, a proliferative overgrowth response is found. The wet weight, DNA and RNA all increased significantly. This proliferative overgrowth response appears to be maximally stimulated at a dose of 200 µg DHT/100 g body weight/day since injections of higher doses of DHT do not produce any significant increases in any parameter. This clearly demonstrates that the normal prostate has the ability to undergo a proliferative overgrowth response if androgen concentrations are increased.

The data presented in Figure 2 also demonstrates that the prostate responds to different levels of DHT with different growth responses. The doses of DHT needed to maintain the prostate are lower (100 µg) than the doses needed to stimulate a proliferative overgrowth response (200 µg). Also, the doses needed for stimulation of these different responses are not massively different, being only a range of two-fold. Therefore, small changes in the cellular levels of DHT may have a key function in determining which type of growth response is induced.

What Controls the Level of Androgens in the Prostate?

Ultimately, the control for prostatic DHT levels is determined by the relationship between the rate of production and removal of this steroid by the gland. The rate of production of DHT is dependent upon the flux of testosterone into the prostate and the activity of Δ^4-3-ketosteroid 5α-reductase: EC 1.3.1.4 (5α-reductase). Once testosterone enters the cells, it can be converted by either the 17β-hydroxy reductive pathway, the 17-keto oxidative pathway or combinations of the two, Figure 3. The first step of the reductive pathway is the 5α-reduction of testosterone to DHT. This irreversible reaction requires NADPH specifically as cofactor and is catalyzed by either the outer nuclear membrane or endoplasmic reticular 5α-reductase enzyme (8). This enzyme will also reduce Δ^4-androstenedione; in fact, the K_m for this steroid is actually lower than for testosterone. The K_m for the 5α-reductase enzyme determined in the prostates for a variety of species is approximately 1 µM for testosterone and 10 µM for NADPH (8). The prostatic levels of testosterone are in the range of 3-7 nM (12, 27, 28) and for NADPH it is 14 µM (11). These concentrations produce an enzyme rate of only 1% of the maximum velocity of the 5α-reductase enzyme. Clearly the rate of production of DHT in vivo is predominantly determined by the concentration of testosterone rather than by the 5α-reductase or NADPH. Once formed, DHT enters a competitive steady-state relationship with: 1) the cytoplasmic receptor, 2) the 3α-hydroxysteroid oxidoreductase, 3) the 3β-hydroxysteroid oxidoreductase, and 4) the 17β-hydroxysteroid oxidoreductase. All of these interactions are reversible and are discussed in detail as follows:

1) Cytoplasmic receptor

It is the binding of DHT to this cytoplasmic androgen receptor protein which is believed to be responsible for the structural changes ("activation")

117

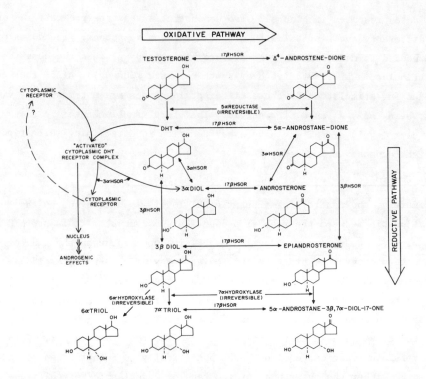

Figure 3. General overview of androgen metabolism in the prostate. 17β HSOR= 17β-Hydroxysteroid oxidoreductase; 3α HSOR = 3α-hydroxysteroid oxidoreductase; 3β HSOR = 3β-hydroxysteroid oxidoreductase.

required to allow the temperature sensitive translocation of the "activated" DHT receptor complex into the prostatic nucleus. This translocated nuclear DHT receptor complex is then thought to bind to acceptor site in the nucleus with the resultant increase in mRNA and DNA synthesis characteristic of the particular androgenic response. Numerous studies have shown that the binding of DHT to the cytoplasmic receptor is a concentration dependent process. Since it is this binding which begins the process of androgen action, it becomes clear that the dynamic competition for DHT between these cytoplasmic receptors and the enzymes metabolizing DHT is fundamental in determining the type of prostatic response illicited by androgens.

2) 3α-Hydroxysteroid oxidoreductase (EC 1.1.1.50)

The activity of 3α-hydroxysteroid oxidoreductase is generally thought to be higher than either the 3β-hydroxysteroid or 17β-hydroxysteroid oxidoreductase

and to be the main pathway for DHT. However, this enzyme is unique in that
while its activity is high and production of 5α-androstane-3α,17β-diol
(3α-diol) from DHT is continuous in homogenates of ventral prostate, these
same results are not seen with mince or slices of the prostate. In slice
or mince experiments, DHT is metabolized to 3α-diol, but the production of
3α-diol plateaus rapidly. The metabolism of DHT does continue to proceed
but via other pathways (Figure 4). The 3α-hydroxysteroid oxidoreductase

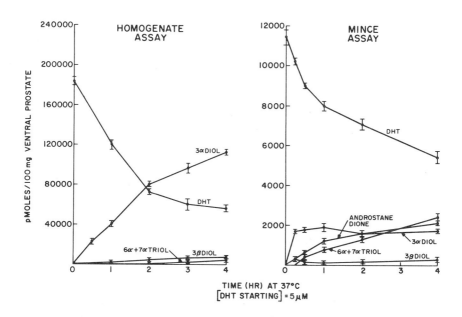

Figure 4. Differences between rat ventral prostate homogenate and mince
           assay for 3α-hydroxysteroid oxidoreductase activity. In homo-
           genate assay, homogenate representing 5 mg ventral prostate was
           incubated with 40 ml of media containing 5 μM ^{3}H-DHT and .5 mM
           NADPH. In mince assays, 100 mg of rat ventral prostate was
           incubated in 2.5 ml of media containing 5 μM ^{3}H-DHT. At various
           times, aliquots were removed, and the levels of various meta-
           bolites were determined.

enzyme thus appears to be under some type of important though little recognized regulation which is lost upon homogenization of the prostate. It is
known that the 3α-hydroxysteroid oxidoreductase is competitively inhibited
by androstanedione (29). It is possible that in mince experiments where
androstanedione is a major metabolite, significant levels of this steroid
are retained by the tissue mince to produce a local concentration sufficient
to inhibit the 3α-hydroxysteroid oxidoreductase. In homogenate experiments

which are supplemented with NADPH, little androstanedione is produced and the 3α-hydroxysteroid oxidoreductase in these assays appear to be maximally active. Recently, this 3α-hydroxysteroid oxidoreductase has been shown in vitro to be able to metabolize DHT when it is bound to the cytoplasmic receptor complex. The product of the reaction is 3α-diol dissociated from the cytoplasmic receptor (25). This interaction may be important in controlling the recycling of receptors in the prostate.

3) 3β-Hydroxysteroid oxidoreductase (EC 1.1.1.51)

The production of 5α-androstane-3β,17β-diol (3β-diol) from DHT catalyzed by the 3β-hydroxysteroid oxidoreductase (3β HSOR) was once thought to be of minor importance in the overall flux of prostatic DHT and also to be irreversible. These assumptions were based upon two observations: 1) the apparent low rate of 3β-diol production from DHT by the prostate (30), and 2) the inability of the prostate to reform DHT when incubated with 3β-diol (19). Recently both of these observations have been shown not to be entirely correct. The reason for the earlier misunderstanding was due to lack of knowledge that 3β-diol is rapidly further metabolized to hydroxylated products (3β-triols) by the prostate (14-17, 22, 26). In the rat prostate, the major metabolite of 3β-diol is 5α-androstane-3β,6α,17β-triol (6α-triol) accounting for approximately 75% of the total 3β-triols. The remaining 25% of the 3β-triols are accounted for by 5α-androstane-3β,7α,17β-triol (7α-triol) (15). The 3β-diol 6α and 7α-hydroxylases responsible for the irreversible production of these 3β-triols are both microsomal NADPH requiring enzymes (16). The products of these enzymes, 6α- and 7α-triol, have no androgenic abilities when tested by the classical bioassays in rats (15). In canine and human prostate, 3β-diol also has been found to be hydroxylated in the 6α- and 7α-position (17, 22, 26). However, in these tissues the major product is 7α-triol and not 6α-triol. The consequences of these interesting species differences are at present totally unclear. What is clear, however, is that the total hydroxylase activity (6α- and 7α-hydroxylation) for 3β-diol is much faster than the activity of the 3β-hydroxysteroid oxidoreductase (3β HSOR) regardless of the species. This means that once 3β-diol is formed, it is rapidly converted irreversibly to hydroxylated products thus minimizing any buildup of 3β-diol. This rapid irreversible metabolism of 3β-diol has direct consequences in relation to both the accurate assaying of prostatic 3β HSOR and the reversibility of this enzyme. First, if the 3β HSOR is to be accurately assayed in the DHT → 3β-diol direction, all the 3β-hydroxy products including the triols must be accounted for. In previous studies, the contribution of the triols to the total 3β-hydroxy-5α-androstane metabolites were neglected and therefore the activities reported for 3β HSOR are probably underestimations of the true activity for this enzyme. Second, the incubation of 3β-diol with prostatic tissue results in a competition for the added 3β-diol substrate between the 3β HSOR (3β-diol → DHT) and the 3β-diol hydroxylases (3β-diol → 3β-triols). Since the 3β-diol hydroxylases are in such large enzymatic excess in relation to the 3β HSOR, this prostatic incubation results in nearly exclusive irreversible conversion of 3β-diol to the triols with minimal formation of DHT, thus giving the appearance that the 3β HSOR itself is irreversible.

4) 17β-Hydroxysteroid oxidoreductase (EC 1.1.1.63)

Each of the reductive metabolites of testosterone possesses a 17β-hydroxyl group which is capable of being oxidized to a 17 ketone group by the 17β-hydroxysteroid oxidoreductase. The corresponding oxidative products (Δ^4-androstenedione, 5α-androstanedione, androsterone, epiandrosterone, and 5α-androstane-3β,7α-diol-17-one) are all able to be reconverted back to their 17β-hydroxy counterparts due to the reversibility of the 17β-hydroxysteroid oxidoreductase.

To summarize, testosterone enters the prostatic cell via passive diffusion and is converted irreversibly via 5α-reductase to the active androgen DHT. DHT can then be converted into a complex mixture of oxidized and reduced biotransformation products. These transformations are catalyzed by reversible enzymes (3α, 3β, 17β-oxidoreductase). This means that all of these metabolites are capable of being converted back to DHT and thus are potentially androgenic. In contrast to the production of androgen metabolites which can be converted back to DHT, 6α- and 7α-triols are unique. These steroid metabolites, which possess no androgenic ability, are unable to be converted back to DHT due to the irreversible nature of the 3β-diol hydroxylase enzymes. This may indicate that these enzymes function as a common final pathway for the termination of androgenic abilities of the C_{19}-androstane steroids. The complex androgen metabolic pathways seen in the prostate may thus serve an important dynamic function to regulate the concentration of intracellular DHT. In the normal intact animal this system may allow sufficient amounts of intracellular DHT to completely maintain the prostate, but insufficient levels to induce continuous proliferative overgrowth on the gland.

121

Therefore the complex prostatic metabolism of androgen itself may represent one form of normal constraint mechanism on the proliferative overgrowth of this tissue. Clearly, it is not, however, the sole mechanism.

It is interesting that the prostate itself apparently possesses the ability to moderate and control the levels of intracellular androgen via their metabolism and thus help control its own response to androgen. This may be very important for two reasons. First, the levels of circulating plasma androgens are not constant. Various groups have clearly shown that there are large fluctuations in plasma androgen levels having both seasonal, episodic, and possibly diurnal variations (2, 3, 7, 19). These changes in the circulating androgen levels could have profound consequences on the prostate if it did not possess some type of ability to moderate this flux. Secondly, a defect in one or several components of this metabolic system could have profound consequences on the response of the prostate to androgen. The net result of such a defect could be critical in developing the correct environment whereby the prostate loses its normal constraint mechanism for proliferative growth, thus allowing neoplastic transformation of the prostate.

Levels of Androgen in Prostatic Neoplasia

The relevance of the preceding statement is demonstrated by the finding that the levels of intracellular DHT in neoplastic diseases of the prostate are significantly higher than normal, Table 2. While no clear-cut cause and effect relationship has definitely been established for the increase in DHT level, these observations do clearly demonstrate that prostatic neoplasia must be associated with definitive changes in the normal prostatic metabolism of androgen. Exactly what the changes are will require further work.

Future Direction

In future work, it will be of major importance to comparatively examine the metabolism of androgen in normal and cancerous prostatic tissue. In such work, it will be critical to examine all the potential pathways for androgen metabolism since all are interconnected and interrelated. Analysis of single enzymes (e.g., 5α-reductase) will be difficult or impossible to interpret due to the interrelationship of androgen metabolism of the prostate. Also, it is clear that there are many subtle forms of cellular control for androgen metabolism which appear to be destroyed or partially lost by homogenization of the gland. Homogenate assays used to study androgen

Table 2

STEROID	HUMAN PROSTATE			CANINE PROSTATE		RAT VENTRAL PROSTATE
	NORMAL	BPH	CANCER	NORMAL	BPH	NORMAL
	(ng/gram wet weight prostate)					
TEST.	$0.9{\pm}0.3^a$ $0.2{\pm}0.1^f$ $0.3{\pm}0.1^h$	$0.9{\pm}0.2^a$ $0.3{\pm}0.1^f$ $0.3{\pm}0.1^h$	$1.2{\pm}0.8^f$ 1.8^h	0.3^d	1.0^d	$2.0{\pm}0.4^e$
DHT	$1.3{\pm}0.5^a$ $2.1{\pm}0.32^b$ $2.0{\pm}0.31^c$ $1.6{\pm}1.0^f$ $1.3{\pm}0.3^h$	$6.0{\pm}1.0^a$ $5.6{\pm}0.93^b$ $5.0{\pm}0.54^c$ $4.5{\pm}1.4^f$ $5.5{\pm}0.5^h$	$3.2{\pm}0.42^c$ $3.9{\pm}0.3^f$ 4.2^h	3.3^d	16.0^d	$2.8{\pm}0.5^e$
5α-DIOL^g	$10.2{\pm}2.4^b$ $1.7{\pm}0.3^f$ $4.3{\pm}0.7^h$	$2.3{\pm}0.35^b$ $0.6{\pm}0.7^f$ $1.5{\pm}0.2^h$	$1.6{\pm}0.8$ 35.0^h			

[a]Siiteri et al. (26) [b]Geller et al. (9) [c]Geller et al. (10)
[d]Gloyna et al. (12) [e]Robel et al. (27) [f]Krieg et al. (18)
[g]5α-diol = 5α-androstane (3α + β), 17β-diol [h]Hammond (13)

metabolism may therefore be of limited value in understanding the overall
picture of the dynamics of androgen metabolism. Prostatic minces or slices
allow the evaluation of androgen metabolism in a more physiological and
integrated manner and are highly recommended for future work on these important questions. As an example of such an approach, the work of Morfin
et al. is excellent (22). It will likewise be very important to determine
intracellular levels of androgen in prostatic cancer tissue to document
whether the increase in DHT levels reported by several groups (10, 18, 13)
is a general observation or highly dependent upon the degree of differentiation of the tumor.

REFERENCES

1. Anderson, K. H. and Liao, S.: Selective Retention of Dihydrotestosterone by Prostatic Nuclei. Nature 219: 277-279, 1968.
2. Bartke, A., Steele, R. E., Musto, N. and Caldwell, B. V.: Fluctuations in Plasma Testosterone Levels in Adult Male Rats and Mice. Endocr. 92: 1223-1228, 1973.
3. Boon, D. A., Keenan, R. E. and Slaunwhite, W. R.: Plasma Testosterone in Men: Variation, But Not Circadion Rhythm. Steroids 20: 269-278, 1972.
4. Bruchovsky, N. and Wilson, J. D.: The Conversion of Testosterone to 5α-androstan-17β-ol-3-one by Rat Prostate in vivo and in vitro. J. Biol. Chem. 243: 2012-2021, 1968.
5. Coffey, D. S., Shimazaki, J. and Williams-Ashman, H. G.: Polymerization of Deoxyribonucleotides in Relation to Androgen-Induced Prostatic Growth. Arch. Biochem. Biophys. 124: 184-198, 1968.
6. DeKlerk, D. P., Coffey, D. S., Ewing, L. L., McDermott, I. R., Reiner, W. G., Robinson, C. H., Scott, W. W., Strandberg, J. D., Talalay, P., Walsh, P. C., Wheaton, L. G. and Zirkin, B. R.: A Comparison of Spontaneous and Experimentally INduced Canine Prostatic Hyperplasia. J. Clin. Invest. (In press), 1979.
7. Faiman, C. and Winter, J. S. D.: Diurnal Cycles in Plasma FSH, Testosterone, and Cortisol in Men. J. Clin. Endocr. 33: 186-192, 1971.
8. Frederiksen, D. W. and Wilson, J. D.: Partial Characterization of the Nuclear Reduced Nicotinamide Adenine Dinucleotide Phosphate: Δ^4-3-Ketosteroid 5α-Oxidoreductase of Rat Prostate. J. Biol. Chem. 246: 2584-2593, 1971.
9. Geller, J., Albert, J., Lopez, D., Geller, S. and Niwayama, G.: Comparison of Androgen Metabolites in Benign Prostatic Hypertrophy (BPH) and Normal Prostate. J. Clin. Endo. Metab. 43: 686-688, 1976.
10. Geller, J., Albert, J., Lopez, D., Geller, S., Stoeltzing, W. and De La Vega, D.: DHT Concentration in Human Prostatic Cancer Tissue. J. Clin. Endo. Metab. 46: 440-444, 1978.
11. Glock, G. E. and McLean, P.: Determination of Oxidized and Reduced Diphosphopyridine Nucleotide and Triphosphopyridine in Animal Tissues. Biochem. Journal 61: 381-388, 1955.
12. Gloyna, R., Siiteri, P. and Wilson, J.: Dihydrotestosterone in Prostatic Hypertrophy. II. The Formation and Content of Dihydrotestosterone in the Hypertrophic Canine Prostate and the Effect of Dihydrotestosterone on Prostate Growth in the Dog. J. Clin. Invest. 49: 1746-1753, 1970.
13. Hammond, G. L.: Endogenous Steroid Levels in the Human Prostate from Birth to Old Age: A Comparison of Normal and Diseased Tissues. J. Endocr. 78: 7-19, 1978.
14. Isaacs, J. T., DeKlerk, D. P. and Coffey, D. S.: Special Properties of 5α-Androstane-3β,17β-Diol on the Growth of the Sex Accessory Tissues. Fed. Proc. 37: 286, 1978.
15. Isaacs, J. T., McDermott, I. R. and Coffey, D. S.: The Identification and Characterization of a New $C_{19}O_3$ Steroid Metabolite in the Rat Ventral Prostate: 5α-Androstane-3β,6α,17β-Triol. Steroids 33: 639-657, 1979.
16. Isaacs, J. T., McDermott, I. R. and Coffey, D. S.: Characterization of Two New Enzymatic Activities of the Rat Ventral Prostate: 5α-Androstane-3β,17β-Diol 6α-Hydroxylase and 5α-Androstane-3β,17β-Diol 7α-Hydroxylase. Steroids 33: 675-692, 1979.

17. Isaacs, J. T., McDermott, I. R. and Coffey, D. S.: The Identification and Characterization of the $C_{19}O_3$ Steroid Metabolites of 5α-Androstane-3β,17β-Diol Produced by the Canine Prostate: 5α-Androstane-3β,6α, 17β-Triol and 5α-Androstane-3β,7α,17β-Triol. Steroids (In press), 1979.
18. Krieg, M., Bartsch, W., Janssen, W. and Voight, K. D.: A Comparative Study of Binding, Metabolism and Endogenous Levels of Androgen in Normal, Hyperplastic, and Carcinomatous Human Prostate. J. Steroid Biochem. 10: (In press), 1979.
19. Levy, C., Marchut, M., Baulieu, E. E. and Robel, P.: Studies of the 3β-Hydroxysteroid Oxidoreductase Activity in Rat Ventral Prostate. Steroids 23: 251-300, 1973.
20. Mock, E. J., Kamel, F., Wright, W. W. and Frankel, A. I.: Seasonal Rhythm in Plasma Testosterone and Luteinising Hormone of the Male Laboratory Rat. Nature 256: 61-63, 1975.
21. Moore, R. A.: Benign Hypertrophy and Carcinoma of the Prostate. In Endocrinology of Neoplastic Diseases (Twombly, G., Packs, G., eds.) London, New York, Oxford Univ. Press, 194-212, 1947.
22. Morfin, R. F., DiStefano, S., Charles, J. F. and Floch, H. H.: Precursors for 6β- and 7α-Hydroxylations of 5α-Androstane-3β,17β-Diol by Human and Hyperplastic Prostates. Biochemie 59: 637-644, 1977.
23. Morfin, R., Leav, J., Charles, J. F., Cavazos, L., Ofner, P. and Floch, H.: Correlative Study of the Morphology and C_{19}-Steroid Metabolism of Benign and Cancerous Human Prostatic Tissue. Cancer 39: 1517-1534, 1977.
24. Noble, R. L.: Sex Steroids as a Cause of Adenocarcinoma of the Dorsal Prostate in Nb Rats, and Their Influence on the Growth of Transplants. Oncology 34: 138-141, 1977.
25. Nozu, K. and Tamavki, B.: Formation, Nuclear Incorporation and Enzymatic Decomposition of Androgen-Receptor Complex of Rat Prostate. J. Steroid Biochem. 6: 1319-1323, 1974.
26. Ofner, P., Vena, R. L., Morfin, R. F.: Steroids 24: 261-279, 1974.
27. Robel, P., Corpechot, C. and Baulieu, E. E.: Testosterone and Androstanolone in Rat Plasma and Tissues. FEBS Letters 33: 218-220, 1973.
28. Siiteri, P. and Wilson, J.: Dihydrotestosterone in Prostatic Hypertrophy. I. The Formation and Content of Dihydrotestosterone in the Hypertrophic Prostate of Man. J. Clin. Invest. 49: 1737-1745, 1970.
29. Sufrin, G. and Coffey, D. S.: Differences in the Mechanism of Action of Medrogestone and Cyproterone Acetate. Invest. Urol. 13: 1-9, 1975.
30. Taurog, J. D., Moore, R. J. and Wilson, J. D.: Partial Characterization of the Cytosol 3α-Hydroxysteroid: $NAD(P)^+$ Oxidoreductase of Rat Ventral Prostate. Biochem. 14: 810-817, 1975.
31. Vermeulen, A., Rubens, R. and Verderick, L.: Testosterone Secretion and Metabolism in Male Senescence. J. Clin. Endocr. 34: 730-735, 1972.
32. Walsh, P. C. and Wilson, J. D.: The Induction of Prostatic Hypertrophy in the Dog with Androstanediol. J. Clin. Invest. 57: 1093-1098, 1976.

STEROID RECEPTORS AND THE REGULATION OF

TRANSCRIPTIONAL EVENTS IN THE PROSTATE*

CHAPTER VIII

Unquestionably, androgen receptors are present in the prostate glands of
all species studied to date. These prostates contain androgen receptors
with a penchant for binding a specific metabolite of testosterone, 5α-
dihydrotestosterone (DHT) (5α-androstan-17β-ol-3-one). Current models
of the mechanism of action of androgens place very heavy emphasis on the
enhancement of transcription as the key event in most androgenic
responses and all available evidence indicates that the androgen receptors
are implicated in the activation of the genome in androgen-responsive
cells. Regrettably, direct corroboration of this concept has yet to be
achieved with fidelity in reconstituted, cell-free systems. The reasons
for this current impasse are many and all are discussed critically here.

(A) A SURVEY OF PRESENT INFORMATION

No-one these days would dispute the view that steroid-binding proteins or
receptors play a mandatory role in the mode of action of all steroid
hormones, their analogues and their antagonists (17). Evidence supporting
the receptor concept can only be described now as compelling. In molecular
terms, androgen target cells are virtually unique in that the conversion
of testosterone to various metabolites is both extensive and biologically
necessary (23). All of the androgen receptors in the accessory sexual
glands studied thus far preferentially bind metabolites of testosterone
rather than the parent or primary androgen itself, the favoured metabolite
is usually 5α-dihydrotestosterone.

As reviewed in great detail elsewhere (23), current evidence is equally
overwhelming that transcriptional events play a critical part in androgenic
responses in the prostate. Following in the wake of the studies by Liao
(19,20) more sophisticated means of assay indicate that androgens (a)
selectively enhance the synthesis of the messenger RNA coding for aldolase
(27), (b) stimulate all the enzymes and factors associated with DNA
replication (29,37), (c) stringently regulate the principal secretory

*W. Ian P. Mainwaring, Department of Biochemistry
9 Hyde Terrace, Leeds LS2 9LS, U.K.

proteins and the synthesis of the corresponding species of poly(A)-rich
messenger RNA (13,24,35,36). Some four years ago, all the signs augured
favourably for a prompt and satisfactory explanation of how androgen
receptor complexes regulate transcription in the prostate. First, it was
possible to simulate quite accurately the transfer of androgen receptor
complexes into purified nuclei and chromatin, in vitro (28,42). Second,
there were reports on the partial purification of the cytoplasmic androgen
receptor in rat prostate (24,25). Third, when admittedly impure
preparations of androgen receptor complex were added to prostate nuclei
or chromatin in reconstituted systems, it was possible to elicit an
enhancement of nuclear RNA synthesis (9,10,26). Since these apparent early
successes, further progress has really been denied all investigators in this
research area. An appraisal of current problems will now be attempted.

(a) Purification of androgen receptor complexes

This problem remains the most pressing limitation on research progress at
present. Unless highly purified preparations of androgen receptor complex
are used, the interpretation of experiments in vitro on transcriptional
events are always open to criticism and to difficulties in interpretation.
For example, just traces of nucleases or unspecified activators and inhibitors
in receptor preparations could create serious experimental artefacts.

The extensive purification of androgen receptors from the prostates of
all species has foundered for two principal reasons (23). First, androgen
receptors appear to be intrinsically more labile than those for other
steroid hormones. This problem is compounded by the very high proteolytic
activity in accessory sexual glands which resists commonly used inactivators,
such as p-methylsulphonyl fluoride. Second, androgen receptors do not
lend themselves to purification by affinity chromatography, despite the
fact that suitable matrices containing immobolized androgens are available
(30,38). This powerful means of protein fractionation has led to the
successful purification of the receptors for oestrogens (4,39), progesterone
(41), and glucocorticoids (12), yet it has been found unsuitable for
androgen receptors. In all the satisfactory procedures published thus far,
there has been a preliminary "work-up" of crude extracts of target tissues
in the absence of the appropriate steroid ligand prior to the affinity
chromatography step. Androgen receptors cannot withstand these early
manipulations, such as precipitation by ammonium sulphate or protamine
sulphate, unless saturating amounts of a 5α-dihydrotestosterone are present.
The latter prerequisite precludes the use of affinity chromatography as a

subsequent purification step.

In view of these difficulties, it may be expedient to gain experience
and suitable technology from studies on other androgen receptors, then
returning to the more difficult task of purifying the androgen receptors
in the prostate. For several reasons, the kidney of the female mouse appears
to be a suitable alternative. This organ contains androgen receptors (1,2),
yet endogenous concentrations of androgens in the female will be low. In
addition, it has been reported that the administration of testosterone to
female mice provokes a rapid and significant increase in RNA synthesis in
the kidney (15,16). Finally, it seems likely that mutant mice, particularly
the testicular feminization mutant or Tfm mouse (16,21,22) may be useful
in unravelling the androgenic regulation of genetic transcription. The Tfm
mouse lacks androgen receptors (1,2) and also fails to respond to androgenic
stimulation in terms of RNA synthesis, de novo (16,22).

(b) Improvements in the translocation of androgen receptors, in vitro
After nearly eighty years of uncertainty and contentious debate, there
have recently been revolutionary proposals on the structure of eukaryotic
chromatin, as embodied in the nucleosome concept (5). It seems that we
may be approaching a better understadning of (a) the distribution of histones
and non-histone proteins within chromatin, (b) how to reconstruct chromatin
accurately from its separated components, (c) the structural features of
chromatin necessary for active transcription, (d) the true complexity of
the synthesis and processing of eukaryotic messenger RNA and finally,
(e) how transcriptional mechanisms are switched on and off.

These important advances may well be germane to the problem of the nature
and distribution of the acceptor sites for steroid receptor complexes in
chromatin. Current evidence suggests a role for both DNA and non-histone
proteins in the acceptor sites, but their distribution and configuration
remains to be clarified. It also may prove possible to explain in structural
terms why the chromatin of androgen target cells has more putative acceptor
sites than that of non-target cells (18,28,43). Such information would
significantly improve the chances of successfully stimulating transcriptional
events in vitro in a manner approaching that in the intact prostate cell.

(c) Fidelity of chromatin transcription in vitro
There is now a consensus that sophisticated means must be employed to
monitor a meaningful activation of transcription under conditions in vitro;
an enhancement of RNA polymerase or DNA polymerase is simply not good enough.

Even in very favourable circumstances where specific eukaryotic genes are amplified, as with the ribosomal RNA genes in oocytes of Xenopus laevis (3), their accurate transcription was for a long time impossible, even with homologous RNA polymerases (14). The faithful transcription of the genes for histones, 5 S ribosomal RNA, chick ovalbumin and rabbit α- and β-globin has now been independently claimed by many laboratories (for review, see 5). It is worth emphasizing that transcription, in vivo, has the following characteristics; asymmetry, initiation with purine nucleoside 5' triphosphates (all phosphates being conserved at the 5' RNA terminus), rigorous strand selection in the DNA template and elongation (5' → 3') from the 3' end of the DNA template. With modern technology, many of these fundamental features of transcription can be faithfully reproduced, in vitro.

Means of analysis for RNA transcripts: It is now possible to purify many poly(A)-rich messenger RNAs from eukaryotic cells and to use them as templates for the synthesis of highly radioactive, complementary DNA counter-parts(for review, see 31). These complementary DNA probes are absolutely essential now for probing the transcription of DNA into messenger RNA in detail. As described below, however, the complementary DNA probes must be used with prudence. An attractive alternative is to use radioactive purine nucleoside 5'-triphosphates to monitor the critical initiation step of RNA transcription (40).

Choice of RNA polymerase: The RNA polymerases of eukaryotes are generally of low activity and can present problems in their accurate assay and in chromatin trsnscription, in vitro. To offset this difficulty, it has become very fashionable to measure transcription, in vitro, using a vast excess of E. coli RNA polymerase, usually in the presence of mercury-contain-ing RNA precursors (7,8). Bearing this heavy metal substituent, the RNA transcript can be readily purified by affinity chromatography on matrices containing immobilized sulphydryl groups. While seemingly elegant, this approach can create surprising artefacts. In particular, the E. coli RNA polymerase can use endogenous RNA in chromatin as a spurious template, forming "nonsense transcripts" which nevertheless are recognized by complementary DNA probes (32,44). Many investigators now report that, despite their lower activity, eukaryotic RNA polymerases transcribe eukaryotic chromatin with more fidelity that the E. coli enzyme (5).

Reconstruction of chromatin : The accurate reassembly of eukaryotic chromatin in terms of accessible genes for transcription has been widely reported (31).

However, this reconstruction may not be as simple as once imagined, as the order of mixing the various components is now recognised as vital for subsequent transcription to be precise (11).

Nature of the template: In the past, most investigators have used chromatin almost exclusively as the DNA template for exogenous RNA polymerase. This practice may also not be too advisable. In one very recent report, the use of purified nuclei as both a source of template DNA and homologous (endogenous) RNA polymerase has been persuasively argued (33).

With these contemporary innovations, and their prudent application, accurate transcription of precise genes, in vitro, is now becoming a practical reality.

(B)   FUTURE PROSPECTS

In the light of these recent advances, investigations on the activation of the prostate genome by androgen receptor complexes can now be tackled anew with greater confidence. Even so, there still remain some problems particular to the chromatin of steroid target cells, including the prostate. First, there are steroid-sensitive ribonucleases associated with such chromatin (6,17) and their activation by the appropriate hormone may yet create some problems. Second, there is an unsolved paradox in relating receptor translocation into the nucleus with the reported enhancement of ribosomal RNA synthesis (17,23). Receptor complexes can seemingly be retained in all nuclear areas but the nucleolus, yet this intranuclear organelle is the sole site of ribosomal RNA synthesis and a ubiquitously important indicator of hormonal stimulation, particularly in the prostate. The question of a regulatory "middle man" between receptor binding and the nucleolar response is therefore very real. Notwithstanding these problems, investigations into the androgenic regulation of genomic transcription could now be entering a new and successful phase.

References:

1. Attardi, B. and Ohno, S.: Cytosol androgen receptor from kidneys of normal and testicular feminized (Tfm) mice. Cell, 2: 205-212, 1974.
2. Bullock, L. P., Mainwaring, W. I. P. and Bardin, C. W.: The physicochemical properties of the cytoplasmic androgen receptors in

kidneys of normal, carrier female (Tfm/+) and androgen-insensitive (Tfm/y) mice. Endocrinology Research Communications, 2: 25-45 1975.

3. Brown, D. D. and Sugimoto, K.: 5 S DNAs of Xenopus laevis and Xenopus mulleri: evolution of a gene family. Journal of Molecular Biology, 78: 397-415, 1973.

4. Coffer, A. I., Milton, P. J. D., Pryse-Davies, J. and King, R. J. B.: Purification of oestradiol receptor from human uterus by affinity chromatography. Molecular and Cellular Endocrinology, 6: 231-246, 1977.

5. Cold Spring Harbor Symposium on Quantitative Biology, Volume XLII, parts 1 and 2, 1977.

6. Cox, R. F.: Chromatin-associated ribonucleases are activated by estradiol in chick oviduct. Journal of Steroid Biochemistry, 9: 697-704, 1978.

7. Dale, R. M. K., Livingston, D. C. and Ward, D. C. The synthesis and enzymatic polymerization of nucleotides containing mercury; potential tools for nucleic acid sequencing and structural analysis. Proceedings National Academy of Sciences, 70: 2238-2242, 1973.

8. Dale, R. M. K. and Ward, D. C.: Mercurated polynucleotides, new probes for hybridization and selective polymer fractionation. Biochemistry, 14: 2458-2469, 1975.

9. Davies, P. and Griffiths, K.: Stimulation of prostatic ribonucleic acid polymerase in vitro by prostatic steroid-receptor complexes. Biochemical Journal, 136: 611-622, 1974.

10. Davies, P. and Griffiths, K.: Similarities between 5α-dihydrotestosterone receptor complexes from human and rat prostatic tissue: effects on RNA polymerase activity. Molecular and Cellular Endocrinology, 3: 143-164, 1975.

11. Gadski, R. A. and Chae, C.-B.: Mode of chromatin reconstitution; elements controlling globin gene transcription. Biochemistry, 17: 869-874, 1978.

12. Govindan, M. V. and Sekeris, C. E.: Purification of two dexamethasone-binding proteins from rat liver cytosol. Biochemistry, 89: 95-103, 1978.

13. Heyns, W., Peeters, B. and Mons, J.: Influence of androgens on the concentration of prostatic binding protein (PBP) and its mRNA in rat prostate. Biochemical Biophysical Research Communications, 77: 1492-1499, 1977.

14. Honjo, T. and Reeder, R. H.: Transcription of Xenopus chromatin by homologous ribonucleic acid polymerase; aberrant synthesis of ribosomal and 5 S ribonucleic acid. Biochemistry, 13: 1896-1899, 1974.

15. Jacob, S. T. Janne, O. and Sajdel-Sulkowska, E. M.: Hormonal regulation of RNA polymerases in rat liver and kidney. In Isoenzymes (Ed. C. L. Maskert), Volume III, p. 9, Academic Press, New York, 1975.

16. Janne, O., Bullock, L. P., Bardin, C. W. and Jacob, S. T.: Early androgen action in kidney of normal and androgen-insensitive (Tfm/y) mice. Biochemica et Biophysica Acta, 418: 330-343, 1976.

17. King, R. J. B. and Mainwaring, W. I. P.: Steroid-Cell Interactions, Butterworths, London, 1974.

18. Klyzsejko-Stefanowicz, L., Chiu, J.-F., Tsai, Y.-H. and Hnilica, L. S.: Acceptor proteins in rat androgenic tissue chromatin. Proceedings National Academy of Sciences, Washington, 73: 1954-1958, 1976.

19. Liao, S., Barton, R. W. and Lin, A. H.: Differential synthesis of ribonucleic acid in prostatic nuclei. Proceedings National Academy of Sciences, Washington, 55: 1553-1600, 1966.

20. Liao, S. and Lin, A. H.: Prostatic nuclear chromatin: an effect of testosterone on the synthesis of RNA rich in cytidyl (3',5') guanosine. Proceedings National Academy of Sciences, Washington, 57: 379-386, 1967.

21. Lyon, M. F., Glenister, P. H. and Lamoreux, M. L.: Normal spermatozoa from androgen-resistant germ cells of chimaeric mice and the role of androgen in spermatogenesis. Nature, 258: 620-622, 1975.

22. Lyon, M. F. and Hawkes, S. G.: X-linked gene for testicular feminisation in the mouse. Nature, 225: 1217-1219, 1970.

23. Mainwaring, W. I. P.: The Mechanism of Action of Androgens, Springer-Verlag, New York, 1977.

24. Mainwaring, W. I. P. and Irving, R. A.: The use of deoxyribonucleic acid-cellulose chromatography and isoelectric focusing for the characterization and partial purification of steroid-receptor complexes. Biochemical Journal, 134: 113-127, 1973.

25. Mainwaring, W. I. P. and Irving, R. A.: Partial purification of steroid-receptor complexes by DNA-cellulose chromatography and isoelectric focusing. Journal of Steroid Biochemistry, 5: 711-716, 1974.

26. Mainwaring, W. I. P. and Jones, D. A.: Influence of receptor complexes on the properties of prostate chromatin, including its transcription by RNA polymerase. Journal of Steroid Biochemistry, 6: 475-482, 1975.

27. Mainwaring, W. I. P., Mangan, F. R., Irving, R. A. and Jones, D. A.: Specific changes in the messenger ribonucleic acid content of the rat ventral prostate gland after androgenic stimulation. Biochemical Journal, 144: 413-426, 1974.

28. Mainwaring, W. I. P. and Peterkin, B. M.: A reconstituted, cell-free system for the transfer of steroid-receptor complexes into nuclear chromatin isolated from rat ventral prostate gland. Biochemical Journal, 125: 285-295, 1971.

29. Mainwaring, W. I. P., Rennie, P. S. and Keen, J.: The androgenic regulation of prostate proteins with a high affinity for deoxyribonucleic acid. Biochemical Journal, 156: 253-264, 1976.

30. Mickelson, K. E., Teller, D. C. and Petra, P. H.: Characterization of the sex steroid binding protein of human pregnancy serum; improvements in the purification procedure. Biochemistry, 17: 1409-1415, 1978.

31. O'Malley, B. W., Towle, H. C. and Schwartz, R. J.: Regulation of gene expression in eucaryotes. Annual Review of Genetics, 11: 239-260, 1977.

32. Orkin, S. H.: In vitro synthesis of a DNA probe for antisense globin sequences. Journal of Biological Chemistry, 252: 5606-5608, 1977.

33. Orkin, S. H.: Fidelity of globin ribonucleic acid synthesis in vitro by isolated nuclei; asymmetric gene expression. Biochemistry, 17: 487-492, 1978.

34. Parker, M. G. and Mainwaring, W. I. P.: Effects of androgens on the complexity of poly(A) RNA from rat prostate. Cell, 12: 401-407, 1977.

35. Parker, M. G. and Mainwaring, W. I. P.: Androgenic regulation of poly(A)-containing RNA sequences in rat ventral prostate. Journal of Steroid Biochemistry, 9: 455-462, 1978.

36. Parker, M. G., Scrace, G. T. and Mainwaring, W. I. P.: Testosterone regulates the synthesis of major proteins in rat ventral prostate. Biochemical Journal, 170: 115-121, 1978.
37. Rennie, P. S., Symes, E. K. and Mainwaring, W. I. P.: The androgenic regulation of the activities of enzymes engaged in the synthesis of deoxyribonucleic acid in the rat ventral prostate gland. Biochemical Journal, 152: 1-16, 1975.
38. Rosner, W. and Smith, R. N.: Isolation and characterization of the testosterone-binding globulin from human plasma; use of a novel affinity column. Biochemistry, 14: 4813-4820, 1975.
39. Sica, V., Parikh, I., Nola, E., Puca, G. A. and Cuatrecasas, P.: Affinity chromatography and the purification of estrogen receptors. Journal of Biological Chemistry, 248: 6543-6558, 1973.
40. Smith, M. M., Reeve, A. E. and Huang, R. C. C.: Transcription of bacteriophage DNA in vitro using purine nucleoside 5'-[γ-S] triphosphates as affinity probes for RNA chain initiation. Biochemistry, 17: 493-500, 1978.
41. Smith, R. G., Iramain, C. A., Buttram, V. C. and O'Malley, B. W.: Purification of human uterine progesterone receptor. Nature, 253: 271-272, 1975.
42. Steggles, A. W., Spelsberg, T. C., Glasser, S. R. and O'Malley, B. W.: Soluble complexes between steroid hormones and target-tissue receptors bind specifically to target-tissue chromatin. Proceedings National Academy of Sciences, Washington, 68: 1479-1482, 1971.
43. Takayasu, S.: Androgen binding to cytosol and nuclei of hamster sebaceous glands. Journal of Steroid Biochemistry, 9: 181-190, 1978.
44. Zasloff, M. and Felsenfeld, G.: Use of mercury-substituted ribonucleoside triphosphates can lead to artefacts in the analysis of in vitro chromatin transcripts. Biochemical Biophysical Research Communications, 75: 598-603, 1977.

STEROID RECEPTORS AND THE REGULATION

OF DNA SYNTHESIS*

CHAPTER IX

Many facets of the physiology and biochemistry of androgen receptors have
received in-depth review in the recent literature (3,14,18,21,27,30). but
few if any critiques have touched upon the subject of the regulation of
DNA synthesis by receptors. This is understandable in view of the contemporary emphasis on the regulation of transcription by hormone receptors, and
the lack of suitable experimental model systems for studying DNA synthesis.
Furthermore, from two accounts of preliminary work concerned with DNA
synthesis and androgen receptors (4,6), the complexities involved in the
design of appropriate experiments can be readily appreciated. On the other
hand, despite such qualification, it is reasonably certain that the rat
ventral prostate remains the tissue of choice for studying most aspects of
androgen action. Involution of glandular tissue can be induced by withdrawing
androgens, and regeneration of tissue can be stimulated by replacing them.
Since the cycles of regression and growth are relatively short and easily
controlled, they lend themselves well to investigation. During such episodes
of physiological change, the rates of DNA synthesis and cell proliferation
undergo marked fluctuations, as do the concentrations of cytoplasmic and
nuclear androgen receptors. A more complete description of these events
will be given in the following parts of this review; attention will be
drawn especially to evidence which seems to support the idea that a functional
receptor apparatus and DNA synthesis are interlocking processes.

A. CONSIDERATIONS IN THE DESIGN OF EXPERIMENTS

1. SIZE OF THE PROSTATE GLAND

In studying the response of rat ventral prostate to androgens, it is customary
to begin an experiment by administering androgens to castrated animals within
a few days of orchidectomy. The timing of the onset of replacemnt therapy
is very important, since the character of the response of prostatic tissue
is largely determined by the number of cells in the gland.

---

*Nicholas Bruchovsky and P. S. Rennie; Department of
Medicine; The University of Alberta; Edmonton, Canada T6G 2G3.
Supported by grants from the National Cancer Institue of Canada and the
Medical Research Council of Canada (MRC MT 3729)

If this number is normal, as in animals castrated less than three days previously, neither DNA synthesis nor cell proliferation can be induced to a significant degree, but secretory activity, as indicated by an increase in wet weight, is stimulated (16). If this number is below normal, as in animals castrated longer than three days previously, both DNA synthesis and cell proliferation are markedly increased in the presence of androgen. However, as soon as the number of cells is restored to the normal value, some homeostatic mechanism shuts off proliferation (16). Secretory activity is very low during the proliferative phase and for the most part seems to commence well after replication has come to a halt (22).

Hence it is evident that, when androgen is to be administered to castrated animals, the duration of castration must be chosen carefully so as to produce the response desired. For studies on the secretory function of the prostate, the animals of choice are short-term castrated animals (1 day or less) or long-term castrated animals whose prostates have completely regenerated after androgen treatment; in these cases, proliferation does not occur. For studies of proliferation, long-term castrated animals (7 days or more) should be used, and only during the period when the cellular complement is below normal. If one uses animals whose prostates are in the process of atrophy (2-6 days after castration), then interpretation of results is difficult, because this is a very unstable period and one cannot be as certain of the responses elicited by hormones (16).

2. THE CONCENTRATION OF ANDROGEN IN PLASMA AND TISSUE

A precipitous fall in the circulating level of testosterone is observed after orchidectomy. The concentration of testosterone is reduced to 20% of the normal value within 30 minutes, and to less than 4% after 120 minutes (10). In contrast, the quantity of androgen in prostatic tissue declines more slowly, being reduced by about 90% over a period of 12 hours (29). The rapidity with which the concentration of androgens in plasma and whole-tissue are restored to precastration levels depends on the dose of hormone and the route of administration. Androgens injected intravenously are delivered to the prostate within a few minutes (7). When they are administered by subcutaneous injection, a common practice, the delivery is undoubtedly much slower. The use of pharmacological amounts of androgen in the range of 1-2 mg daily per adult animal may partly compensate for the low rate, but it is fair to say that the ideal protocol for replacing androgens remains to be established. In planning the type of replacement therapy, one must also take into account that the prostate responds differentially to high and low doses of androgen (22).

B. PHYSIOLOGY OF THE PROSTATE BEFORE INVOLUTION

1. DNA SYNTHESIS

Decreases in plasma and whole-tissue levels of androgen at first have no effect on the number of cells in the prostate. However, between days 4 and 7 after orchidectomy, the gland regresses to 20% of its normal size (15). Although the withdrawal of hormone does not produce any gross changes in prostatic structure for 3 to 4 days, there is nevertheless an immediate effect on the rate of DNA synthesis. In fact, one of the earliest biochemical manifestations of orchidectomy is a rapid decline in incorporation of radio-active thymidine into DNA to 25% of normal within 24 hours. This rate is maintained until day 4 when a further decline occurs; by day 6 incorporation has dropped to 5% of normal, after which this minimal level is maintained (15).

2. ANDROGEN RECEPTOR DYNAMICS

The kinetics of the disappearance of nuclear receptor after orchidectomy have been studied by Blondeau et al (4) and Van Doorn et al (29). Both groups observe a rapid decline in the quantity of receptor to a low or negligible level after 24 hours. This is matched by an increase of similar velocity and magnitude in the concentration of cytoplasmic receptor (28,29). Throughout the interval, the net concentration of receptor in the cell remains almost constant (Table 1). Owing to these observations, and also the fact that no receptor inactivating factors are detected in the nucleus, Van Doorn et al (29) infer that the appearance of cytoplasmic receptor follows from the release of nuclear receptor into the cytoplasm. The possibility that the change in cytoplasmic binding might be due to depletion of endogenous dihydrotestosterone from the binding sites on receptors is considered by Grover and Odell (12). However, such reasoning implies that the cytoplasmic receptor is a static molecule when evidence runs contrary to this notion. Indeed, the intravenous administration of as little as 7 nmoles of dihydro-testosterone to 24-hour castrated rats stimulates a massive shift of cytoplasmic receptor back into the nucleus well within 60 minutes (Table 1 and reference 8). This observation is clearly in keeping with the view that the receptor population of the cell is capable of being recycled between the cytoplasmic and nuclear compartments with great rapidity (28).

TABLE 1. Concentration of androgen receptors in prostatic tissue

Experiment	Number of receptors per cell[a]		
	Nucleus	Cytoplasm	Total
normal rat	20,700	4,400	25,100
24 hour castrated rat	1,500	20,100	21,600
24-hour castrated rat given dihydrotestosterone	20,600	2,700	23,300
7-day castrated rat	0	3,000	3,000

[a]Data condensed from references 8,28, and 29.

The change in distribution of receptors brought about by orchidectomy is not accompanied by any major alteration in the total number of receptors in the cell for at least 24 hours (Table 1). However, commencing at 24 hours and continuing to about the 7th day, there is a striking 90% decrease in the cellular content of receptors (13,20,24,29, and Table 1). Spontaneous regeneration of receptor after the 6th day has been reported (24) but the finding has not been confirmed (4,5).

3. POTENTIAL CORRELATIONS

Both the concentration of nuclear receptors and the rate of DNA synthesis decline in parallel after orchidectomy, and presumably both are restored to normal by the administration of androgens. However, such treatment within the first 24 hours will simply prevent prostatic regression; it will not stimulate new rounds of cell division. During this time, the total number of receptors in the cell remains constant, implying that the quantity of receptors may be a factor in limiting the responsiveness of prostatic cells. A temporary change in the location of the bulk of receptors seems to have little or no effect on the outcome of androgen therapy.

C. PHYSIOLOGY OF THE PROSTATE AFTER INVOLUTION

1. DNA SYNTHESIS

Coffey et al (9) were the first to define the time course of DNA synthesis
in regenerating rat prostate. These investigators report that the treatment
of 7-day castrated rats with testosterone proprionate produces a large but
transitory increase in the incorporation of radioactive thymidine into prostatic
DNA both in vitro and in vivo, which is paralleled by an elevation and
decline in DNA polymerase activity. DNA content increases to a maximum within
2 weeks and cannot be augmented by further treatment for as long as 25 days;
in contrast, prostatic weight continues to increase without interruption,
owing to excessive secretion by overstimulated epithelial cells. These
findings were subsequently confirmed and extended by other researchers
(15,16,17,23). Taken together, the evidence indicates that prostatic regeneration is characterized by a series of very specific events in long-term
castrated rats. Only the responses in the 7-day castrated rat will be described
here.

The amount of dihydrotestosterone required to stimulate cell proliferation
in the atrophic prostate is 100 to 400 μg per 100 g body weight per day.
There is a latent period of 24 to 36 hours after the beginning of treatment
before the incorporation of radioactive thymidine into nuclear DNA can be
detected in vitro. The incorporation then increases rapidly to a maximum
by the 3rd day of about 200 times the rate for untreated controls and 10
times the normal rate. Between days 4 and 10, the rate falls precipitously
to below the normal value, and by day 14 it has decreased to the level observed
in control untreated castrates despite continued administration of hormone
(9,15,16).

The number of cells per prostate and prostatic wet weight is raised significantly above the control values by 36 hours after the beginning of treatment,
and increases rapidly between day 2 and day 5. By day 5 these parameters
have reached the normal levels. After this time the rate of increase in cell
number declines to 25% of the former value, whereas weights continue to increase
linearly until at least day 14.

Because the period of DNA synthesis between days 2 and 4 is so sharply
defined, other androgen induced responses can be divided into those which
precede, parallel or follow replication. Prior to replication, there is
a marked increase in the synthesis of androgen receptor (29) and also in

138

the activities of ornithine decarboxylase (25) and nuclear phosphokinase (1,2). During replication, activities of thymidine kinase (23) and superhelical DNA nicking-closing enzyme (11) are increased. Following DNA replication there is a reduction in the activity of receptor-inactivating factors (29) and secretory acid phosphatase is induced (22, 26). The sequence of response appears to depend in part upon the dose of androgen (22). To what extent androgen receptors might be involved will be considered next.

2. ANDROGEN RECEPTOR DYNAMICS

The method of choice to clarify the relationship between androgen receptors and prostatic responses might be one furnishing a direct measurement of the concentration of cytoplasmic and nuclear receptors while the sensitivity of the cell to androgen is changing. Using this rationale, Van Doorn et al. (29) assayed the quantity of androgen receptors in the regenerating prostate at regular intervals over a 14-day period of growth. Beginning seven days after orchidectomy, rats were treated with daily injections of dihydrotestosterone to stimulate DNA synthesis and cell proliferation and restore the prostate to its normal size. The principal findings can be summarized as follows: Within 12 hours of the first injection, the number of molecules of nuclear receptor increases from 0 to 5000 per cell and continues to increase to a maximum of 12,000 per cell at two days. The value is maintained for the next three days and then falls to 9000 per cell by day seven of treatment. There is a further gradual decline to about 8000 per cell over the remaining period of seven days. During the same time-course of tissue regeneration, the apparent number of cytoplasmic receptors remains small and constant.

The flux in the amount of nuclear receptor is not in phase with the changes in rate of DNA synthesis. DNA synthesis is initiated well after the number of nuclear receptors at 9000 per cell is almost at a maximum. More significantly, the negative-feedback inhibition of DNA synthesis observed between days three and four of treatment occurs in the presence of a constant amount of nuclear receptor. On the basis of these two observations, Van Doorn et al. conclude that any effect of nuclear receptor on DNA synthesis must be indirect, and that other factors besides nuclear receptor are probably responsible for switching DNA synthesis on and off.

The decline in the number of nuclear receptors between days 5 and 14 of treatment parallels the decrease in the rate of DNA synthesis, probably because the synthesis of nuclear receptor is confined to dividing cells. Between days two and five of treatment, 50-60% of the total cell population of the prostate is progressing through the cell cycle at all times (17). In preparing for division, these cells apparently double their complement of nuclear receptor, giving rise to the marked elevation in the average number from 8000 per cell to 12,000 per cell. The dependence of receptor synthesis de novo on cell proliferation is further demonstrated by a distinct parallelism between the number of nuclear receptors per prostate and the number of cells per prostate. Also, on day five of treatment when cell proliferation is sharply curtailed by the negative-feedback effect, the net synthesis of nuclear receptor becomes negligible.

Since the rate of DNA synthesis in the regenerating prostate is proportional to the number of cells entering the S-phase (15), Van Doorn et al. (29) assumed that there should be a correlation between the rate of DNA synthesis and the formation of nuclear receptor. The results of their experiments show that both DNA synthesis and nuclear receptor formation increase as a function of dose of dihydrotestosterone, and maximal stimulation in each case is achieved at a dose of about 400 μg per 100 g body weight. These results indicate clearly that synthesis of nuclear receptor is coupled to cell proliferation and that the average number of receptors per cell in a given cell population is strongly influenced by the growth fraction.

3. POTENTIAL CORRELATIONS

In the regenerating prostate, the appearance of receptors in the nucleus precedes the initiation of DNA synthesis and cell proliferation by several hours. Because the concentration of cytoplasmic receptor does not exceed 3000 molecules per cell (Table 1), the appearance of nuclear receptor can be accounted for by the synthesis de novo of receptor protein, as demonstrated by two lines of evidence. First, the average number of nuclear receptors is proportional to the growth fraction in the regenerating prostate, signifying that nuclear receptor is synthesized during the proliferative response at the beginning of the G1 phase of the cell cycle; this deduction is consistent with the observed lag period between the appearance of receptor in the nucleus and the onset of DNA synthesis. Second, since the number of nuclear receptors per prostate parallels the number of cells per prostate, the synthesis of nuclear receptor must proceed during cell proliferation. This conclusion is also confirmed by the finding that the synthesis of nuclear receptor and the rate of DNA synthesis in regenerating prostate are both dependent on dose of dihydrotestosterone. Under these conditions of cell replication, the cytoplasmic synthesis of nuclear receptor is not in synchrony with either the onset or shutdown of DNA synthesis. Hence, it is extremely unlikely that nuclear receptor contributes directly to the initiation of DNA synthesis or to its cessation. A more general correlation between receptor synthesis and cell proliferation is nevertheless obvious.

D. DNA CONTENT AND ANDROGEN RECEPTORS IN HUMAN PROSTATE

Both benign hyperplasia and carcinoma of the human prostate are pathological conditions in which the fraction of cells undergoing mitotic division is probably greater than in normal prostate. Furthermore, it is reasonable to expect that any increase in the growth fraction might be associated with a higher concentration of nuclear androgen receptor. Two observations based on the data presented in Table 2 lend support to this line of thinking.

TABLE 2. DNA content and androgen receptors in human prostate

Tissue	Concentration of nuclear receptor[a]		
	pg DNA / nucleus	molecules / nucleus	fmoles / mg DNA
normal	[b]14.9 ± 1.7 (4)	1000 ± 200 (5)	110
hyperplasia	18.3 ± 1.6 (12)	1400 ± 300 (11)	130
carcinoma	28.5 ± 3.0 (6)	1900 ± 200 (5)	110

[a]Condensed from reference 19 and N. Bruchovsky, unpublished data.

[b]Mean ± S.E. for number of experiment in parentheses.

Firstly, the nucleus of the cancerous cell on the average contains almost twice as much DNA as the nucleus of the normal cell. Secondly, the concentration of nuclear receptor is directly proportional to DNA content. Thus, the correlation between DNA synthesis and the formation of receptor in rat ventral prostate evidently holds, in a general way, for human prostate as well.

E. CONCLUSIONS

On the basis of the information reviewed above, the following conclusions seem justified.

It is virtually impossible to stimulate DNA synthesis and cell proliferation in the presence of a normal number of receptors per cell and a normal number of cells per gland. A reduction in the total number of receptors per cell precedes and accompanies the autophagic involution of prostatic tissue induced by orchidectomy. The regressed prostate contains only a small number of androgen receptors per cell and is sensitive to androgenic stimulation. In regenerating prostate, the synthesis of nuclear androgen receptor commences several hours before the onset of DNA synthesis and cell proliferation, apparently because receptor is synthesized in early GI phase. Receptor synthesis is closely coupled to cell proliferation, but whether receptor is directly involved in the control of DNA replication is uncertain. Lastly, the concentration of nuclear receptor in well-differentiated prostatic carcinoma appears to be elevated in proportion to the DNA content of the nucleus; this change is consistent with the observed relationship between the synthesis of receptor and cell proliferation.

REFERENCES

1. Ahmed, K. and Ishida, H.: Effect of testosterone on nuclear phosphoproteins of rat ventral prostate. Molec. Pharmacol. 7, 323-327, 1971.
2. Ahmed, K. and Wilson, M. J.: Chromatin-associated protein phosphokinases of rat ventral prostate. Characteristics and effects of androgenic status. J. Biol. Chem. 250, 2370-2375, 1975.
3. Baulieu, E-E., Atger, M., Best-Belpomme, M., Corvol, P., Milgrom, E., Robel, P., Rochefort, H. and De Catalongne, D.: Steroid hormone receptors. Vitamin. Horm. 33, 649-736, 1975.
4. Blondeau, J. P., Corpechot, C., LeGoascogne, C., Baulieu, E-E. and Robel, P.: Androgen receptors in the rat ventral prostate and their hormonal control. Vitamin. Horm. 33, 319-345, 1975.
5. Bruchovsky, N. and Craven, S.: Prostatic involution: effect on androgen receptors and intracellular androgen transport. Biochem. Biophys. Res. Comm. 62, 837-843, 1975.

6. Bruchovsky, N., Lesser, B., Van Doorn, E. and Craven, S.: Hormonal effects on cell proliferation in rat prostate. <u>Vitamin. Horm.</u> <u>33</u>, 61-102, 1975.

7. Bruchovsky, N., Rennie, P. S. and Vanson, A.: Studies on the regulation of the concentration of androgens and androgen receptors in nuclei of prostatic cells. <u>Biochim. Biophys. Acta</u>, <u>394</u>, 248-266, 1975.

8. Callaway, T., Bruchovsky, N. and Rennie, P. S.: Effects of antiandrogenic compounds on translocation of prostatic androgen receptor. Endoctrine Society (U.S.A.) Program and Abstracts 60th Annual Meeting, p. 298, 1978.

9. Coffey, D. S., Shimazaki, J. and Williams-Ashman, H. G.: Polymerization of deoxyribonucleotides in relation to androgen-induced prostatic growth. <u>Arch. Biochem. Biophys.</u> <u>124</u>, 184-198, 1968.

10. Coyotupa, J., Parlow, A. F. and Kovacic, N.: Serum testosterone and dihydrotestosterone levels following orchidectomy in the adult rat. <u>Endocrinology</u> <u>92</u>, 1579-1581, 1973.

11. Filipenko, J. D.: Androgen effects on NC enzyme and chromatin structure in rat ventral prostate. M.Sc. thesis, University of Alberta, Canada, p. 50, 1978.

12. Grover, P. K. and Odell, W. D.: Correlation of <u>in vivo</u> and <u>in vitro</u> activities of some naturally occurring androgens using a radioreceptor assay for 5α-dihydrotestosterone with rat prostate cytosol receptor protein. <u>J. Steroid Biochem.</u> <u>6</u>, 1373-1379, 1975.

13. Jung, I. and Baulieu, E-E.: Neo-nuclear androgen receptor in rat ventral prostate. <u>Biochimie</u>, 53, 807-817, 1971.

14. King, R. J. B. and Mainwaring, W. I. P.: Steroid cell interactions. University Park Press, Baltimore, 41-101, 1974.

15. Lesser, B. and Bruchovsky, N.: The effects of testosterone, 5α-dihydrotestosterone and adenosine 3', 5'-monophosphate on cell proliferation and differentiation in rat prostate. <u>Biochim. Biophys. Acta</u> <u>308</u>, 426-437, 1973.

16. Lesser, B. and Bruchovsky, N.: Effect of duration of the period after castration on the response of the rat ventral prostate to androgens. <u>Biochem. J.</u> <u>149</u>, 429-431, 1974.

17. Lesser, B. and Bruchovsky, N.: The effects of 5α-dihydrotestosterone on the kinetics of cell proliferation in rat prostate. <u>Biochem. J.</u> <u>142</u>, 483-489, 1974.

18. Liao, S.: Cellular receptors and mechanisms of action of steroid hormones. <u>Int. Rev. Cytol.</u> <u>41</u>, 87-172, 1975.

19. Lieskovsky, G. and Bruchovsky, N.: Assay of androgen receptor in human prostate. <u>J. Urology</u>, 1978, in press.

20. Mainwaring, W. I. P. and Mangan, F. R.: A study of the androgen receptors in a variety of androgen-sensitive tissues. J. Endocrinol. <u>59</u>, 121-139, 1973.

21. Mainwaring, W. I. P.: The mechanism of action of androgens. Springer Verlag, New York, 1977.

22. Rennie, P. S., Bruchovsky, N. and Hook, S. L.: Androgenic regulation of a tissue specific isoenzyme of acid phosphatase in rat ventral prostate. <u>J. Steroid Biochem.</u> <u>9</u>, 585-593, 1978.

23. Rennie, P. S., Symes, E. K. and Mainwaring, W. I. P.: The androgenic regulation of the activities of enzymes engaged in the synthesis of deoxyribonucleic acid in rat ventral prostate gland. <u>Biochem. J.</u> <u>152</u>, 1-16, 1975.

24. Sullivan, J. N. and Strott, C. A.: Evidence for an androgen-independent mechanism regulating the levels of receptor in target tissue. <u>J. Biol. Chem.</u> <u>248</u>, 3202-3208, 1973.

143

25. Takyi, E. E. K., Fuller, D. J. M., Donaldson, L. J. and Thomas, G. H.:
    Deoxyribonucleic acid and polyamine synthesis in rat ventral prostate.
    Effects of age of the intact rat and androgen stimulation of the
    castrated rat with testosterone, 5α-dihydrotestosterone and 5α-
    androstane-3β,17β-diol. Biochem. J. 162, 87-97, 1977.
26. Tenniswood, M. P., Abrahams, P. P., Bird, C. E. and Clark, A. F.:
    Effects of castration and androgen replacement on acid phosphatase
    activity in the adult rat prostate gland. J. Endocrinol., 77, 301-
    308, 1978.
27. Tymoczko, J. L., Liang, T. and Liao, S.: Androgen receptor
    interactions in target cells: biochemical evaluation, in "Receptors
    and Hormone Action", vol. II (B. W. O'Malley and L. Birnbaumer, eds.)
    Academic Press, New York, 121-156, 1978.
28. Van Doorn, E. and Bruchovsky, N.: Mechanisms of replenishment of
    nuclear androgen receptor in rat ventral prostate. Biochem. J. 174,
    9-16, 1978.
29. Van Doorn, E., Craven, S. and Bruchovsky, N.: The relationship
    between androgen receptors and the hormonally controlled response of
    rat ventral prostate. Biochem. J. 160, 11-21, 1976.
30. Williams-Ashman, H. G. and Reddi, A. H.: Actions of vertebrate sex
    hormones. Ann. Rev. Physiol. 33, 31-82, 1971.

THE APPLICATION OF CELL CULTURE TECHNIQUES TO HUMAN PROSTATIC CARCINOMA*

CHAPTER X

Introduction

Theoretically, cell-culture techniques should be particularly useful for
the study of human tumors. These techniques offer many potential advantages,
for example: 1) the milieu surrounding the cells can be precisely defined;
2) growth can be easily monitored by simple cell counts; 3) known and unknown
influences of host factors can be studied; 4) cultures can be endocrinologi-
cally manipulated; 5) culture can be utilized as a source of tumor antigens;
and 6) stromal-epithelial cell interactions can be studied since theoretically
epithelial cells can be grown with or without adding stroma or stromal factors.
Although still valid, these optimistic potential considerations have been
found to have severe limitations in the practical experience of a large number
of researchers in this field. Interest in this area has been steadily increasing since the initial report in 1917 by Burrows, Burns, and Suzuki (5)
who first reported the growing of a monolayer of cells from an explant of
human prostatic adenocarcinoma.

The further development of cell culture of prostatic tissues is in many respects characteristic of the state of achievement of the application of in
vitro techniques to other human tumors. Few advancements have been made in
cell culture studies of human neoplasia which are not paralleled by studies
of human prostatic carcinoma. In this respect a review of this subject is
also characteristic for the situation of cell culture of human malignancy
in general.

At the time of this review although there has been an intense amount of effect
(3,20,24,41,42,43,48,52,54,63) in the area of cell culture of human prostatic
adenocarcinoma, there has been little convincing data obtained. This tends
to induce a rather pessimistic view on the future significance of this type
of research. However, there are some recent advances which clearly indicate
future directions for research of this type which should be followed with
strong effort and support.

Technical considerations

Applicable standard cell-culture techniques include those of short term monolayer or suspension cultures have been achieved. Long term strains have been
found to grow best in monolayer, long term suspension cultures have not been
reported to be established.

*Fritz H. Schroeder, and K. Oishi, Institute of Urology, Erasmus University,
Rotterdam. H. U. Schweikert, Medizinische Poliklinik, University of Bonn.

Short term cultures have been established in various media by the use of the explant technique. Fresh tissue is minced with scissors or crossed scalpels and suspended in medium under standard tissue culture conditions.

Mailing of operative specimens in medium with delays up to 48 hours from removal of tissue and initiation of primary cultures does not seem to negatively influence later growth in monolayer in our own experience. Initiation of cultures from autopsy specimens has also been successful (51). Tissue culture plastic ware is used by all investigators. Our own experience with the use of regular bacterial plastic dishes was discouraging. Humidified CO_2 incubators are generally used but do not seem to be essential (57).

Media used include serum clots (5,41), chicken embryo extracts and fowl serum (63), Eagles minimal essential medium (MEM) (24), Hank's solution plus serum (54), Hams F10 (48), basal medium Eagle (BME) (3), F12K (20), RPMI 1640 and Hams F12 (42), or Dulbecco's modified Eagles's (43). A clear advantage of one medium over another has not been documented. It was our impression that Ham's F10 was superior to BME and MEM. No reports are available on initiation of primary cultures in medium without serum. A recent report suggests that combinations of hormones may be suitable to replace serum in tissue culture media (13). Frequent medium changes do not seem to be important for the initiation of primary cultures. Fetal calf serum (FCS) and/or horse serum were used at various concentrations.

Subcultures of primary cultures have been obtained by most investigators by the use of proteolytic enzymes such as trypsin, viokase and collagenase in calcium and magnesium free buffer solutions with or without versene. Old primary cultures require long incubation times with the enzymes.

Cell cultures have more recently been initiated by seeding of cells obtained from mechanical (55) or proteolytic disruption of tissue (53). This technique, if successful, offers the advantage of a quantitative primary culture allowing the study of plating efficiency. In our own hands unfortunately this technique is only occasionally successful. Cells very infrequently stick to the bottom of the culture vessel.

One of the difficult problems associated with short term monolayer cultures of prostatic tissues lies in the presence of several different cell types in the primary outgrowth and the subcultures. Some of these cell types, epithelial-like cells and fibroblastic cells can be identified microscopically.

In subcultures usually the epithelial cells are overgrown by the faster growing

fibroblasts and tend to disappear. Some authors have attempted to suppress
this process based on the idea that the epithelial-like cells may be the
desired cells for study of normal and cancerous prostatic tissue. Selective
killing of fibroblasts as presumably autonomous, hormone independent cells
by the use of selective radio-sensitization with 5-BUdR, fractioned subcultur-
ing (48), use of selective properties of horse serum for growth of epithelial
cells (47,58), the use of explants kept in organ culture for some time to
initiate primary cultures (61) or the use of collagenase for tissue preparation
(43) has been unreliable in enriching cultures with epithelial cells. A reproducible technique which establishes pure short term epithelial cultures
has not yet been described.

Franks (12) described a technique for the mechanical separation of stroma
and epithelium by squeezing fragments of benign prostatic hyperplasia. He
was never able to grow epithelium obtained by this technique in culture and
concluded that stroma was necessary for growth of prostatic epithelial cells.
This technique and the techniques of enzymatic dissociation of prostatic tissue
(40) or the combination of both (30) can be used to obtain almost pure epithelium or stromal cells. Little work has been done to define the usefulness
of these cell suspensions as suspension cultures. This modality seems to
be very promising and will be discussed later more extensively.

Long term cell-lines from prostatic tissue are rare. At present, one cell
line from benign prostatic hyperplasia (11) and 4 permanent lines grown from
prostatic carcinoma tissue, have been reported (4,18,25,32,51). Some of these
lines are possibly the results of contamination of primary- or subcultures
with HeLa cells. A review of the original papers on these cell-lines reveals
no common technical features which may allow reproduction of successful cultivation of long term lines. The techniques used for subcultivation of these
lines are routine tissue culture techniques. Long term lines allow cloning,
kinetic studies in vitro and after heterotransplantation, genetic studies,
immunological studies and mass production of cells for biochemical purposes.
Such research has been carried out and will be discussed later.

Characterization of prostatic cells
Information obtained in cell-culture studies of human tumors has oncological
value only if it reflects the characteristics of the tumor in vivo. Cells
growing in cultures from such tumors must therefore be characterized and
their similarity with the tumor cell itself or other cells associated with
it must be established. After demonstrating that features known to be charac-

147

teristic for a given tumor in vivo have been identified in culture, it may then be safe to assume that observations made in culture do reflect the in vivo behaviour of the tumor.

In the case of prostatic carcinoma a number of parameters are available which may be used in the identification and characterization of cells growing in vitro. Some are valid, some others are misleading.

The cells which may potentially grow from explants of native prostatic carcinoma tissue include stromal elements such as smooth muscle, fibroblasts, metastatic prostatic epithelial cells and prostatic carcinoma cells. These four cell types have in fact been identified. Growth of other cell types has not been excluded.

Morphology

Morphology by light microscopy is notoriously misleading in identifying cells in culture. Electron microscopy has been carried out and has confirmed the epithelial character of the epithelial-like cells (4,59). However, marked differences were found when the cells were compared to prostatic epithelium in vivo. Another step in the morphological characterization of epithelial-like cells was made by histological examination of the prostatic tissue explants after various time in culture. It could be shown that the explants become epithelialized by flat epithelium originating from metaplastic benign prostatic epithelium, and not by the malignant fraction of the explants (61). Time course histological examination of explants over 3 weeks has shown that this epithelialization results by proliferation of the basal acinar epithelial layer and of ductal epithelium. Epithelialization of the explant surface also coincides in time with outgrowth of cells in monolayer. This suggests that the epithelial-like cells seen in primary cultures are in fact derived from benign epithelium (45). In a study of 18 prostatic carcinomas in a similar way proliferation of the carcinomatous part was never seen in more than 1500 histological slides in our laboratory (14). This suggested to us that prostatic cancer cells will not grow under standard culture conditions used. Two reports in the literature seem to prove successful plating of prostatic cancer cells from a lymph node metastasis (55) and from a brain metastasis (52). In the first instance formalin inhibition of acid phosphatase was used to prove the prostatic origin of the metastatic cells, in the second case cultures have led to a permanent line with some prostatic characteristics (DU 145).

Genetic studies

Genetic studies have been carried out on aspiration biopsies from metastatic carcinoma of the prostate. Cells were found to be hypotriploid and interestingly a y-chromosome could not be identified in native cells from bone marrow (35). Tavares found in a retrospective histocytophotometric study diploidy and tetraploidy as well as quadroploidy and hexaploidy (56) in prostatic carcinoma cells in histological specimens.

In short term cell-cultures chromosomal counts were carried out by Jellinghaus (16) on three prostatic carcinomas. Uniformly diploidy was found just as in primary cultures of prostatic hyperplasia. These studies again confirmed to us that prostatic cancer cells probably do not grow in primary cultures.

Most available permanent lines (11,32,51) have been studied extensively with genetic techniques. All lines are hypotriploid with aneuploid subpopulations. Marker chromosomes have been described. The line EB 33 does not have a y-chromosome; a y-chromosome was lost from early to later passages of the MA160 line. In some of the lines (EB 33 and MA160) HeLa marker chromosomes have been identified (27,28) suggesting that these lines may be HeLa derivatives. This suspicion is contradicted by a number of findings characterizing both lines as non-HeLa but of possible prostatic origin (21,44,46,60). These findings will be discussed later.

Biochemical parameters

Biochemical parameters have been used for the identification of prostatic epithelial cells in culture. It has long been known that prostatic epithelium contains large amounts of acid phosphatase and that only small amounts of this enzyme are present in stroma. Histochemical techniques have been used by almost all workers in the field to differentiate epithelial-like cells and fibroblasts. Quantitative studies of predominantly epithelial and predominantly fibroblastic cultures have shown that epithelial cultures contain about 10 times more acid phosphatase (48). Hormonal effects on acid phosphatase in cultured cells from prostatic tumors have been studied by several investigators (2,47). Studies from our laboratory (2) suggest that extraction of steroid hormones from the serum used in tissue culture media reduces acid phosphatase in cells in primary cultures and in cells of the cell line EB 33. Induction of the enzyme by androgens or other steroids in vitro has however never been proven quantitatively. Immunoflorescence techniques which have recently become available (10,17,38) are powerful tools in identifying prostatic acid phosphatase. The use of phosphorylcholine as a histochemical

149

substrate is probably sufficient specific if no cells of other organs than prostate are present in cultures (44). Comparison of the immunofluorescence and phosphorylcholine technique has confirmed this and led to the exclusive use of phosphorylcholine for identification purposes in our laboratory (30).

Other enzymes including β-glucuronidase (29) and lactic dehydrogenase (50) have been used to identify prostatic epithelium. Other chemical and potential immunological markers are zinc, the polyamines (spermine and spermidine) and enzymes of the steroid metabolism. Recently carcino-embryonic antigen (CEA) has been shown to be a marker for prostatic epithelium (62).

Androgen dependency

Since _in vivo_ prostatic tissue is androgen dependent, the androgen sensitivity of prostatic cells in primary culture has been examined. The fact that primary epithelial cultures can be initiated in medium from which steroids had been extracted with charcoal or methylene chloride was a discouraging experience (47). Brehmer and co-workers (3) have shown that plating efficiency of mixed cell populations from benign prostatic hyperplasia is decreased with testosterone concentrations increasing from 1.0 - 10.0 µg/ml medium. The plating efficiency of cells from two prostatic carcinomas remained unaffected under the same conditions. Testosterone was in these experiments found to act synergistically to diethylstilbestrol (DES). The interpretation of these results is difficult. Similar observations made by Lasnitzki (21) with MA160 cells suggest that the effect of testosterone at these pharmacological doses may be toxic.

Attempts to induce androgen stimulated increase in the cell number in primary cultures has also failed. The pattern of growth in these mixed cell populations is unpredictable, irregular, and cannot be shown to be androgen sensitive.

Kinetic studies

Kinetic techniques based on cell counts are easily applicable to permanent cell lines. The influence of hormonal manipulations on growth can easily be studied in these lines. Such studies have been carried out but will be discussed later (31). Cells from permanent lines can be heterotransplanted into nude mice; their kinetics can be studied in vivo (33,46). Cloning by single cell plating for selection of functional sublines is a powerful tool which can also be applied to permanent lines. This has been carried out for the EB 33 line by Okada and Laudenbach (31).

Little attention has been given to the fibroblastic cells growing out of

150

prostatic explants. It is likely that these cells represent stromal elements, but it is not precisely known which ones. As will be shown later, fibroblast cultures of prostatic tumors present a unique opportunity to study stromal properties, i.e. testosterone metabolism.

Results in short term cultures

In reviewing the data available from the literature on short term monolayer culture of prostatic epithelial and carcinoma cells, one has to make the disappointing statement that no major contribution has been made which has any impact on better understanding of pathogenesis, host-tumor relationship or treatment of this tumor. This probably means that studies of epithelial cells in short term cultures should be abandoned until better techniques have become available. Some advance in this direction can possibly be seen in the preliminary attempts of Kaighn to isolate growth factors from serum and epidermis (19).

Recently, the possibility that cultures overgrown by fibroblasts (which were discarded for years) might be used to study stromal properties of prostatic tumors was investigated in our laboratory in cooperation with the Medizinische Poliklinik of the University of Bonn. The metabolism of ^{3}H-testosterone added to cultures of fibroblasts from 3 benign prostatic hyperplasias, 3 prostatic carcinomas and 2 non-genital skin specimens was studied (49). Characteristic differences were found in time course experiments. Some of the results are shown in Fig. 1 A-C. Testosterone was much more rapidly metabolized by fibroblasts from BPH, about 90% had disappeared after 2 hours. A peak of androstenedione after 2 hours suggests a high activity of 17 β-steroid dehydrogenase. After 24 hours DHT and the androsterones are the predominant metabolites. Fibroblasts from all three carcinomas metabolize testosterone at a much slower rate but still faster than those from non-genital skin (fig. 1, B-C). These findings compare favourably with similar results found in organ culture (22,23) of BPH and in the study of stromal and epithelial fractions obtained by tissue dissociation (8,30). The latter studies by Cowan suggest that testosterone metabolism takes place almost exclusively in the stroma. The stroma could therefore have the function of metabolizing steroids into metabolites needed by the prostatic epithelium. This is speculation, but the available facts clearly indicate the direction of future efforts. Also, the different steroid metabolism found in fresh preparations of epithelial cells from prostatic adenoma is a finding which allows keen speculation and needs further investigation.

Figure 1.

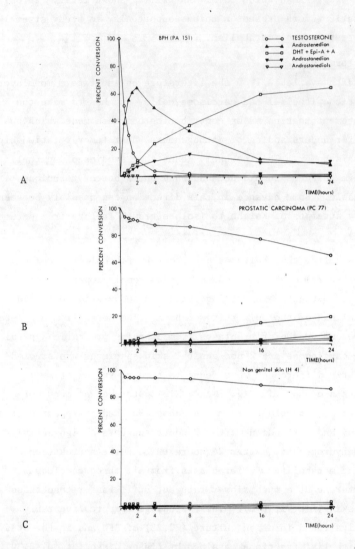

Testosterone metabolism in fibroblasts grown from BPH, prostatic carcinoma and non-genital skin.

Unfortunately it remains impossible to obtain similarly large amounts of
epithelial cells from BPH even less so from carcinoma of the prostate with
culture techniques. For this reason, tissue dissociation by mechanical and
enzymatic techniques with subsequent application of cell separation techniques
should be further evaluated. Oishi and Romijn in Rotterdam were successful
in obtaining reproducibly 20 x 10^6 epithelial cells per gram of BPH tissue.
80-90% of these cells are acid phosphatase positive with histochemical stain-
ing using phosphorylcholine as substrate. Viability after tissue dissociation
is above 90% and remains so for 10 days (22) when cells are kept in suspension
culture under standard conditions. These techniques do allow separate studies
of epithelial and stroma cells from prostatic tumors especially when lymphnode
specimens containing metastases are included.

Long term cell-lines

A total of five long term cell-lines developed from primary cultures of human
prostatic tissue have been reported (11,18,25,32,51). One, the line MA160
(11) was derived from benign prostatic hyperplasia and will therefore be
left out of discussion. A recent review of all facts known about the MA160
cells has been published by Webber and suggests that they have little in
common with human BPH and may be the result of HeLa contamination (60).

The line HPC 36 was reported by Lubaroff in 1977 (25). Only very preliminary
attempts at characterization have been made on this line. The cells have
an epithelial appearance but are morphologically non-homogeneous. Acid
phosphatase has been demonstrated with non-specific techniques. The line is
transplantable in "nude" mice and forms solid tumors.

The line DU145 was developed from a brain metastasis of a solid prostatic
carcinoma and was reported by STONE and co-workers in 1978 (51). Its origin
from a metastasis makes it more likely to be derived from prostatic carcinoma
cells. The cells grow in soft agar suspension and have been in culture con-
tinuously for more than 2 years at the time of publication. The doubling
time was found to be 34 hours and has remained constant. Electron/microscopical
studies have revealed a striking similarity of the cultured cells with the
original tumor. The cells contain very little formaline   resistant acid
phosphatase as did the tumor of origin. Karyotypic analysis has revealed
a y-chromosome. The modal chromosome number is 64; three marker chromosomes
were identified. Hormone dependence of growth could not be shown. The line
grows in "nude" mice and forms solid tumors. The presence of a y-chromosome
precludes the possibility of HeLa origin of this line. However, the properties

described have little in common with clinical prostatic carcinoma.

It is very doubtful that this line will contribute more to the understanding of prostate cancer than any of the other lines. The findings obtained with DU 145 are most discouraging and cast doubt on the usefulness of long term prostatic carcinoma cell lines in the research concerning this tumor.

The line PC 1 reported by Kaighn in 1978 has not been characterized sufficiently to be discussed further (18). It is apparently kept in frozen stock and used for experiments studying the growth requirements of prostatic cells.

The cell-line EB 33 grown from a human prostatic adenocarcinoma has been studied most extensively (32). It will therefore be used to demonstrate what can be done in terms of characterization of a permanent line. The most pertinent results obtained will be discussed.

Morphology

Morphologically EB 33 cells are polygonal in shape and have varying numbers of large nucleoli. The cells appearance is epithelial with the nucleus being located in the centre of the cells. The polarity of the prostatic epithelial cell is lost. There is no evidence of secretion. EB 33 cells appear to be very similar to prostatic epithelial cells growing in primary cultures of human adenomas and carcinomas.

The epithelial character of EB 33 cells is confirmed by electron microscopy. Pseudovilli are present at the margins of cells. Cytoplasmic organelles can be identified, but there is again no evidence of secretory activity. No comprehensive EM studies of EB 33 cells have been done. They have not yet been compared to HeLa cells, epithelial cells from primary cultures, or any possible prostatic cells of origin (32).

The original tumor was a moderately differentiated carcinoma with two different architectural patterns. Adenocarcinoma was prevalent, but solid carcinoma in cords and sheets was also found. When EB 33 cells were transplanted into "nude" mice subcutaneously, fast growing, solid tumors resulted. Histologically these tumors are solid carcinomas with large, anaplastic nuclei and many mitoses. There is no similarity to the tissue of origin (33).

The morphological picture of these heterotransplants does not contribute to the characterization of EB 33 cells as prostatic carcinoma cells. The histological picture reflects alterations acquired in vitro which may be described by the term "malignant transformation in vitro".

Biochemical characterization

Acid phosphatase has been demonstrated in EB 33 cells by histochemical, eletron microscopical, biochemical and immunochemical methods (32,38,39).

An attempt to show androgen dependence of acid phosphatase by incubation of EB 33 cells in androgen-free and androgen enriched culture medium did reveal very suggestive, but non-significant results. Histochemical techniques proved to be inadequate for this study. It became evident however, that HeLa cells contain much less acid phosphatase. They served as a negative control. This subject warrants another study with more adequate biochemical or immunological techniques.

Pontes, Rose and co-workers (38,39) have shown the presence of human prostatic acid phosphatase in EB 33 cells by indirect immunofluorescence. After extensive testing with non-related tissues these authors feel that their antibody is specific for prostatic acid phosphatase. Their findings present a strong argument for the prostatic origin of the EB 33 cell line. Recently the metabolism of testosterone was studied in EB 33 cells and was found to be identical with fibroblasts from non-genital skin (15).

Endocrinological characterization and growth kinetics

As a first step EB 33 cells were grown in androgen-free culture medium (H) and in the full media containing 1.0 µg of testosterone (T) (H+T) or 5α-dihydrotestosterone (DHT) (H+DHT) per ml of medium. Androgen-free media was prepared after extraction of steroids from the sera with activated charcoal (AC) and/or dichloromethane (DCM). This was the subject of a previous report (32). No difference in growth was seen in both media.

Subsequently the possiblity was investigated that the EB 33 line might be a heterogeneous mixture of autonomous and androgen-dependent cells. To identify a possible hormone dependent subpopulation, 111 clonal cell lines were established by single cell plating. 23 clones revealed a suppression of growth of more than 50% in androgen-free media. Complete growth curves of the most sensitive clones were obtained by plotting averages of four daily cell counts on the ordinate against time on the abscissa. With this technique the significant depression of growth in vitro by extraction of steroids from the culture media was confirmed. However, the addition of T or DHT to the extracted media only compensates for a small part of the growth suppression obtained (Fig. 2) (31).

In order to obtain a better statistical evaluation and to rule out non-specific

Figure 2.

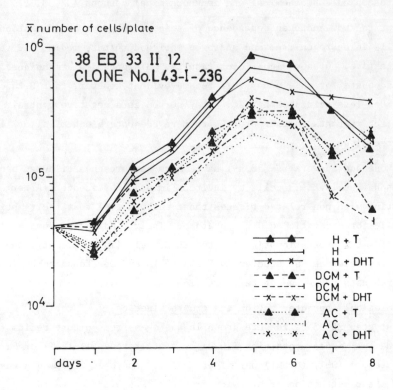

Growth of cloned EB 33 cells in androgen-free and androgen-enriched media. Clone used for experiment (No. L43-I-236) was found to require androgen for maximal growth.

    H = Normal non-extract media
    DCM = dichloromethane extracted media
    AC = activated charcoal extracted media

effects of extracted media, cloned and uncloned EB 33 cells were transplanted into castrated "nude" mice which were or were not injected with DHT. The daily measurement of the resulting tumors over a 40 day period again produced growth curves. HeLa cell transplants served as controls. Major differences were found between HeLa cells and EB 33 clones. HeLa cells grow faster initially, but their exponential phase of growth is about 50% shorter. These findings are statistically highly significant. Uncloned EB 33 cells (84 EB 33) and HeLa cells show no difference of growth in castrated mice with or without injections of 1.0 μg of DHT/gram of body weight. Under similar conditions sensitive clones of the EB 33 line (L 108 EB 33) grew significantly faster with DHT substitution than without. The slope of the regression lines is significantly different at $p \leq 0.01$. DHT stimulates the growth of some clones of EB 33 cells in "nude" mice (Fig. 3)(46).

Genetics

Genetic studies of EB 33 cells were carried out by three different laboratories. They revealed the human origin of the Eb 33 line (16). Modal chromosome numbers vary in low and high passages but are usually hypotriploid. Hypotriploidy is common in human carcinomas and was also found in human prostatic carcinomas (35,56). An isochromosome 17 may be a marker for prostatic carcinoma (35). EB 33 has not been screened for this.

No y-chromosome was detected by two independent investigators using the quinacrine orange and Giemsa banding techniques (9,46). The lack of a y-chromosome in EB 33 cells is not a disturbing finding. Several reports suggest that the loss of a y-chromosome is a common event in cell lines derived from male donors (36,37) and may also depend on age. Also, in the only genetic analysis of prostatic carcinoma cells obtained directly by aspiration from bony metastases no y-chromosome was found (35). The lack of y-chromosomes may be characteristic for prostatic carcinoma.

Dr. Nelson-Rees has identified in EB 33 cells of passage 31 and 62 four marker chromosomes which are considered to be characteristic for HeLa cells. Subsequently he has classified the EB 33 line as a HeLa derivative (26). Fogh has recently confirmed his findings (9). This classification is also based on the lack of a y-chromosome and on the presence of the mobility pattern A of glucose 6-phosphate dehydrogenase. Since HeLa cells are maintained in the laboratory where EB 33 cells were originated, the possiblity of cross-contamination cannot be excluded. However, it is felt that the functional parameters discussed earlier which established the identity of the EB 33 cell

157

Figure 3.

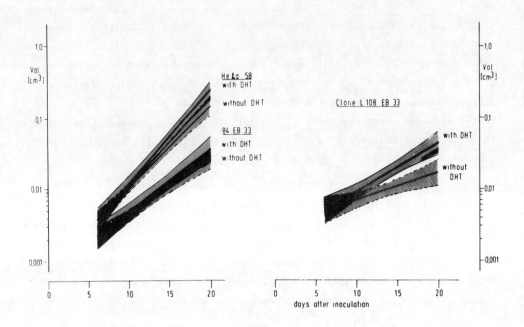

Growth kinetics of tumors resulting from EB 33 clonal transplants into castrated "nude" mice with and without injection of DHT. Control: HeLa cells.
DHT injection 1μg/gram body weight/day.

with the tissue of origin rank much higher than these genetic findings.
Experience with chromosomal alterations in cell culture appears to be too
limited to establish reliable markers. The possibility that the rearrange-
ments of chromosomes found in HeLa cells are common in permanent lines or
may even represent a pre-requisite for permanent growth has not been sufficiently excluded.

Immunological characterization

The immunological findings obtained with EB 33 cells are the subject of
several reports from this laboratory (1,34). However, it should be mentioned
here that rabbit anti-EB 33 antibodies still kill EB 33 cells after absorption
with HeLa cells. Preliminary experiments have shown that lymphocytes from
some prostatic cancer patients kill EB 33 cells. Only reduced killing was
found with the lymphocytes of numerous unrelated sex and age matched control
persons. These findings suggest that EB 33 cells carry membrane antigens
that differ from HeLa cells and may be present in prostatic cancer.

In conclusion

The morphological and biochemical parameters thus far studied are either
incomplete or contribute little to the overall characterization of the EB 33
line.

Endocrinological parameters, cell and tumor kinetics, and immunological data
present evidence that EB 33 cells indeed originated from prostatic epithelium.
The fact that the enhancement of growth with testosterone or dihydrotestosterone alone does not produce a very pronounced effect in vitro, is not at
all disturbing. Hormonal dependence of prostatic epithelium is expected to
be a much more complex process.

Other lines of research

Some other new directions of research should at least be mentioned in this
review. Heidelberger and his associates have made a strong effort to induce
growth of rat prostatic cells in culture by using methylcholanthrene to obtain
growth by transformation of cells. Permanent fibroblast lines have resulted
which produced only fibrosarcomas when transplanted back into the animals
of origin (7).

Prostatic carcinomas of laboratory animals such as the Dunning (R-3327) tumor
or the spontaneous tumor found in old Wistar rats kept under germ-free conditions (6) may be ideal models to explore the role cell culture can indeed
play in the exploration of prostatic tumors.

Summary and future aspects

On the whole, attempts to use tissue culture techniques in research related to prostatic cancer have been disappointing. They have contributed minimally to the understanding of this tumor and to its better management. Some long term cell lines have been produced and explored. This work has brought along interesting information about the behavior of human cells in vitro which has little in common with the pattern of growth and the functional characteristics of prostatic cancer in vivo.

Still, some aspects of the work in cell culture remain attractive, and we believe that short term culture after tissue fractionation and cell separation is a very promising field of work. The suspension cultures are however not suitable for studies of growth parameters. Production of separate cell populations from stroma, normal epithelium and carcinoma cells already allows the study of their endocrinological and functional characteristics separately. Knowledge about stromal-epithelial interactions will result. Mass production of clearly defined suspensions of prostatic carcinoma cells may be a useful source of antigen and help to further investigate the immunology of prostatic cancer.

Finally, the finding of a very rapid testosterone metabolism in fibroblasts grown from BPH and the large difference found in similar cultures from prostatic carcinoma is a significant finding which will need to be followed up.

References

1. Ackermann, R., Okabe, T., Hempel, K., and Schroeder, F. H.: Membrane antigens of a cell-line from human prostatic carcinoma. National Cancer Institute Monograph on the Immunology of Urogenital Cancer, in press.
2. Ban, R. W., Cooper, J. F., Imfeld, H. and Foti, A.: Hormonal effects on prostatic acid phosphatase synthesis in tissue culture. Investigative Urology, 11: 308, 1974.
3. Brehmer, B., Marquardt, H. and Madsen, P. O.: Growth and hormonal response of cells derived from carcinoma and hyperplasia of the prostate in monolayer cell-culture. A possible in vitro model for clinical chemotherapy. Journal of Urology, 108: 890, 1972.
4. Brehmer, B., Riemann, J. F., Broodworth, J. M. B., Jr. and Madsen, P. O.: Electron microscopic appearance of cells from carcinoma of the prostate in monolayer tissue culture. Urological Research, 1: 27, 1973.
5. Burrows, M. T., Burns, J. E. and Suzuki, Y.: Studies on the growth of cells: The cultivation of bladder and prostatic tumors outside the body. Journal of Urology, 1: 3, 1917.
6. Chang, C. F. and Pollard, M.: In vitro propagation of prostate adenocarcinoma cells from rats. Investigative Urology, 14: 331, 1977.

7. Chen, T. T. and Heidelberger, C.: Malignant transformation of cells derived from mouse prostate in the presence of 3-Mehtylcholanthrene. Journal of the National Cancer Institute, 42: 915, 1969.

8. Cowan, R. A., Cowan, S. K., Grant, J. K. and Elder, H. Y.: Biochemical investigations of separated epithelium and stroma from benign hyperplastic prostatic tissue. Journal of Endocrinology, 74: 111, 1977.

9. Fogh, J.: Personal communication by letter, 1978.

10. Foti, A. G., Herschman, H. and Cooper, J. F.: A solid-phase radioimmunassay for human prostatic acid phosphatase. Cancer Research, 35: 2446, 1975.

11. Fraley, E. E., Ecker, S. and Vincent, M. M.: Spontaneous in vitro neoplastic transformation of adult human prostatic epithelium. Science, 170: 540, 1970.

12. Franks, L. M., Riddle, P. N., Carbonell, A. W. and Grey, G. O.: A comparative study of the ultrastructure and lack of growth capacity of adult human prostate epithelium mechanically separated from its stroma. Journal of Pathology, 100: 113, 1970.

13. Hayashi, I., Larner, J. and Sato, G.: Hormonal growth control of cells in culture. In Vitro, 14: 23, 1978.

14. Heinemeyer, H. M.: Prostatatumoren in Organkultur und Heterotransplantation. Inaugural-Dissertation, Universitat Wurzburg, 1978.

15. Hoehn, W., Schweikert, H. U. and Schroeder, F. H.: Testosteron-metabolismus in kultivierten menschlichen Prostata-Zellen (Abstract). Urological Research, 1978, in press.

16. Jellinghaus, W., Okada, K., Ragg, C., Gernardt, H. and Schroeder, F. H.: Chromosomal studies of human prostatic tumors in vitro. Investigative Urology, 14: 16, 1976.

17. Joebsis, A. C., De Vries, G. P., Anholt, R. R. H. and Sanders, G. T. B.: Demonstration of the prostatic origin of metastases. An immunohistochemical method for formalin fixed unbedded tissue. Cancer, 41: 1788, 1978.

18. Kaighn, M. E.: Characteristics of human prostatic cell cultures. Cancer Treatment Reports, 61: 147, 1977.

19. Kaighn, M. E.: Characteristics of human prostatic cell cultures. Cancer Treatment Reports, 61: 147, 1977.

20. Kaighn, M. E. and Babcock, M. S.: Monolayer cultures of human prostatic cells. Cancer Chemotherapy Reports, 59: 59, 1975.

21. Lasnitzki, I.: Human benign prostatic hyperplasia in cell and organ culture. In: Benign prostatic hyperplasia, NIH Monograph, Washington, 1975.

22. Lasnitzki, I. and Mizuno, T : Induction of the rat prostate gland by androgens in organ culture. Journal of Endocrinology, 72: 47, 1977.

23. Lasnitzki, I., Whitaker, R. H. and Withycombe, J. R. F.: The effect of steroid hormones on the growth pattern and RNA- snythesis in human benign prostatic hyperplasia in organ culture. British Journal of Cancer, 32: 168, 1975.

24. Lerch, V. L., Todd, J., Lattimer, J. K. and Tannenbaum, M.: A technique for the study of human prostatic epithelial cells in vitro by time-lapse cinematography. Journal of Urology, 104: 564, 1970.

25. Lubaroff, D. M.: Development of an epithelial tissue culture line from a human prostatic adenocarcinoma. Journal of Urology, 118: 612, 1977.

26. Nelson-Rees, W. A.: Personal communication, letter of May 30, 1975.

27. Nelson-Rees, W. A., Flandermeyer, R. R. and Hawthorne P. K.:
    Banded marker chromosomes as indicators of intraspecies cellular
    contamination. Science, 184: 1093, 1974.
28. Nelson-Rees, W. A., Zhdanov, V. M., Hawthorne, P. K. and
    Flandermeyer, R. R.: HeLa-like marker chromosomes and type A
    variant glucose-6-phosphate dehydrogenase isoenzyme in human cell
    cultures producing Mason-Pfizer monkey virus like particles.
    Journal of the National Cancer Institute, 53: 751, 1974.
29. Nilsson, T., Schueller, E. and Staubitz, W.: β-glucuronidase
    activity of the epithelial cells and stromal cells in prostatic
    hyperplasia. Investigative Urology, 11: 145, 1973.
30. Oishi, K., Romijn, J. C., Joebsis, A. C. and Schroeder, F. H.: Cell
    separation and characterization of epithelial cells from human
    benign prostatic hyperplasia. Investigative Urology, submitted for
    publication 1979.
31. Okada, K., Laudenbach, I. and Schroeder, F. H.: Human prostatic
    epithelial cells in culture: clonal selection and androgen
    dependence of cell-line EB 33. Journal of Urology, 115: 164, 1976.
32. Okada, K. and Schroeder, F. H.: Human prostatic carcinoma in cell
    culture: Preliminary report on the development and characterization
    of an epithelial cell-line (EB 33). Urological Research, 2: 111,
    1974.
33. Okada, K., Schroeder, F. H., Jellinghaus, W., Wullstein, H. K. and
    Heinemeyer, H. M.: Human prostatic adenoma and carcinoma:
    Transplantation of cultured cells and primary tissue fragments in
    "nude mice". Investigative Urology, 13: 395, 1976.
34. Okabe, T., Ackermann, R., Wirth, M. and Frohmueller, H.: Cell-
    mediated cytotoxicity in patients with cancer of the prostate.
    Investigative Urology, submitted for publication.
35. Oshimura, M. and Sandberg, A. A.: Isochromosome 17 in prostatic
    cancer. Journal of Urology, 114: 249, 1975.
36. Peterson, W. D., Jr., Simpson, W. F. and Ecklund, P. S.: Diploid
    and hetereoploid cell-lines surveyed for y-chromosome fluorescence.
    Nature, 242: 22, 1973.
37. Pierre, R. V. and Hoagland, H. C.: Age associated aneuploidy: loss
    of y-chromosome from human bone marrow cells with aging. Cancer,
    30: 889, 1972.
38. Pontes, J. E., Choe, B., Rose, N. and Pierce, J. M.: Immunochemical
    identification of prostatic epithelial cells in culture. Presented
    at the 73rd Annual Meeting, American Urological Association, 1978.
39. Pontes, J. E., Choe, B., Rose, N. and Pierce, J. M.: Indirect
    immunoflorescence for identification of prostatic epithelial cells.
    Journal of Urology, 117: 459, 1977.
40. Pretlow, T. G., II: Disaggregation of prostates and purification
    of epithelial cells from normal and cancerous prostates using
    sedimentation in an isokinetic density gradient of ficoll in tissue
    culture medium. Cancer Chemotherapy Reports, 59: 143, 1975.
41. Roehl, L.: Prostatic hyperplasia and prostatic carcinoma studied
    with tissue culture technique. Acta Chirurgica Scandinavica,
    Suppl. 240, 1959.
42. Rose, N. R., Choe, B. K. and Pontes, J. E.: Cultivation of
    epithelial cells from the prostate. Cancer Chemotherapy Reports,
    59: 147, 1975.
43. Sanford, E. J., Geder, L., Jones, R. E., Rohner, T. J. and Rapp, F.:
    In vitro culture of human prostatic tissue. Urological Research,
    5: 207, 1977.

44. Serrano, J. A., Wasserkrug, H. L., Serrano, A., Paul, B. D. and Seligman, A. M.: The histochemical demonstration of human prostatic acid phosphatase with phosphorylcholine. Investigative Urology, 15: 123, 1977.

45. Schroeder, F. H.: Endokrinologische und morphologische Untersuchungen am Prostata-Carcinom in vitro. Habilitationsschrift, Medizinische Fakultat der Universitat des Saarlandes, Homburg/Saar, 1971.

46. Schroeder, F. H.: EB 33, an epithelial cell-line from human prostatic carcinoma? A review. National Cancer Institute Monograph on Immunology of Urological Cancer, in press.

47. Schroeder, F. H. and Mackensen, S. J.: Human prostatic adenocarcinoma in cell culture. The effects of androgen-free culture medium. Investigative Urology, 12: 176, 1974.

48. Schroeder, F. H., Sato, G. and Gittes, R. F.: Human prostatic adenocarcinoma: Growth in monolayer tissue culture. Journal of Urology, 106: 734, 1971.

49. Schweikert, H. U., Schroeder, F. H. and Hein, H. J.: Testosterone metabolism of fibroblasts grown from prostatic carcinoma, benign prostatic hyperplasia and non-genital skin. Investigative Urology, submitted for publication.

50. Srinivasan V., Keil E., Villalba, R., Baron, T. and Clark, S. S.: Lactic dehydrongenase isoenzymes in benign and malignant prostatic tissues. Investigative Urology, 11: 224, 1973.

51. Stone, K. R., Mickey, D. D., Wunderli, H., Mickey, G. H. and Paulson, D. F.: Isolation of a human prostate carcinoma cell line (DU 145). International Journal of Cancer, 21: 274, 1978.

52. Stone, K. R., Paulson, D. F., Bonar, R. A. and Reich, C. F., III: In vitro culture of epithelial cells derived from urogenital tissues. Urological Research, 2: 149, 1975.

53. Stone, K. R., Stone, M. P. and Paulson, D. F.: In vitro cultivation of prostatic epithelium. Investigative Urology, 14: 79, 1976.

54. Stonington, O. G. and Hemmingsen, H.: Culture of cells as a monolayer derived from the epithelium of the human prostate: A new cell growth technique. Journal of Urology, 106: 393, 1971.

55. Stonington, O. G., Szwec, N. and Webber, M.: Isolation and identification of the human malignant prostatic epithelial cell in pure monolayer culture. Journal of Urology, 114: 903, 1975.

56. Tavares, H. S., Costa, J. and Costa, Maia, J.: Correlation between ploidy and prognosis in prostatic carcinoma. Journal of Urology, 109: 676, 1973.

57. Vincent, M.: Personal communication of April 15, 1970.

58. Webber, M. M.: Effects of serum on the growth of prostatic cells in vitro. Journal of Urology, 112: 798, 1974.

59. Webber, M. M.: Ultrastructural changes in human prostatic epithelium grown in vitro. Journal of Ultrastructure Research, 50: 89, 1975.

60. Webber, M. M., Hornan, P. K. and Bouldin, T. R.: Present status of MA160 cell-line. Prostatic epithelium or HeLa cells? Investigative Urology, 14: 335, 1977.

61. Webber, M. M. and Stonington, O. G.: Stromal hypocellularity and encapsulation in organ cultures of human prostate: Application in epithelial cell isolation. Journal of Urology, 114: 246, 1975.

62. Williams, R. D., Bronson, D. L., Elliott, A. Y., Gehrke, C. W., Kuo, K. and Fraley, E. E.: Biochemical markers of cultures human prostatic epithelium. Journal of Urology, 119: 768, 1978.

63. Wojewski, A. and Przeworska-Kaniewicz, D.: The influence of stilbestrol and testosterone on the growth of prostatic adenoma and carcinoma in tissue culture. Journal of Urology, 93: 721, 1965.

CHAPTER XI.   REGULATION OF PROSTATE GROWTH IN ORGAN CULTURE*

INTRODUCTION

The use of animal prostates or human prostatic tissues in organ culture as
a means of establishing regulatory parameters affecting and/or controlling
the growth, physiology and pathology of this gland has a number of advantages
as well as shortcomings vis-a-vis in vivo conditions. The interpretation
of results must take these factors into consideration (Table 1). Most impor-
tantly, in organ culture the various tissue components, their anatomical
relationship and function and their histological structure are essentially
preserved and can be readily followed for prolonged periods in vitro. For
the purposes of this Workshop, whose primary interest resides in cancer of
the prostate in the human, the outstanding advantage of organ culture is
the fact that human prostatic tissue can be studied under in vitro conditions;
and the effects of hormones or drugs determined, inasmuch as data obtained
in animals or with their tissues often cannot be extrapolated to the human
condition. Though complex and difficult even under in vivo conditions, the
putative shortcoming of organ culture is the inability to monitor the exocrine
activity of the prostate, probably the gland's most essential function.

The utilization of organ culture environment for growth and differentiation
of embryonic organs or fragments of adult tissues and some of the basic techniques for this approach were applied more than 50 years ago by Strangeways

---

Abbreviations used in text:

T - testosterone

DHT - dihydrotestosterone

VP - ventral prostate

CA - cyproterone acetate

E_2 - estradiol-17β

MCA - methyl cholanthrene

BPH - benign prostatic hyperplasia (or hypertrophy)

ER - endoplasmic reticulum

DES - diethylstilbestrol

TeBG - testosterone binding globulin

EBP - estrogen binding protein

PBP - progesterone binding protein

*Avery A. Sandberg, Roswell Park Memorial Institute, Buffalo, N.Y., U.S.A.
Supported in part by a grant (CA-15436) from the National Cancer Institute

TABLE I

Shortcomings and Advantages of Organ Culture of Prostatic Tissue

Shortcomings

1. Tissues in organ culture can only be maintained for relatively short periods of time (several weeks).

2. Complications resulting from infected tissues rather common, particularly human tissues.

3. Removal from the effects of the circulation and systemic effects (e.g., pituitary, testes, etc.).

4. In the case of the human, infrequent availability of prostatic tissue and untoward effects of the surgery (e.g., coagulated tissue during transurethral resection).

5. Lack of control for ingress or egress of substances to and from the cells, respectively.

6. In the case of cancer, parameters such as spread and metastases cannot be observed vs. events studied in vivo.

7. Inability to monitor exocrine activity of the gland vs. studies in vivo.

Advantages

1. Lack of systemic effects.

2. Maintenance of stromal/epithelial ratio and other anatomic relationships vs. lack of these in tissue culture.

3. Events can be observed.

4. Ready manipulation of environment.

5. Ease of sampling.

6. Tissues can be divided into a number of specimens affording a means of studying events chronologically.

7. Testing of drugs directly on prostatic tissues.

8. Only way in which human prostatic tissue can be studied repeatedly.

and Fell (48). The application of organ culture to prostatic tissue has found wide use in the past 2 decades or so. During the initial stages of application of organ culture techniques to the in vitro growth to prostatic tissues much effort was spent in defining the medium and various substances, particularly hormones, necessary for the maintenance of anatomic and functional integrity in vitro. The ultimate application of organ culture is to the field of carcinogenesis of the prostate and the testing of drugs potentially useful in prostatic disease. In this presentation no attempt will be made to present the details of the various methodologies used, since they can be found in the appropriate publications (11,23-26,35). The utilization of prostatic organ culture has led to a clarification of testosterone (T) metabolism in this gland and the key role played by its reduction product (DHT) in the maintenance of epithelial anatomy and control of mitosis.

A. STUDIES OF ANIMAL PROSTATES IN ORGAN CULTURE

1. The crucial role of T, DHT and other androgenic substances.

Prostatic tissue in organ culture rapidly deteriorates in solutions not containing additives, the most crucial of which is T. The presence of T in the serum or plasma in certain media probably accounts for the survival of prostatic tissue in organ culture. The conversion of T to DHT by 5α-reductase is an essential step for the survival of prostatic tissue, since the 5α-reduced product is the active androgen in all mammalian prostates studied to date.

When prostatic tissue (rat VP) is grown in organ culture without hormones the epithelial cells undergo changes resembling those seen in vivo after castration. Large autophagic vacuoles, residual bodies and dilations of rough endoplasmic reticulum (ER) were noted in 2 days of culture and by 4 days the ER was markedly decreased and no secretory vacuoles were visible. The treatment of explants with T results in an apparent intensification of the morphological equivalents of secretion. Besides the well developed rough ER and Golgi complex, numerous large secretory vesicles with flocculent content are observed. These observations are compatible with the concept that T promotes the formation and probably also the excretion of the secretion in the epithelial cells and that it also prevents partially the appearance of signs of cellular degeneration.

It has also been shown that in the absence of T, the epithelium of the rat VP in organ culture becomes flattened, the acini unfolded and the stroma more cellular. These changes can be prevented or reversed by the addition

167

of T to the culture medium, but it may be important that they are more marked in organs from immature animals (22).

Studies on the metabolism and effects of T in organ culture primarily of the rat VP, have led to the following observations (3,4,36): 1. Only the 5α metabolites of T and not the 5β ones are physiologically active; 2. DHT controls cellular division in the prostatic epithelium; 3. T maintains epithelial height and secretory activity and keeps stroma at a minimum; 4. DHT is more active than T in provoking epithelial hyperplasia, which is seen only after high doses of T; 5. 3β-androstanediol fully maintains epithelial height and stimulates secretory activity but does not cause hyperplasia and 6. T action in the prostate may be related to its conversion to different active metabolites.

These findings confirm in organ culture what has been described in vivo, though the levels of T or DHT necessary for these effects are somewhat more optimally defined by organ culture systems than in vivo (10^{-6} to 10^{-9} M concentrations of T and DHT). The ability of prostatic tissue to convert T to DHT with subsequent binding of the DHT by receptors keeps the activity of intracellular T low and promotes passive diffusion down an arbitrary gradient from blood, particularly in bloods containing binding proteins for these androgens (28). The activity of androstenedione in rat VP may be attributed to the formation of active 5α-reduced metabolites inside the cells (37). CA appears to counteract the action of T in organ culture (7,43).

The presence or absence of human or animal serum in the incubation medium has led to differences in the response of the prostatic tissue to either endogenous and/or exogenous T or DHT. The most likely explanation resides in the ability of TeBG present in such serum to "tie up" the androgen with the result that in the presence of serum much less free or unbound T is available to the prostatic gland than when serum is not present (27). Of course, the influence of the serum will depend on its source, since some animals do not contain TeBG whereas others do, the level of the TeBG (39), such as its greatly increased concentrations during pregnancy and, of course, the concentration of T, DHT and possibly other androgens in the culture medium. Both in vivo and in vitro the presence in serum of binding proteins for corticosteroids (transcortin), estrogens (TeBG, EBP) and progesterone (transcortin, PBG) may seriously influence not only the activity of these steroids but also that of T and/or DHT.

2. Estrogens

In explants derived from 6-week-old rats, E_2 suppressed the growth of columnar cells completely. Combined with T, E_2 reduced the T effect from 70% to 15% columnar cells. The remainder consisted of flat or cuboidal cells with little or no secretory activity. The response of glands from 9-month-old rats differed strikingly. E_2 was less effective than in the young organ and did not increase the regression seen in controls kept in nonsupplemented medium. If combined with T, E_2 did not inhibit the T effect and the proportion of columnar cells in T-treated explants equalled that in explants exposed to both steroids (25).

3. Prolactin

Apparently, prolactin enhances the effects of T, e.g., epithelial cell size is augmented with a marked enlargement of the supranuclear area resulting in the appearance of very tall columnar cells; cell proliferation is promoted leading to increased formation of new alveoli.

It was found that doses of prolactin which augment T effect did not increase the uptake of T or the formation of DHT. It is possible that the prolactin effect is mediated _via_ an increased adenyl cyclase activity.

The enhancing effect of prolactin on T is more pronounced in the glands of older animals (24,25).

4. Polyamines

Edwards et al. (9) using the ventral and dorsal prostates of mice maintained as explants in organ culture showed regressive changes with complete necrosis by the fifth day, if the explants were cultured in a control medium (embryo extract in chicken plasma). When cultured in the presence of T plus the control medium, the explants continued to maintain their epithelial height and stromal characteristics after five days; however, by the seventh day regressive changes similar to those seen in explants cultured in the absence of T were observed. With spermine and spermidine in the medium along with insulin and T, the stromal and epithelial integrity of the explants was kept intact for 14 days. When either T or spermine was omitted from the list of additives, survival and maintenance of normal morphology was greatly impaired. Omission of spermidine did not affect the results, if the other substances were added.

Spermine and spermidine are present in extremely high concentrations in rat prostate explants when compared to numerous other tissues from rodents

and other animals. When rat prostatic fluid is analyzed similar high
concentrations of these polyamines are present. Though some evidence
exists that these polyamines promote clonal growth of cells in culture,
that these factors can replace others in the culture medium (e.g., fetuin)
and that they can stimulate DNA synthesis and cell growth in human
fibroblast cultures, their exact role in prostatic physiology remains to
be elucidated. Polyamines have been reported to stimulate protein and
polypeptide synthesis in vitro; possibly, one of their actions in the
prostate may be related to that area. In some other studies, inhibition
of cells with spermine and spermidine in culture has been also
demonstrated, indicating the rather conflicting nature of the possible
effects of these polyamines on cellular growth.

   5. Vitamin A

       Vitamin A is an important factor for the maintenance of secretory
epithelia including that of the prostate and though the in vivo induction
of a deficiency of this vitamin in animals takes a prolonged period of
time, changes can be very readily observed in organ culture. Thus, VP
glands of mice grown in media composed of plasma and serum which contained
physiological amounts of the vitamin did not alter their growth pattern or
increase secretory activity when the vitamin A was added (24).
Cultivation in completely defined media not containing the vitamin
resulted in the appearance of widespread, irregularly distributed foci of
squamous metaplasia after ten days in vitro. Excessive keratin formation
and the mingling of squamous and normal secretory epithelium, considered
typical of vitamin A deficiency, were observed. Addition of vitamin A to
the defined medium completely prevented the squamous changes and fully
preserved the secretory character of the epithelium.

   6. Adrenal Steroids

       The role of adrenal secretory products in prostatic anatomy and
physiology are difficult to establish in vivo, though their overall
effects may be studied under such conditions. Studies in organ culture
have shown that cortisol counteracts the prostatic regression in all
cultures to which it was added. Some details of the action of adrenal
steroids in organ culture are shown in Table 2 (21).
Cortisol and to a lesser extent prednisolone caused an increased
incorporation of labeled precursors into the DNA and protein of the rat
VP and an augmentation of the effects of T exceeding a simple summation

170

TABLE II

SUMMARY OF THE MAIN EFFECTS OF HYDROCORTISONE AND TESTOSTERONE

ON THE VENTRAL PROSTATE GLAND OF THE RAT GROWN IN VITRO

	Height of epithelium	Folding	Secretory activity	Number of alveoli	Stroma
Before explanation	Cuboidal, columnar	Present	Present	-----	Scanty
Natural medium: Controls	Flat	Absent	Absent	Severely reduced	Markedly increased
Hydrocortisone	Cuboidal, columnar	Absent	Present	Unchanged	Absent
Testosterone	Flat (centre) cuboidal, columnar (periphery)	---	Present (periphery)	Slightly reduced	Slight increase
Semi-defined medium: Controls	Flat cuboidal	Absent	Reduced absent	Unchanged	Absent
Hydrocortisone	Cuboidal, columnar	Absent	Present	Unchanged	Absent
Testosterone	Cuboidal	Slight	Present	Unchanged	Slight increase

Table taken from Lasnitzki (21).

of the responses to individual hormones (43). The most characteristic
feature of cortisol treated epithelial cells was the copious supply of
rough ER. Of some interest was the formation of endoplasmic reticulum
whorls which would not be observed in control and T treated tissues.
Cortisol was shown to promote the formation of juvenile secretory
vesicles.

7. Insulin (Table 3)

The stimulatory effects of insulin on the prostate in organ
culture are probably a reflection of an enhanced uptake by and possibly
effects of T or DHT in prostatic epithelial cells. It is doubtful
whether insulin has a prostatic effect in the absence of T or DHT. The
presence of these steroid hormones in the explants and/or serum appears
to be sufficient for the stimulatory effects of insulin (11,30). Insulin
delayed the onset of degeneration of the epithelial cells but marked
degenerated changes were, however, noted on day six. There were no
specific ultrastructural characteristics which could be interpreted as
specific for insulin action in the epithelial cells (16).

B. STUDIES IN DOG PROSTATE

It has been reported that the 17α- rather than the 17β-DHT is the
active androgen in the dog prostate (46,47). Epitestosterone and DHT
were partially successful in maintaining epithelial height of the dog
prostate in organ culture. The only substance that sustained epithelial
height and secretory activity while keeping stromal cells at a minimum was
5α-androstane-3α,17α-diol (17α-DHT) (46,47). It should be pointed out,
however, that the preponderant metabolic pathway taken by T in the dog is
in the 17β direction (50). Apparently, the canine prostatic receptor
interacts primarily with 17α-DHT.

Fischer et al. (10) showed that dog prostatic explants cultivated in organ
culture for a minimum of nine days showed decreased viability in the
presence of high concentrations of T, whereas those cultivated at lower
levels of T appeared similar to control explants in T free medium.

C. STUDIES WITH HUMAN PROSTATIC TISSUES

1. Studies with BPH tissues

The utilization of organ culture for studying parameters of human
noncancerous and cancerous prostatic tissues is of relatively recent
vintage.

172

TABLE III

Effects of Insulin in Organ Culture of Prostatic Tissues

Prostate Source	Effects	Reference
Mouse VP	Irregular hyperplasia in 5-7 days in the absence or presence of serum	Franks, 1961
Mouse VP	T and insulin necessary to restore gland and to cause increase in secretory epithelium Uptake of T influenced by insulin Augmentation of citric acid Production related to synthesis of an enzyme (?) for which insulin must be present	Lostroth, 1971
Rat VP	Insulin caused incorporation of labeled precursors into RNA and protein Caused an augmented effect in the presence of T	Santti & Johansson, 1973
Rat VP	Delayed the onset of degeneration	Ichihara et al. 1973
BPH tissue	Insulin plus placental lactogen plus T stimulatory; some stimulation with insulin plus E_2	Dilley & Birkhoff, 1977

173

Schrodt and Foreman (44) were apparently the first to explant human prostatic tissue (BPH) in organ culture. The tissue was grown in Trowell medium (49) on agar rafts supported on grids of tantalum mesh. In most explants the morphology of the epithelium and stroma was well maintained during the first three days and in some explants up to nine days. In older cultures the secretory epithelium was often low columnar and occasionally underwent squamous metaplasia. The fine structure resembled that of fresh tissue, including abundant rough ER and secretory vesicles and granules. Exposure to T-propionate (50 μg/ml of medium) caused severe epithelial necrosis.

In another study (32) in which BPH slices were cultured for a period of a week in Eagle's basal medium supplemented with insulin and bovine serum, no morphological responses to T or DES were observed. The authors drew attention to a possible source of a misinterpretation of results based on the uptake of labeled thymidine into the DNA of organ culture tissues, i.e., the possibility that reduplication of the DNA at the explant surface may be balanced by necrosis deep in the explant with the result that the total amount of DNA in explants may remain relatively stable.

Harbitz et al. (13) extended the above studies to several other hormones and examined the effects of T, DHT, E_2, progesterone and CA on BPH tissue grown in Trowell medium. They found that the epithelium and its enzymes were well maintained in androgen free medium and, further, that none of the hormones altered epithelial morphology, the normal enzyme pattern or DNA synthesis.

When explants of BPH tissues were grown in a chemically defined medium (Trowell T8) for periods of 2-12 days, the fibromuscular stroma survived less well than the acinar epithelium (12). This author also showed that in a chemically defined medium DNA synthesis in acinar epithelium and edge cells, shown autoradiographically by the incorporation of ^{3}H-thymidine into cell nuclei, was regularly present in explants cultured for four days. The incorporation of ^{3}H-uridine was demonstrable in acinar epithelium as well as in stromal cells after six days in vitro. In these short term experiments the glandular epithelium retained the histological features of BPH and the ability to synthesize DNA and RNA despite diffuse degeneration of the fibromuscular stroma. The author indicated that the organ culture technique utilizing chemically defined medium should have considerable value for the study of the diseased human prostate and its responses to defined external influences.

Shipman et al. (45) showed that BPH tissue grown in organ culture appeared to be less sensitive than rat VP to withdrawal of hormonal support, in that the changes which occur during culture of BPH were more typical of a repair mechanism of injury than of a castration effect. Cell kinetics were investigated using labeled deoxyuridine and vincristine; both approaches demonstrated a spontaneous surge in proliferative activity of BPH reaching a peak at about day four. In contrast, proliferative activity in rat prostate tended to fall off over the period of 2-8 days of culture.

Mc Rae et al. (33) have indicated that the failure of T to influence BPH tissue in organ culture may be attributed to three possible reasons. Firstly, the tissue in organ culture may not behave as it does in vivo, even though it has been shown in organ culture that the BPH tissue does take up and metabolize T in a way similar to normal animal tissues, both quantitatively and qualitatively. Secondly, BPH tissue may not be hormone dependent at all and, hence, may not be susceptible to influences by T. Thirdly, the length of time that the cultures have been maintained may be insufficient to demonstrate morphological changes under the influences of T. It may be that more appropriate biochemical measurements are needed to demonstrate dependence of BPH tissues over these relatively short periods of time. These same authors in developing an organ culture method for human prostatic tissue suggested on the basis of results in preliminary investigations that T does influence DNA and acid phosphatase production even in the absence of a morphological change of BPH tissue in organ culture.

The findings on BPH tissues in organ culture and the relative independence of such tissues of hormonal controlling factors are of relevance to the problem of cancer of the prostate. For under suitable conditions, satisfactory growth or maintenance of human BPH can be achieved in vitro. Although the tissue is derived from different patients and cultivated by different techniques the findings reveal nevertheless a generally consistent pattern. In contrast to the rodent prostate, tissue from benign BPH grows or is relatively well maintained in androgen free medium. It is unlikely that this property has been acquired during cell transformation or cell selection or is due to a loss of steroid receptors, since it occurs in organ cultures explanted shortly after removal from

175

the patients (26).

2. Other considerations of BPH tissue in organ culture

In androgen deprived target tissues one of the first consequences of T treatment is an increase in RNA synthesis that precedes the increase in DNA synthesis and the restoration of normal morphology. RNA synthesis is, therefore, a sensitive criterion of hormonal effects and attempts were made to correlate the action of T, DHT, 3β-androstanediol and E_2 on epithelial structure with that on RNA synthesis (26). In nonsupplemented medium and in the presence of hormones, the BPH epithelium multiplied to form several layers projecting into the lumen. In the controls, the cells showed some evidence of squamous metaplasia. Testosterone and DHT prevented the latter and preserved the secretory character of the epithelium; in addition, DHT increased the proliferation of the epithelium beyond that seen in controls and in the other experimental explants. In contrast to the androgens, E_2 caused much cellular breakdown including the loss of the secretory cells lining the alveolar lumen.

The cytological changes were reflected in variations of RNA synthesis. The incorporation of labeled uridine into RNA was determined by autoradiography separately in epithelium and smooth muscle and expressed as the percentage of labeled cells in the average number of grains per cell. In the epithelium the uptake was increased by T and DHT, reduced by E_2, and not affected by 3β-androstanediol. In smooth muscle the number of labeled cells was similar to that in controls and androgen treated explants and decreased by E_2, but the grain counts per cell were raised by the androgens and again reduced by E_2. Thus, although the growth of the tissue in organ culture appeared independent of androgens, the explants continue to exhibit hormone responsiveness under the conditions of these experiments utilizing human BPH tissue.

The hormonal study of BPH in organ culture is based not only on cell growth but includes maintenance of epithelium and its function as important criteria of hormonal action. While the data relating to androgen independence of growth and epithelium maintenance are in good agreement, those concerned with hormonal response to BPH in organ culture are still controversial. MacMahon and Thomas (32) and Harbitz et al. (13) reported a failure of steroid hormones to modify the morphology of the epithelium or its enzymes. In contrast, alteration of epithelial growth or morphology and changes in RNA synthesis by T, DHT and E_2 were

176

demonstrated by Lasnitzki (26). In this context, two points deserve
special attention. First, unlike DHT which seems to play a similar role
in the human tissue as in the rat prostate, 3β-androstanediol is ineffective
and may, therefore, have no function in the maintenance of the human
hyperplastic epithelium. Second, the changes of RNA synthesis induced by
the steroid hormones in smooth muscle cells suggest that, like the
epithelium, they are also hormone responsive. Since the muscle forms a
substantial part of the stroma, the finding is important and should be
considered in the evaluation of hormonal effects and their application to
the clinical state.

When BPH prostates were maintained in organ culture for periods of up to
eight days, there was an increased number of cells with histochemically
demonstrable acid phosphatase for a short period of time in culture
(four-six days); however, by eight days such cells decreased in number
(19).

Dilley and Birkoff (8) studied the effect of various combinations of
insulin and other hormones on glandular BPH tissue maintained in organ
culture for four days. Six of nine specimens were stimulated 80% or more
by insulin plus placental lactogen plus T, but only one was stimulated by
insulin plus T. Four of the ten were stimulated by insulin plus E_2.
Histologic and autoradiographic results indicated that all growth occurred
in the epithelium.

Chung and Coffey (7) demonstrated the formation of androgen glucuronides
by normal human prostatic and BPH tissue minces when incubated with
labeled T. Apparently, the normal gland tends to synthesize T-glucuronide,
whereas the hypertrophic one appears to make mostly DHT-glucuronide. The
total amount of steroid glucuronides formed in the two types of tissue was
similar, i.e., 1.5% of the total androgen accumulated in the tissues.
However, the ratio of total DHT to total T-glucuronide found in BPH was
15, which is about 20 times as much as observed in the normal prostatic
tissue. The antiandrogen CA markedly inhibited the formation of the
androgen glucuronide by the BPH tissue, with only slightly decreased
accumulation of the steroids in the tissue.

Studies with prostatic cancers
McMahon et al. (31) studied tissues from cancers of the prostate in organ
culture. In the presence of T, differentiation of the cells occurred
accompanied by an increased mitotic index. DES produced no changes.

177

Bard and Lasnitzki (2) studied the uptake and metabolism of T, androstenedione and DHT by BPH and prostatic carcinomas in organ culture. DHT was a major metabolite of both T and androstenedione in the benign tissue and androstanediols of DHT. Over half the carcinomas produced less DHT from T than did the BPH tissue. Carcinomas from the older patients showed an enhancement of 17β-hydroxysteroid dehydrogenation. There was no relationship between these differences in metabolism of T and the degree of differentiation of the carcinomas. Estradiol decreased the production of DHT, both from T and androstenedione, and at lower androgen concentrations increased the production of androstanediols from T, androstenedione and DHT. The uptake of DHT but not of the other two androgens was stimulated by E_2.

Some of the carcinomas were still hormone responsive in vitro (32). One tumor from a patient treated with DES was relatively differentiated and showed alveoli lined with crowded small cells. In DES-treated explants the cells were larger and less basophilic and the interalveolar stroma was increased. Additions of T to the medium strikingly increased the differentiation of the tissue. The epithelial cells were much taller than in the tumor in vivo owing to a striking increase in cytoplasmic height; there were fewer but larger alveoli per unit area. The second carcinoma from an untreated patient was anaplastic and consisted of densely packed cells separated by fine strands of fibers. Treatment of the cultures with DES for four days did not change this growth pattern, but T produced effects which could be interpreted as attempts at differentiation. The cells were larger and in some regions became arranged in a pattern suggesting alveolar formation. The promotion of differentiation by T in the carcinomas was unexpected but highly interesting and awaits further corroboration.

D. EFFECTS OF CARCINOGENS AND OTHER AGENTS ON PROSTATIC TISSUES IN ORGAN CULTURE

The advantages offered by prostatic tissue in organ culture as a means of studying the effects of carcinogens and/or the changes involved in the genesis of malignant transformation are obvious. The ease of observation and sampling of the tissue to ascertain the effects of carcinogens, the ability to add substances to the medium with possible anticarcinogenic activity and the readiness with which concentrations and combinations of various substances can be manipulated are but few of these advantages.

Major disadvantages are the inability to study metastatic spread or to ascertain whether the transformed tissue has the ability to grow as a tumor _in vivo._

Noyes (34) indicated that in long term organ culture of normal (?) human prostatic tissue, functional and morphologic normality of the glandular epithelium is essentially maintained. MCA at a level of 4 μg/ml in the culture fluid apparently induced morphologic changes that were not observed in untreated cultures. The changes observed after exposure to the carcinogen for 15-20 days included hyperplasia and anaplasia of the glandular epithelial cells with large variation in nuclear size and shape. Even though the author suggested that the changes have a neoplastic potential, it should be indicated that in the past when such preparations were injected into animals, tumors did not develop.

Vitamin A is necessary for the maintenance of normal differentiation and function of secretory epithelium and this applies to the prostate. Thus, in organ cultures of mouse prostates grown in a vitamin A deficient medium the epithelium underwent squamous metaplasia; the addition of the vitamin to the culture medium prevented this change (23-26). In one study (29) the authors tested the effects of vitamin A and its analogues on MCA induced changes in the mouse prostate in organ culture. The compounds studied included retinol, retinoic acid and two analogues of retinoic acid with virtually no growth promoting vitamin A activity. When the prostates of mice were grown in organ culture for seven-nine days and the MCA added to the culture medium, the latter stimulated the alveolar epithelium to become hyperplastic, such epithelium frequently displaying the first stages of squamous metaplasia or undergoing parakeratosis. All vitamin A related compounds were highly active in inhibiting the effects of MCA. When added together with the carcinogen, the vitamin A compounds inhibited epithelial cell multiplication and maintained normal differentiation, thus counteracting the hyperplastic and metaplastic changes induced by MCA. Since all four compounds were highly active in antagonizing the effects of MCA, it is apparent that the anticarcinogenic activity of vitamin A is not correlated with the growth promoting activity of the vitamin. Apparently, the vitamin A effects are not due to their surface active properties.

Chopra and Wilkoff (5,6) determined the effect of β-retinoic acid (RA) on carcinogen induced hyperplasia of mouse prostate glands in organ culture resulting from the addition of MCA or its analogue MNNG, the latter not requiring activation. The development of hyperplasia was inhibited when RA was added simultaneously with MCA or MNNG. However, RA had no significant effect on cell proliferation in untreated control cultures. The elimination of the carcinogen from the hyperplastic cultures after eight days of treatment did not reverse hyperplasia of the alveolar epithelium. When the withdrawal of MCA of MNNG was followed by treatment of the cultures with RA, hyperplasia was markedly reversed within 96 hours. Thus, RA actively inhibited and reversed the effect of MCA and MNNG, two carcinogens that may have different mechanisms of action. Ascorbic acid had no effect on prostate carcinogenesis in organ culture (1).

Lasnitzki (20) had carried out extensive research on the morphological effects produced by polycyclic hydrocarbons and hormones in organ cultures of mouse and rat prostate glands. Those pieces of prostate cultivated in plasma clots and not treated with the test compounds, maintained for periods of up to two weeks a differentiated appearance consisting of a single layer of epithelial cells surrounding the alveoli. When these prostate fragments were treated with microgram quantities of oncogenic hydrocarbons, the epithelial cells underwent hyperplasia and squamous metaplasia, which the author considered as preneoplastic changes.

In order to ascertain whether the above morphological effects were associated with malignancy, the organ culture technique of Lasnitzki was adapted to liquid media using the VP from inbred C3H mice (14). In addition to the hyperplasia and squamous metaplasia following exposure to MCA, pleomorphism of the epithelial cells and invasion through the basement membrane were observed. Some of the slides were read as malignant by pathologists. Disappointingly, however, when nearly 900 of these hydrocarbon-treated pieces from the organ cultures were implanted into isologous mice under a variety of conditions, no tumors were produced. Thus, these profound morphological alterations were not associated with detectable malignancy. Therefore, it was concluded that morphological transformations cannot be seriously considered as being malignant unless tumor formation can be consistently detected in suitable hosts. However, when established cell lines were obtained from some of the morphologically altered hydrocarbon-treated organ cultures they did give rise to sarcomas on inoculation into C3H mice (14).

Despite the fact that the morphological changes produced by chemical oncogens in organ culture cannot be equated with malignancy, studies of this sort are considered useful. The changes seen histologically in these cultures often parallel premalignant changes seen in vivo. Thus, observation of organ cultures is particularly valuable in the case of epithelial tissues, since when chemical oncogenesis in cell culture has been successful, the tumors ultimately produced in animals have almost invariably been in sarcomas.

A profound inhibitory effect on growth of rat VP explants was shown to be produced by estracyt, which was more pronounced than that seen after E_2. When the nitrogen mustard was linked to position-17 of DHT no inhibition of the parameters, including incorporation of ^{3}H-thymidine into the explants of the rat VP, were observed (15).

E. ORGAN CULTURE AS A TEST SYSTEM FOR DRUGS POTENTIALLY USEFUL IN
    PROSTATIC CANCER

In an attempt to develop test systems for drugs potentially useful in cancer of the prostate a number of in vivo and in vitro preparations and systems have been used (38-42), including organ culture (17-18). The latter approach offers the advantage in that human prostatic cancer tissues can be utilized and the drugs tested directly on such tissues. The advantages of this approach are limited, however, by the fact that even though a positive result in organ culture probably indicates that a drug might be useful under clinical conditions, the ineffectiveness of a drug does not necessarily imply that such an agent may not be effective in vivo. Such an ineffective drug may have to undergo metabolic conversion in vivo to a more active form, e.g., flutamide (38,39). Primary reliance in this organ culture system has been placed on two indices: the histology of the glandular tissue and the relative level of 5α-reductase activity. The activity of the latter enzyme has been used as an index of drug effect both in vivo and in vitro (38-42) and though some human cancers of the prostate may not contain much 5α-reductase activity, most of the cancers studied have had such enzymatic activity, though the levels vary from one tumor to another. A distinct advantage of the organ culture system is the fact that very small amounts of tissue are required and that a combination of various drugs can be tested in a relatively short period of time.

Examples of the use of prostatic organ culture to study a number of parameters, including the effects of drugs, are shown in Figures 1-9.

Figure 1.

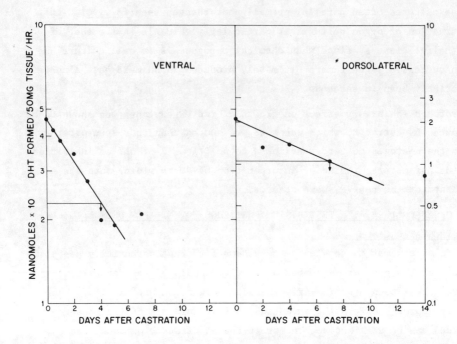

Rate of loss of 5α-reductase activity in rat prostate following castration. Groups of three 400 gm adult wistar rats were orchiectomized. Ventral and dorsolateral lobes of the prostate were removed at various times after surgery and triplicate determinations of the enzyme activity were performed, using homogenates equivalent to 50 mg of tissue. The decrease in 5α-reductase activity, particularly in the VP, indicates dependence of the enzyme on testicular secretion, primarily T.

Figure 2.

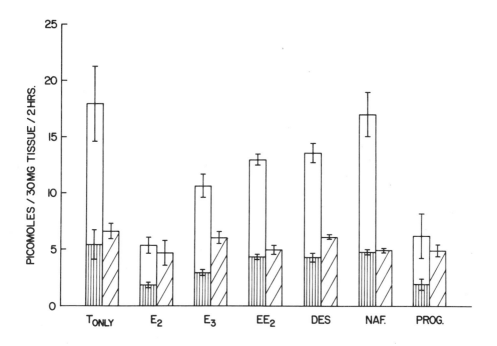

Effect of estrogenic agents on T metabolism in human prostate in organ culture. After 1 day in control medium, explants prepared from a specimen of human prostate (BPH) were maintained for 2 days in media containing 0.5 μM T or T plus an estrogenic agent (1 μg/ml). On the final day, tissues were exposed to ^{3}H-labeled T for 2 hrs. Metabolites of T were extracted and analyzed. E_2, estradiol-17β; E_3, estriol; EE_2; ethynyl estradiol; DES, diethylstilbestrol; NAF., nafoxidine; PROG., progesterone. In this and the following figures the ordinates show the picomoles of DHT formed from T. E_2 and progesterone were particularly effective in inhibiting 5α-reductase. In this and in Figs. 3,4,7 and 8 the 5α-reductase activity is indicated by a summution of the open bars (DHT formation) plus the striped bars (A-diol). The oxidative pathway is indicated by the hatched bars (Δ^4-A-dione).

Figure 3.

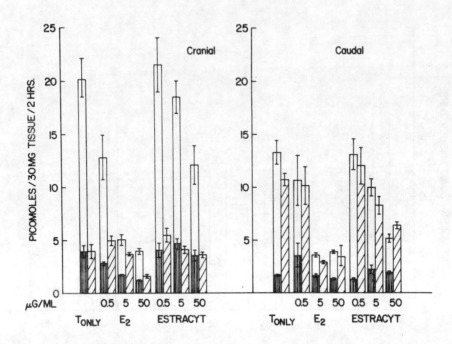

Comparison of the effect of E_2 and estracyt on T metabolism in baboon prostate in organ culture. After 1 day in control medium, explants prepared from cranial and caudal lobes were maintained in media containing 0.5 μM T or T plus 0.5, 5 and 50 μg/ml of E_2 or estracyt. On the final day, tissues were exposed to ^{3}H-T for 2 hrs. Values are means ± s.e. for triplicate determinations. E_2 was more effective in inhibiting 5α-reductase.

Figure 4.

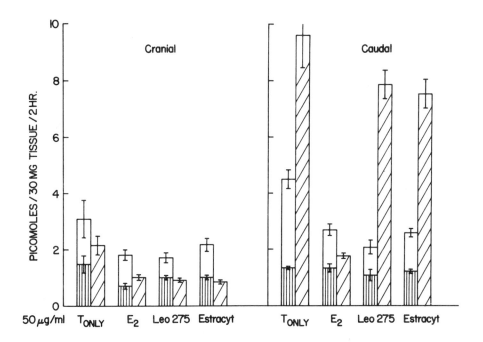

Effect of E_2, Leo 275 (estramustine) and estracyt on testosterone metabolism in baboon prostate in organ culture. Experiment was performed as described in Fig. 3. E_2, Leo 275 and estracyt were each present at a concentration of 50μg/ml. Values are means ± s.e. for triplicate determinations. E_2 was more effective an inhibitor of 5α-reductase than either drug.

Figure 5.

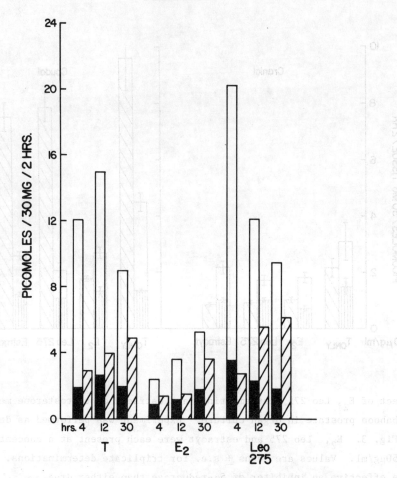

Comparison of the effect of E_2 and Leo 275 on T metabolism in human prostate in organ culture. All media contained 0.5 μM T. E_2 concentration was 6 μg/ml. Leo 275 concentration was 10 μg/ml (equivalent to 6 μg/ml of E_2). Explants in duplicate dishes were exposed to media containing 1.2 nM [³H]-labeled T for the following periods: 2-4 hrs., 10-12 hrs. and 28-30 hrs. Metabolites were extracted and analyzed by TLC. Open bar, DHT; closed bar, A-diol; hatched bar, Δ^4-A-dione. As in the case of baboon prostate (Figs. 1 and 2), E_2 was a more effective inhibitor of 5α-reductase than Leo 275.

Figure 6.

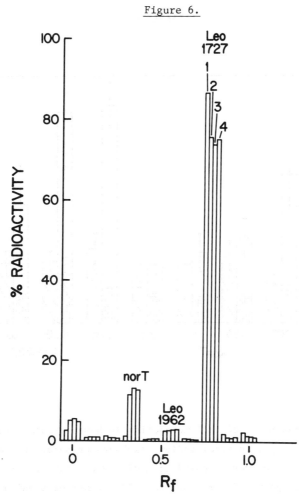

Metabolites of Leo 1727 (a conjugate of a nitrogen mustard with nor-testos-
terone) recovered from incubation with human prostatic tissue. Minces (100
mg) were prepared from specimens of adenocarcinoma and BPH. Incubation mix-
tures (5 ml) contained 0.5 µM T and 0.2 mM ^{3}H-Leo 1727. Experiment included
controls that contained no tissue. After 1 hr. at 37, reactions were termin-
ated by homogenization and addition of 25 ml ethanol. Metabolites were extracted and analyzed on TLC. All steps were performed in the dark or in diffuse light. Values are averages of duplicate determinations. 1 = stock solution, 2 = medium, 3 = BPH tissue, 4 = cancerous tissue. Some hydrolysis (ca.
15%) occurred in the presence of the medium, BPH tissue and cancerous tissue.

Figure 7.

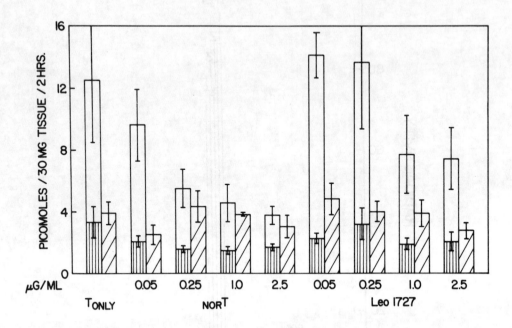

Effect of nor-T and Leo 1727 on T metabolism in human prostate in organ culture. After 1 day in control medium, explants prepared from a specimen of human prostate (BPH) were exposed to media containing 0.5 μM T or T plus 0.05, 0.25 and 1.0 μg/ml of nor-T or Leo 1727. Experiment was performed as described in Fig. 2. Values are means ± s.e. for triplicate determinations. Nor-T appeared to be a more effective inhibitor of 5α-reductase than Leo 1727.

Figure 8.

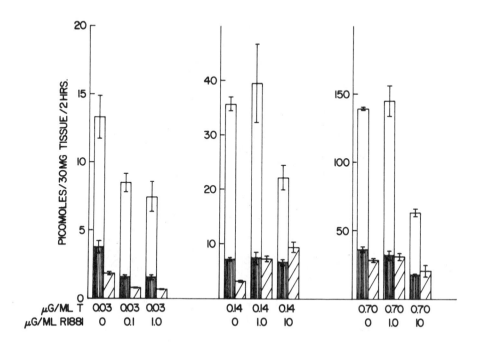

Effect of R1881 (anti-androgen) on T metabolism in baboon ventral prostate in organ culture. After 1 day in control medium, explants were maintained for 2 days in media containing varying concentrations of R1881 at 3 different concentrations of T.

Figure 9.

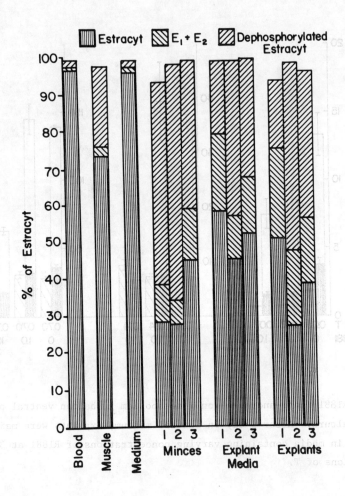

Percentage of labeled estracyt (estramustine phosphase, a phosphorylated conjugate of E_2 with a nitrogen mustard) dephosphorylated and hydrolyzed (shown as E, plus E_2) by various human fluids and tissues, including 3 adenocarcinomas of prostate in organ culture. Explant media were examined after period of culture was completed (18).

F. CONCLUDING REMARKS

From a review of the behavior of prostatic tissue in organ culture it is apparent that such an approach can be utilized to study parameters controlling histologic and functional integrity of such tissue, particularly of normal constituency. The essential independence of hormonal control, or for that matter, of other controls by BPH and possibly cancerous tissue might be due either to the presence of large amounts of DHT and possibly other active androgens within such tissue or the attainment of some independent status by such tissue outside the body. The somewhat variable effects of T on BPH and prostatic cancer tissues remain to be further ascertained and clarified. Certainly, the response of such tissues is minimal when compared to that of normal animal prostates under similar conditions. It is possible that the human tissues reflect an advanced stage of independence from direct hormonal control, as evidenced by the minimal effects of T and other agents in organ culture conditions. However, organ culture offers the distinct advantages of utilizing human prostatic cancer tissues in vitro and the ability to test various drugs either singly or in combination against such tissues and establishing the sensitivity of such tissue to these drugs. Since in all probability human prostatic tissues, particularly cancerous, differ morphologically and/or biochemically from one case to another, such a system offers an important avenue of ascertaining the effects of drugs directly on each cancer, with the amount of tissue required for such testing being rather small. Hence, one can envision the ultimate testing of each cancer with a battery of drugs under organ culture condition in order to ascertain the agent most likely of effectiveness against a particular cancer.

References

1. Bal, E. and De Lustig, E. S.: Prostate carcinogenesis in vitro. Unresponsiveness to ascorbic acid. Medicina 36: 23-28, 1976.
2. Bard, D. R. and Lasnitzki, I.: The influence of oestradiol on the metabolism of androgens by human prostatic tissue. J. Endocr. 74: 1-9, 1977.
3. Baulieu, E. E., Lasnitzki, I. and Robel, P.: Metabolism of testosterone and action of metabolites on prostate glands grown in organ culture. Nature, 219: 1155-1156, 1968.
4. Baulieu, E. E., Lasnitzki, I. and Robel, P.: Testosterone, prostate gland and hormone action. Biochem. Biophys. Res. Comm., 32: 575-577, 1968.
5. Chopra, D. P. and Wilkoff, L. J.: Inhibition and reversal by β-retinoic acid of hyperplasia induced in cultured mouse prostate tissue by 3-methylcholanthrene or n-methyl-n'-nitro-n-

nitrosoguanidine. J. Nat. Cancer Inst., 56: 583-589, 1976.

6. Chopra, D. P. and Wilkoff, L. J.: Reversal by vitamin A analogues (retinoids) of hyperplasia induced by n-methyl-n-nitro-n-nitrosoguanidine in mouse prostate organ cultures. J. Nat'l. Cancer Inst., 58: 923-930, 1977.

7. Chung, L. W. K. and Coffey, D. S.: Androgen glucuronide II. Differences in its formation by human normal and benign hyperplastic prostates. Invest. Urol. 15: 385-388, 1978.

8. Dilley, W. G. and Birkhoff, J. D.: Hormone response of benign hyperplastic prostate tissue in organ culture. Invest. Urol., 15: 83-86, 1977.

9. Edwards, W. D., Bates, R. R. and Uspa, S. H.: Organ culture of rodent prostate. Effects of polyamines and testosterone. Invest. Urol., 14: 1-5, 1976.

10. Fischer, T. V., Burkel, W. E., Kahn, R. H. and Herwig, K. R.: Effect of testosterone on long-term organ cultures of canine prostate. In Vitro, 12: 382-392, 1976.

11. Franks, L. M.: The growth of mouse prostate during culture in vitro in chemically defined and natural media, and after transplantation in vivo. The effects of insulin and normal human serum. Exp. Cell Res., 22: 56-72, 1961.

12. Harbitz, T. B.: Organ culture of benign nodular hyperplasia of human prostate in chemically-defined medium. Scand. J. Urol. Nephrol, 7: 6-13, 1973.

13. Harbitz, T. B., Falkanger, B. and Sander, B.: Benign prostatic hyperplasia of the human prostate exposed to steroid hormones in organ culture. Arch. Path. Microbiol. Scand., Sect. A Suppl. 248: 89-93, 1974.

14. Heidelberger, C.: Chemical oncogenesis in culture. Adv. Cancer Res., 18: 317-366, 1973.

15. Hisaeter, P. A.: Incorporation of 3H-thymidine into rat ventral prostate in organ culture. Influence of hormone-cytostatic complexes. Invest. Urol., 12: 479-489, 1975.

16. Ichihara, I., Santti, R. S. and Pelliniemi, L. J.: Effects of testosterone, hydrocortisone and insulin on the fine structure of the epithelium of rat ventral prostate in organ culture. Z. Zellforsch, 143: 425-438, 1973.

17. Kadohama, N., Kirdani, R. Y., Murphy, G. P. and Sandberg, A. A.: 5α-reductase as a target enzyme for anti-prostatic drugs in organ culture. Oncology, 34: 123-128, 1977.

18. Kadohama, N., Kirdani, R. Y., Murphy, G. P. and Sandberg, A. A.: Estramustine phosphate: Metabolic aspects related to its action in prostatic cancer. Urology, 119: 235-238, 1978.

19. Kreisberg, J. I., Brattain, M. G. and Pretlow, T. G., II: Studies on human hyperplastic prostates maintained in organ culture. Invest. Urol., 15: 252-255, 1977.

20. Lasnitzki, I.: Growth pattern of the mouse prostate gland in organ culture and its response to sex hormones, vitamin A and 3-methylcholanthrene. In: Biology of the Prostate and Related Tissues, NCI Monograph 12, 1963, 381-403.

21. Lasnitzki, I.: The effect of hydrocortisone on the ventral and anterior prostate gland of the rat grown in culture. Endocrinology, 30: 225-233, 1964.

22. Lasnitzki, I.: Action and interaction of hormones and 3-methycholanthrene on the ventral prostate gland of the rat in vitro. I. Testosterone and methycholanthrene. J. Nat. Cancer Inst., 35: 339-348, 1965.

23. Lasnitzki, I.: The rat prostate gland in organ culture. In: Some Aspects of the Aetiology and Biochemistry of Prostatic Cancer, Third Tenovus Workshop (Griffiths, K. and Pierrepoint, C. G., Cardiff, eds.) 1970, 68-73.

24. Lasnitzki, I.: The prostate gland in organ culture. In: Male Accessory Sex Organs. Structure and Function in Mammals. (Brandes, D., ed.) Academic Press, New York, 1974, 348-382.

25. Lasnitzki, I.: The effect of hormones on rat prostatic epithelium in organ culture. In: Normal and Abnormal Growth of the Prostate. (Goland, M., ed.) Charles C. Thomas, Publisher, Springfield, Illinois, 1975, 29-54.

26. Lasnitzki, I.: Human benign prostatic hyperplasia in cell and organ culture. (Grayback, . T., Wilson, J. D. and Scherbenske, M. J., eds.) DHEW Publication No. (NIH) 76-1113, 1975, 235-248.

27. Lasnitzki, I. and Franklin, H. R.: The influence of serum on uptake, conversion and action of testosterone in rat prostate glands in organ culture. J. Endocr., 54: 333-342, 1972.

28. Lasnitzki, I., Franklin, H. R. and Wilson, J. D.: The mechanism of androgen uptake and concentration by rat ventral prostate in organ culture. J. Endocr., 60: 81-90, 1974.

29. Lasnitzki, I. and Goodman, D. S.: Inhibition of the effects of methylcholanthrene on mouse prostate in organ culture by vitamin A and its analogs. Cancer Res., 34: 1564-1571, 1974.

30. Lostroh, A. J.: Effect of testosterone and insulin in vitro on maintenance and repair of the secretory epithelium of the mouse prostate. Endocrinology, 88: 500-503, 1971.

31. McMahon, M. J., Butler, A. V. J. and Thomas, G. H.: Morphological responses of prostatic carcinoma to testosterone in organ culture. Br. J. Cancer, 26: 388-394, 1972.

32. McMahon, M. J. and Thomas, G. H.: Morphological changes of benign prostatic hyperplasia in culture. Br. J. Cancer, 27: 323, 1973.

33. McRae, C. U., Ghanadian, R., Fotherby, K. and Chisholm, G. D.: The effect of testosterone on the human prostate in organ culture. Br. J. Urol., 45: 156-162, 1973.

34. Noyes, W. F.: Effect of 3-methycholanthrene (NSC-21970) on human prostate in organ culture. Cancer Chemo. Rep. 1, 59: 67-71, 1975.

35. Robel, P. and Baulieu, E. E.: Biologie experimentale.-Irrigation continue appliquee a la culture organotypique. C. R. Acad. Sc. Paris, 274: 3295-3298, 1972.

36. Robel, P., Lasnitzki, H. and Baulieu, E. E.: Hormone metabolism and action: testosterone and metabolites in prostate organ culture. Biochimie, 53: 81-96, 1971.

37. Roy, A. K., Baulieu, E. E., Feyel-Cabanes, T., Le Goascogne, C. and Robel, P.: Hormone metabolism and action: II. Androstenedione in prostate organ culture. Endocrinology, 91: 396-403, 1972.

38. Sandberg, A. A.: Potential test systems for chemotherapeutic agents against prostatic cancer. Vit. Hor., 33: 155-188, 1975.

39. Sandberg, A. A.: Regulation of plasma steroid binding proteins. In: Endocrinology, proceeding of the fifth international congress of endocrinol. Hamburg, July 18-24, 1976. (James, V. H. T., ed.) Excerpta Medica, Amsterdam 1: 452-457, 1977.

40. Sandberg, A. A. and Gaunt, R.: Model systems for studies of prostatic cancer. Semin. Oncol., 3: 177-187, 1976.

41. Sandberg, A. A., Kirdani, R. Y., Yamanaka, H., Varkarakis, M. J. and Murphy, G. P.: Potential test systems for drugs against prostatic cancer. Cancer Chemother. Rep., 59: 175-184, 1975.

42. Sandberg, A. A., Muntzing, J., Kadohama, N., Karr, J. P., Sufrin, G., Kirdani, R. Y. and Murphy, G. P.: Some new approaches to potential test systems for drugs against prostatic cancer. Cancer Treat. Rep., 61: 289-295, 1977.

43. Santti, R. S. and Johansson, R.: Some biochemical effects of insulin and steroid hormones on the rat prostate in organ culture. Exp. Cell Res., 77: 111-120, 1973.

44. Schrodt, G. R. and Foreman, C. D.: In vitro maintenance of human hyperplastic prostate tissue. Invest. Urol., 9: 85-94, 1971.

45. Shipman, P. A. M., Littlewood, V., Riches, A. C. and Thomas, G. H.: Differences in proliferative activity of rat and human prostate in culture. Br. J. Cancer, 31: 570-580, 1975.

46. Sinowatz, F. and Pierrepoint, C. G.: Hormonal effects on canine prostatic explants in organ culture. J. Endocr., 72: 53-58, 1977.

47. Sinowatz, F., Chandler, J. A. and Pierrepoint, C. G.: Ultrastructural studies on the effect of testosterone, 5α-dihydrotestosterone, and 5α-androstane-3α,17α-diol on the canine prostate cultured in vitro. J. Ultrastruct. Res., 60: 1-11, 1977.

48. Strangeways, T. S. P. and Fell, H. B.: Experimental studies on the differentiation of embryonic tissues growing in vivo and in vitro. Proc. Roy. Soc., B 100: 273-280, 1926.

49. Trowell, O. A.: The culture of mature organs in a synthetic medium. Exp. Cell Res., 16: 118-147, 1959.

50. Yamamoto, Y., Osawa, R., Kirdani, R. Y. and Sandberg, A. A.: Testosterone metabolites in dog bile. Steroids, 31: 233-247, 1978.

SPONTANEOUS ANIMAL MODELS FOR PROSTATIC CANCER*
CHAPTER XII

Need for Animal Models of Prostatic Cancer

Until recently, the development and evaluation of basic concepts
concerning the nature of prostatic cancer have been limited by the
availability of well characterized and appropriate experimental animal
models. The ultimate system for testing concepts of abnormal growth of
the human prostate would, by definition, involve human investigations.
Unfortunately, many important factors cannot be controlled with clinical
material and these include, genetic and immunological differences, time
of initial onset of the disease, tumor load and distribution, variability
of tumor cell types, compliance, precise control of hormonal and
therapeutic levels, and a host of other biological and clinical factors
In addition, ethical,cost and time considerations make it essential that
we evaluate animal models to determine if they are appropriate to
elucidate basic principles of prostatic cancer.

Required Properties of Animal Models for Prostatic Cancer

Selecting a single animal model for prostatic cancer may not be
realistic because the human cancer counterpart is itself a variable and
multifaceted disease. Each type of human tumor is often characterized
by a wide spectrum of diversity in relation to pathology, state and
variability of cellular differentiation, uniformity of growth rate, and
differences in therapeutic responsiveness to hormonal, non-hormonal, and
radiation treatment. Indeed, many of these variations can even be
observed in a single patient within the course of his disease. Because
of the variability in the types of human prostatic cancer, it is possible
that more than one animal model may be required to correspond to these
different states of prostate cancer. Even though we are aware of these
variations within human and animal prostatic cancer, we can refer to the
more typical clinical picture and strive towards an animal model with
similar properties and response. These idealized properties for an
animal model of prostatic cancer are summarized in Table 1.

---

*John T. Isaacs and Donald S. Coffey. James Buchanan Brady Urological
 Institute, Department of Urology, The Johns Hopkins University School
 of Medicine, Baltimore, Maryland 21205. This work supported by
 Grant Number CA15416, awarded by the National Cancer Institute, DHEW.

TABLE 1

SOME IDEALIZED PROPERTIES OF ANIMAL MODELS OF PROSTATIC CANCER

1.) Spontaneous in origin.

2.) Developed in aged animals.

3.) Proven origin from prostatic tissue.

4.) Adenocarcinoma, slow growing tumor.

5.) Histological similarity to human prostatic cancers.

6.) Biochemical profile similar to prostate.

7.) Malignant and metastatic patterns to bone and lymph nodes.

8.) Elevates serum prostatic acid phosphatase levels.

9.) Hormone sensitive.

10.) Capable of responding to castration and estrogen therapy followed

by relapse to hormone insensitive state.

11.) Immunological parameters

A.) Developed in syngeneic animals.

B.) Transplantable or easily induced.

C.) Contains tumor specific antigens.

12.) Large numbers of animals are available for statistical

considerations.

13.) Similar therapeutic response to human prostatic cancer

A.) Correlates with past therapy

i) hormonal therapy

ii) non-hormonal therapy

iii) radiation sensitivity

B.) Accurately predicts response to future modalities of human

therapy.

14.) Wide diversity of tumor types (differentiation, hormonal response,

etc.) corresponding to human tumor variability.

196

Species and Origin

The etiology of human prostatic cancer is still unknown, and while external factors such as carcinogens and viruses are possible causative factors, they have nevertheless failed to be proven as direct etiological agents. Efforts must continue to resolve the roles of these potentially important factors, but as yet, they still remain very speculative. The only firm evidence is that prostatic cancer develops spontaneously in aged males who were not castrated prepubertally; therefore, this should be a prime prerequisite for the animal model. Some of the animals developing spontaneous prostatic cancer are listed in Table 2. The dog develops spontaneous prostatic cancer with age (15) and a few old rats have likewise produced prostatic adenocarcinomas which can be propagated by transplantation. The most popular include the rat prostatic adenocarcinoma of Dunning R-3327 (7,14,18,30,32,33,34) and the Pollard tumors (22-26).

Older primates have not been adequately studied in large numbers to determine the true spontaneous incidence of either prostatic cancer or spontaneous benign prostatic hyperplasia. This is due in part to the great expense of maintaining large numbers of aged primates and to the difficulty in permitting them to age sufficiently in captivity to develop these diseases. It is also very difficult to capture large numbers of older males for study. Because of evolutionary considerations, the ideal animal model for prostatic cancer might be the higher primates, and it is anticipated that increasing interest in animal models for abnormal prostatic growth will soon involve these important species.

Methods of Characterizing Animal Models of Prostatic Cancer

Organ: In animal models, it is essential to establish the specific organ of tumor origin. In the human, it is believed that prostatic cancer primarily develops in the outer regions of the prostate. The dog and human have no clearly defined anatomical prostatic lobes, and it is difficult to draw clear analogies to homologous lobes in rats and other species although it is obvious that the histology of the dorsal lobe of the rat is more similar to the overall normal human prostate than is the large ventral lobe which is almost devoid of stromal elements. Although the dog and man have no clearly defined anatomical lobes, they may nevertheless have different functional zones or areas of different embryological origins. This has not been established but is the basis of

197

TABLE 2

PROSTATIC ADENOCARCINOMAS IN ANIMALS

SPECIES	YEAR	INVESTIGATORS	TUMOR
SPONTANEOUS			
Rat	1961	W. F. Dunning (7)	From dorsal prostate of aged (22 months) Copenhagen rat; syngeneic, androgen-dependent; transplantable
	1973	M. Pollard P. H. Luckert (22,25)	Aged, germ-free Lobund Wistar: ? lobe prostate; hormone-sensitive; transplantable
	1975	S. A. Shain B. McCullough A. Segaloff (27,28)	Aged AxC rats; ventral prostate; no metastases; not transplanted
Hamster	1960	J. G. Fortner J. W. Funkhauser M. R. Cullen (9)	Aged Syrian golden hamster; transplantable; tumor has been lost
Dog	1968	I. Leav G. V. Ling (15)	Aged (>8 years) mongrels; metastases; no occult tumor
Mastomy	1965	K. C. Snell H. L. Stewart (31)	Aged female African rodent prostate
Monkey	1940	E. T. Engel A. P. Stout (8)	Aged Macaca mulatta
HORMONE INDUCED			
Rat	1977	R. L. Noble (19,20)	Induced by sex hormone manipulation
XENOGRAFT HUMAN TO MOUSE			
Nude Mouse	1978	HOEHN FOEBSIS SCHROEDER (12)	Moderately differentiated human prostatic adenocarcinoma carried in nude mouse

198

several active studies. It is important to know why prostatic cancer in humans is primarily limited to specific areas of the prostate and why the aged prostates of other species are devoid of these tumors.

Histology: Many carcinogen induced animal prostatic tumors are squamous carcinomas, and therefore are not similar to the human prostatic adenocarcinomas. In contrast, the spontaneous canine and rat tumors, both Dunning R-3327 and Pollard, are adenocarcinomas. Therefore, the epithelial nature of the animal tumor must be established by both light and electron microscopic analysis and should be substantiated by appropriate histochemical similarities to the prostate epithelium. The presence of microvilli and secretory granules help establish the epithelial nature. Nuclear analysis should indicate the pleomorphic nature of a cancer nucleus and karyotyping is required for species identity and continued identification of the transplanted cells.

Biochemical Studies: Several biochemical markers have been used in concert to identify cells of prostatic origin and while no single test is completely definitive they do, when taken together, provide an overall biochemical profile of the tumor and prostate. In addition, many markers are decreased or lost as cells become malignant or dedifferentiated to a more anaplastic nature. In all cases, the monitoring of the biochemical profile usually provides an identity of the state of the tumor. There are many biochemical factors associated with prostatic tissue and some of the more important include:

A) ENZYMES AND ISOZYME PATTERNS

Acid and alkaline phosphatase; Leucine aminopeptidase; β-glucuronidase; Arginase, Lactic dehydrogenase; Fibrinolysin; 5α-reductase; 3α-and 3β-hydroxysteroid dehydrogenase; 3β-diol-6α and 7α-hydroxylase.

B) SMALL MOLECULES

High ratio of dihydrotestosterone to testosterone; Pattern of steroid conjugates; Zinc, cadmium; Spermine and spermidine; Citric acid; Fructose.

C) RECEPTORS, CYTOPLASMIC AND NUCLEAR

Dihydrotestosterone (DHT); 17β-estradiol; Nuclear uptake of DHT.

D) TISSUE SPECIFIC AND SECRETORY PROTEINS

Electrophoretic profiles; Tissue and tumor specific antigens.

199

Elevated serum acid phosphatase levels have provided one of the useful biomarkers of metastatic human prostatic cancer. This is primarily due to the extremely high tissue levels of acid phosphatase that under normal conditions enter the secretions of the prostate; however, from metastatic prostatic adenocarcinoma cells the enzyme enters directly into the general circulation raising the serum levels and providing an enzymatic marker. The prostatic tissue levels of acid phosphatase are the highest in humans and decrease in other species. For example, the level per unit of tissue in the mouse prostate is only 1/6,000 of that of the human prostate. Relative prostatic tissue levels of acid phosphatase activity are: man, 1,200; baboon, 1,100; Rhesus monkey, 130; dog, 60; rat, 1.0 and mouse, 0.20. Therefore, the extent of elevation of the serum levels of prostatic acid phosphatase in animal tumor models would be dependent on five factors: 1.) the levels of acid phosphatase in the animal prostate from which the tumor was derived, 2.) state of maintained differentiation of the tumor, 3.) the location of the tumor implant and metastasis, 4.) the overall tumor load in the animal, and 5.) the specificity of the assay and the stability of the enzyme in serum. Therefore, all animal tumor models may not exhibit the elevation in serum prostatic acid phosphatase.

Metastatic Pattern: Factors controlling the extent and route of metastasis of human tumors are still poorly understood. Human prostatic cancer invades locally and metastasizes primarily to the lymph drainage and bone. Spontaneous tumors in the prostates of animals such as the dog follow similar patterns of metastasis and also produce elevated serum acid phosphatase values (15). Many other animal tumors such as the Dunning R-3327 and Pollard tumors are transplanted subcutaneously, and would, by necessity follow different routes of metastasis from that of spontaneous prostatic tumor although the end result may be nearly the same. Site of injection of the tumors (subcutaneous, intraperitoneal, intraprostatic), number of cells and state (free cell suspension or small tumor tissue implants), hormonal treatment, and drug therapy can have marked effects on metastasis (24).

Hormonal Response: The tumor should be hormonally sensitive requiring the presence of androgens for full growth and demonstrate growth inhibition following castration, estrogen or androgen deprivation (castration or estrogen therapy), but in humans it is generally concluded that hormonal therapy is not curative and subsequent relapse occurs in essentially all cases as a hormone insensitive state develops. There are very few exceptions and, therefore, this feature should be one of the most important requirements of an appropriate animal model for prostatic cancer since the model should mimic the most consistent and important clinical response seen with the human cancer (29). At present, the treatment of prostatic cancer is limited severely by the hormone insensitive state that almost invariably follows favorable response to hormonal treatment. At present, we have no insight into the mechanism of induction of hormone insensitivity in humans. The mechanism of the development of this hormonal insensitivity appears to have been resolved for the first time for prostatic cancer in an animal model (29,30). The mechanism appears to be a phenomenon of pre-existing resistant cell selection (clone selection) as opposed to a conversion or induction of hormone sensitive cells to an insensitive state. There is some reason to believe that human prostatic cancer may also be multifocal in nature (4).

Immunological Parameters: Tumor immunology is increasing as an important consideration in both cancer biology, etiology, and immunotherapy. Although many easy expectations for immunotherapy of cancer have not been realized, there is still great potential for immunological approaches as we increase our basic understanding of immunology. Tumor associated antigens have been detected in membrane extracts from human prostatic cancer (2,3). Similar tumor membrane antigens have also been detected in the Dunning R-3327 rat prostatic adenocarcinoma (5,16). These studies emphasize the need for further immunological studies in prostatic cancer, and this can best be studied in tumor models in syngeneic animals. Syngeneic animals are essentially immunologically identical and will accept transplants between animals of the group.

It is important to consider, however, that many of the transplantable animal tumors could conceivably have picked up viral particles or foreign elements during the years of continuous transplantation. These foreign factors could complicate immunological studies since they may appear as tumor associated antigens but not to the host or original tumor cell.

Growth Rate and Cell Kinetics: Human prostatic cancer is a relatively slow growing tumor although the time for one cell to double has not been determined. It is estimated that the tumor doubling time may be greater than one month which is not uncommon for many human solid tumor adenocarcinomas. Preliminary DNA labeling studies indicate a small fraction of the prostate cancer cells in active DNA synthesis which indicates a low ^{3}H-thymidine labeling index. One individual tumor cell must divide or double approximately 30 times to grow to a number of tumor cells of one billion (10^9) which is a total tumor volume of 1 c.c. and is about the minimal size for early clinical detection. For example, a single original tumor cell doubling each month would require a minimum of two and a half years to grow to a tumor volume of 1 c.c. (1 division/mo.) (30 divisions) = 30 months. These cell kinetic considerations have been discussed for prostatic cancer (34).

Most animal tumors are rapidly growing with division times in hours or days. These systems would not mimic the very slow growing human prostatic cancer. The Dunning R-3327 rat prostatic adenocarcinoma is the only slow growing model available at this time and has a tumor volume doubling time of 20 days (14,30).

While slow growing animal tumor models may be more similar to the human situation, they nevertheless limit the number of investigations because they require long times for the inoculated tumors to grow out to detectable sizes and another long period of time before the cancers terminate the animals. This limitation requires large colonies of animals under study for an extended period of time.

Tumor Stability, Diversity, and Characterization: Many tumors change properties with growth and diversity can develop; while this also appears to occur with human prostatic cancer, it can nevertheless cause difficulties in transplantable tumors where the tumor type, growth rate, and histology can often change. It is, therefore, easy to lose a transplantable tumor line through irreversible changes or to develop multiple sublines which has occurred with the Dunning and Pollard rat prostatic tumors. This diversity can be helpful in developing a broad range of cancer types with specific properties that more closely mimic a specific type or grade of human prostatic cancer. Nomenclature of many of these transplantable animal tumors refers to an inherited or earlier designated tumor line number which may now have changed properties with continued transplantation. This is why standardization of reporting and identity is essential, but as of now has not been realized. Very few of these animal tumor lines have been properly characterized and reported. Continuing this policy will only cause added and unnecessary confusion.

TRANSPLANTABLE DUNNING RAT PROSTATIC ADENOCARCINOMAS R-3327 SERIES

(R-3327 A, B, C, D, E, F, G, H, HI, and AT)

Source and History: In August, 1961, Dr. W. F. Dunning of the
University of Florida observed a spontaneous tumor of the prostate which
presented at necropsy in a Copenhagen male rats from the 54th brother x
sister generation of line 2331 (7). The rat was a 22 month old retired
breeder and the tumor occupied a large portion of the lower abdominal
cavity and appeared to involve primarily the dorsal prostate gland. This
primary tumor was classified as a papillary adenocarcinoma and no
metastases were identified. Ten milligram grafts of the soft tumor
tissue were transplanted to ten rats, four of the same inbred line as the
host of the primary tumor and 6 F_1 hybrids from a male Copenhagen x
Fischer female cross. The transplanted tumors grew very slowly and
became palpable on the 60th day. Histological analysis of this
transplanted tumor on the 245th day indicated glandular formation and
cellular material corresponding to a normal dorsal-type gland of the rat
prostate. The tumor was positive to periodic acid - Schiff (PAS) stain
and negative to the dithizone stain typical of dorsal type glands.
Samples of heart blood from the rat did not indicate an elevated serum-
acid phosphatase level. These findings were reported by Dr. Dunning in
1963. The tumor has been transplanted subcutaneously for 17 years in
over 20 passages. The mean animal survival in a 13 year period (1961-
1974) was reported by Dr. Dunning to be 356 days (maximum 670 days,
minimum 141 days). The survival data were obtained after transplanting
one cubic millimeter of solid tumor subcutaneously.

This R-3227 tumor remains histologically a well-differentiated
adenocarcinoma. In 1974, Voigt and Dunning (32) reported on the hormone
sensitivity and metabolism of testosterone in the tumor line. In an in
vivo study they were able to demonstrate the 5α-reduction pathway in this
tumor line. In addition, they observed differences in the growth rate
between males and castrates, thus establishing the hormone dependency of
the R-3327 tumor.

Dr. Dunning isolated eight different tumors which she designated A
through H. In 1975, Voigt, Feldman, and Dunning reported on the
development of R-3327A line which is an androgen insensitive squamous cell
carcinoma which is derived from the established line R-3327 (33). This
androgen insensitive tumor, R-3327A, has a growth rate of approximately

ten times that of R-3327. This tumor developed in the fifth transfer
generation in 1965 and has now been transferred over sixty times. The
androgen insensitive squamous cell carcinoma grows well in castrates,
females, and males. This tumor did not have the ability to metabolize
testosterone by the 5α-reduction pathway. In addition, it appeared that
the R-3327 had the androgen receptor in the cytoplasm while this receptor
was absent from the hormone insensitive line (R-3327A) (33).

Dunning has not reported the characteristics of the other R3327 lines
B through H. Following Dr. Dunning's retirement R-3327 lines designated
D through H are now maintained in the laboratory of Dr. Alice Claflin of
the University of Miami (5). The G tumor has been reported to be a
rapidly growing undifferentiated carcinoma which is hormone dependent.
Transplanting 2 x 10^7 cells of the G tumor into intact males produces a
palpable tumor within three weeks (5). The H tumor line is a well
differentiated adenocarcinoma which grows much slower.

In 1976, an anaplastic tumor line developed spontaneously from the
R-3227H. This anaplastic tumor is stable and is hormone insensitive and
grows at a very rapid rate, doubling in volume approximately every 48
hours. This line has been characterized and designated R-3327-AT (14,
30).

In 1977, the hormone sensitive R-3327H was placed in a castrate and
a small fraction of cells grew, thus establishing a new line which was
hormone insensitive, a differentiated adenocarcinoma which was slow
growing (14).

In summary, the following nomenclature exists for the Dunning R-3327
tumors:

Nomenclature of the R-3327 tumor lines

R-3327A	A rapidly growing, hormone insensitive, squamous cell carcinoma.
R-3327B through F	These five sublines not fully described or characterized.
R-3327G	Rapidly growing, undifferentiated, hormone dependent line.
R-3327H	Slow growing, well differentiated adenocarcinoma with active acini, hormone dependent, well characterized (14,30).

| R-3327-HI | Hormone insensitive (HI), slow growing andenocarcinoma. This line established in 1977 from hormone insensitive clones of cells which were present originally in the R-3327H. These are the fraction of cells that grew out when the R-3327H was grown in a castrate animal for a long period (14). This tumor tissue contains small acini which are lined by active epithelial cells and the tumor has been characterized (14). |
| R-3327-AT | Rapidly growing, hormone insensitive, anaplastic tumor developed in 1976 (30). This tumor has been characterized (14). |

Characteristics of the Dunning Tumors: Recent studies indicate that the Dunning R-3327H transplantable rat prostatic adenocarcinoma appears to be an appropriate animal model for studying prostatic cancer. A detailed characterization of this tumor at the morphologic, biochemical, and therapeutic levels has been accomplished (14,30,36). Electron micrographic, histologic, and histochemical studies clearly establish the adenocarcinoma nature of this tumor. The histology of the R-3327H tumor (Figure 1) is similar to well-differentiated human prostatic cancer. The biochemical and enzymatic profile of the tumor indicates its origin from the rat dorso-lateral prostate. The cell kinetics and growth rates of this tumor following a variety of hormonal manipulations (castration, estrogens, androgens, and antiandrogens) have established that 70%-90% of the cells in this tumor require androgens for their growth, Table 3. However, 10%-30% of the cells are capable of growth in the absence of androgens. Both cell types are present in the initial tumor inoculum and these different cell types possess similar growth rates (14,30,36).The predominance of the androgen-sensitive cells accounts for the relatively greater size of the tumor achieved in the intact male animal at a given growth time. After the tumor is well established in an intact animal, subsequent estrogen therapy or castration resulted in a marked diminution in tumor volume. This was followed by a subsequent relapse to a predominant state of androgen insensitivity. This therapeutic relapse following androgen deprivation represents the continued growth of the clone of cells, which were hormone insensitive (14,30,36).This may mimic the relapse phenomenon observed in the hormone control of human prostatic cancer. The component

Figure 1. Histology of the R-3327 tumor sublines: Left panel 60X; center panel 410X, right panel 6300X.

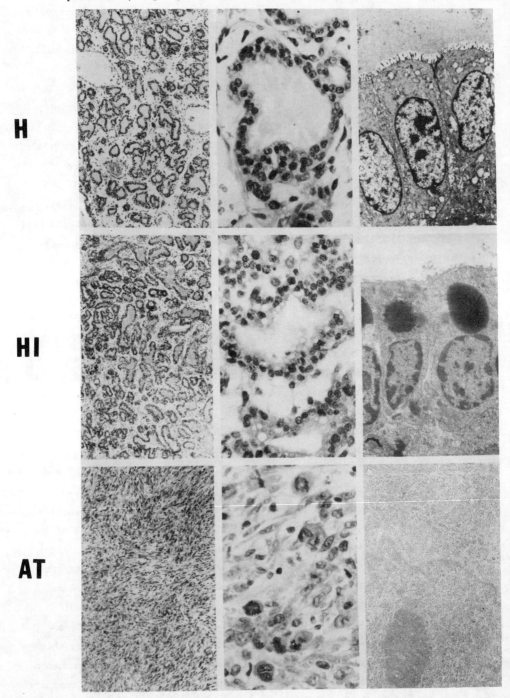

TABLE 3

EFFECTS OF HORMONE MANIPULATION ON THE SIX-MONTH GROWTH OF 1.5 X 10^6 TUMOR CELL INOCULATION OF THE DUNNING R-3327-H TUMOR LINE

HORMONAL STATUS		TUMOR WEIGHT		TOTAL CELL NUMBER		FOLD INCREASE IN INITIAL CELL INOCULUM	% OF INOCULATED CELLS GROWING	CELL DOUBLING TIME
Animal	Six Month Treatment	Absolute (Grams)	Relative	Absolute (10^8)	Relative			
Intact	None	3.47 ± 1.48	100	6.48 ± 2.7	100	432	93	20.9
Intact	Androgen (TP)	4.25 ± 1.10	122	6.40 ± 1.7	99	427	74	18.7
Intact	Estrogen (DES)	0.41 ± 0.06	12	0.65 ± 0.21	10	43	8	20.2
Intact	Antiandrogen (Flutamide)	0.60 ± 0.19	16	1.20 ± 0.32	18	80	16	20.3
Castrate	None	0.31 ± 0.07	8	0.68 ± 0.16	10	45	29	24.8
Castrate	Androgen (TP)	5.26 ± 1.69	151	8.73 ± 3.0	134	582	83	19.8

All animals injected with identical subcutaneous inoculations containing 1.5 X 10^6 viable tumor cells. Animals treated daily as indicated with testosterone propionate (TP), 20 mg/day; diethylstilbestrol (DES), 100 µg/kg/day; flutamide, 50 mg/kg/day.

composed of hormone insensitive cells has been permitted to grow in a
castrate male and a new slow-growing, well-differentiated hormone
insensitive subline of the tumor has been established and has been noted
R-3327-HI.

The R-3327-HI tumor is androgen insensitive but is well
differentiated (Figure 1). This is in contrast to the anaplastic tumor
(R-3327-AT) which is poorly differentiated, grows rapidly, and is androgen
insensitive (Figure 1). These three tumors have been the most
characterized (14) of all the animal tumors for prostatic cancer and
these properties are summarized in Table 4.

In addition, steroid receptor studies have been initiated on these
tumors (11,17,33) (see Table 5). In addition, a new enzymatic index has
been developed to characterize these three tumor types (36). The index
is based on the determination of the specific activity (activity/unit
amount of DNA) of six enzymes in each of the three tumors (R-3327H; HI
and AT) and comparing them on a relative basis to the activity in the
normal dorsolateral prostate (Table 6). A ratio is established using the
product of the relative activity of three enzymes (3α-hydroxysteroid
dehydrogenase; leucine amino peptidase; and lactic dehydrogenase) divided
by the product of another group of three enzymes (5α-reductase; 3β-diol
hydroxylase and alkaline phosphatase). The value of this ratio is termed
the RELATIVE DIFFERENTIATION INDEX and is presented in Table 7. The
relative values for each individual enzyme shown in Table 6 are the
average relative values taken from Table 6 and they compare the three
values in the numerator and three in the denomination as indicated. The
test of the ability of this relative differentiation index to discriminate
the three tumor types is shown in Figure 2. Ten tumors of each type
(R-3327H; HI or AT) were analyzed separately for the activity of each of
the six enzymes. The individual relative differentiation index was
determined for each of the thirty tumors and the individual values are
shown in Figure 2. There was no overlap of individual values between the
tumor types. Thus, it is possible to determine the hormone sensitivity
and type of tumor by determining the relative differentiation index. If
such an index could be established for the different types of human
prostatic cancer, it could be of great clinical value.

Therepeutic Studies: Castration or estrogen therapy does not cure
animals bearing the R-3327-H tumor but if the tumor size is small there is
an increase in survival time (1, 18, 30, 34). The anaplastic tumor

208

TABLE 4

COMPARATIVE PROPERTIES OF THREE TRANSPLANTABLE
DUNNING R-3327 PROSTATIC TUMORS IN RATS.

NUMBER	R-3327-H (Hormone Sensitive)	R-3327-HI (Hormone Insensitive)	R-3327-AT (Anaplastic Tumor)
TYPE	Well differentiated prostatic adenocarcinoma.	Well differentiated prostatic adenocarcinoma.	Anaplastic prostatic tumor. Not a squamous cell carcinoma.
ORIGIN	Spontaneous tumor discovered by W. Dunning in 1961 in a male Copenhagen rat. Stable for 17 years with subcutaneous transplantation.	Subline developed at Johns Hopkins in 1977 from carrying R-3327-H in castrate males.	Subline developed at Johns Hopkins. Spontaneous in 1976 from the R-3327-H.
HISTOLOGY	Large well developed acini filled with secretions.	Smaller acini with less secretions.	No acini. Sheets of anaplastic cells. Pleomorphic nuclei.
ANDROGEN	Hormone sensitive. Maximum growth in intact adult males. Heterogeneous, 80% of cells are hormone sensitive and 20% are hormone insensitive.	Hormone insensitive. Growth rate equal in both intact and castrate males.	Hormone insensitive. Growth rate equal in both intact and castrate males.
GROWTH RATE	Slow	Slow	Fast
TUMOR DOUBLING TIME	15-20 days	15-20 days	2 days
METASTATIC RATE	Approximately 1%.	Probably 1%.	Slow local invasion to lymph nodes, but no distant metastasis detected.
BIO-CHEMICAL PROFILE	Enzyme profile of tumor similar to dorsal lateral prostate tissue. Moderate activity of 5α-reductase. Androgen and estrogen cytoplasmic receptors present.	Moderate levels of 5α-reductase. Decrease in level of androgen cytoplasmic receptor, but no decrease in estrogen receptor. Appearance of progesterone receptor.	Low biochemical correlation to normal lobes of rat prostate. Low in 5α-reductase activity. Androgen receptor absent.

TABLE 5

STEROID CYTOPLASMIC RECEPTORS IN THE NORMAL RAT PROSTATE AND IN THE DUNNING PROSTATIC TUMOR

	ANDROGEN RECEPTOR (R-1881)		ESTROGEN RECEPTOR (Estradiol)		PROGESTERONE (R-5020)	
	Affinity $(10^{-10}M)$	Capacity (femtomoles/g)	$(10^{-10}M)$	(femtomoles/g)	$(10^{-10}M)$	(femtomoles/g)
Dorsal-Lateral Prostate	7	1,660	10	130		Not Detected
Dunning Tumor Androgen Sensitive R-3327-H	7	4,550	5	1,880		Not Detected
Dunning Tumor After Relapse To Castrate R-3327-HI	7	1,730	4	1,400	10	690

Data taken from the studies of Heston, Menon, Tananis and Walsh (11).

Assays by sucrose density gradient and Scatchard plots.

TABLE 6

COMPARATIVE ENZYMATIC ACTIVITIES IN THE DUNNING TUMORS COMPARED TO THE NORMAL RAT PROSTATE

ENZYME	UNITS OF ACTIVITY	ENZYME SPECIFIC ACTIVITY (numbers in parentheses are average relative values)			
		NORMAL DORSOLATERAL PROSTATE	R-3327-H ANDROGEN SENSITIVE	R-3327-HI ANDROGEN INSENSITIVE	R-3327-AT ANAPLASTIC
3α-Hydroxysteroid Dehydrogenase (3α-DH)	pmoles/hr/100 μg DNA	1,228 ± 171 (1.0)	618 ± 129 (0.50)	1,267 ± 129 (1.03)	1,876 ± 246 (1.53)
Leucine Amino Peptidase (LAP)	nmoles/min/100 μg DNA	7.14 ± 0.86 (1.0)	4.29 ± 0.16 (0.60)	8.71 ± 3.39 (1.22)	8.19 ± 0.99 (1.15)
Lactic Dehydrogenase (LDH)	nmoles/min/100 μg DNA	2,071 ± 143 (1.0)	1,798 ± 189 (0.86)	2,954 ± 265 (1.43)	4,485 ± 370 (2.16)
5α-Reductase (5α-RED)	pmoles/hr/100 μg DNA	32.2 ± 10.9 (1.0)	17.0 ± 5.4 (0.53)	12.7 ± 3.16 (0.39)	1.3 ± 0.5 (0.04)
3β-Diol Hydroxylase (3β-HYD)	pmoles/hr/100 μg DNA	250 ± 100 (1.0)	180 ± 60 (0.72)	100 ± 35 (0.40)	90 ± 15 (0.36)
Alkaline Phosphatase (ALK P)	nmoles/min/100 μg DNA	258 ± 18.6 (1.0)	197 ± 3.15 (0.76)	74 ± 12.5 (0.28)	20 ± 8.5 (0.08)

TABLE 7

DETERMINATION OF THE RELATIVE PROSTATIC DIFFERENTIATION INDEX

TISSUE ANALYZED	GROWTH RATE	ANDROGEN RESPONSE	HISTOLOGICAL DIFFERENTIATION	EQUATION[a]	AVERAGE PROSTATIC DIFFERENTIAL INDEX[b] (RANGE)
Normal Dorsolateral Prostate	Very Slow	Sensitive	Well	$\dfrac{(1.0)(1.0)(1.0)}{(1.0)(1.0)(1.0)} =$	1.00 (0.8 - 3)
R-3327-H Tumor	Slow	Sensitive	Well	$\dfrac{(0.50)(0.60)(0.86)}{(0.53)(0.72)(0.76)} =$	0.89 (0.7 - 4)
R-3327-HI Tumor	Slow	Insensitive	Well	$\dfrac{(1.03)(1.22)(1.43)}{(0.39)(0.40)(0.28)} =$	41.4 (26 - 100)
R-3327-AT Tumor	Slow	Insensitive	Poor Anaplastic	$\dfrac{(1.53)(1.15)(2.16)}{(0.04)(0.36)(0.08)} =$	2533 (2337 - 9260)

[a]Equation, product of relative enzyme activities; $\dfrac{(3\alpha\ DH)(LAP)(LDH)}{(5\alpha\ RED)(3\beta\text{-}HYD)(ALK\ P)}$. Range of individual values in parentheses.

[b]Average equation values from ten determinations.

Figure 2.

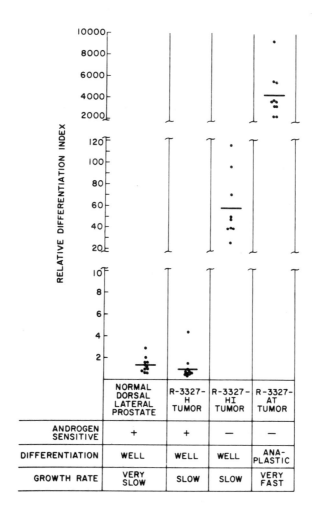

Scattergram of the Relative Differentiation Indexes determined individually
for each sample tumor are compared to the normal dorsolateral prostate
of the appropriate tissue groups. Each group N=10.

(R-3327-AT) has been studied for the development of adjuvant therapy
techniques and beneficial effects have been reported (34). Similarly,
the rapidly growing R-3327-G tumor has been used to screen therapeutic
agents for their effects on tumor growth (1).

POLLARD TRANSPLANTABLE PROSTATIC ADENOCARCINOMAS IN LOBUND WISTAR RATS

In 1973, Dr. Morris Pollard at the University of Notre Dame reported
that spontaneous tumors were observed in germ free, random bred Lobund Wistar
rats in increasing frequencies and numbers as the rats advanced in age beyond
24 months. Most of these tumors involved endocrine organs and/or their
target organs (22-26). The tumors were predominantly benign, but some
with malignant characteristics were noted in individual animals over age
30 months. Among eighty germ free male Lobund Wistar rats over 30 months
of age, were 9 with prostate adenocarcinomas. It is possible that the germ
free status of the animals was not an essential consideration but only
permitted the animals to survive to the old age without the complications
of bacterial infection. All of the animals also had benign liver tumors
of unknown etiology. The tumors were free of virus particles and carcinogen
effects have not been established. The prostate tumors retained their
original structural characteristics of combined epithelial and connective
tissue cells. In addition, a few animals who were treated with estrogens
for 8 weeks had a decrease in the tumor size by about 50%. Three of the
spontaneous prostate carcinomas were transplanted subcutaneously and
propagated in a series of conventionally random bred Lobund Wistar rats.
These animals also developed lymph node and pulmonary metastases. Three
Pollard tumor lines (I, II, and III) have been established in Lobund
Wistar strain. The cells have been grown in vitro as cell monolayers
and when inoculated back into either males or females grew extremely
rapidly, forming back the histology of the original adenocarcinoma. A
special feature of these tumors is their ability to rapidly metastasize
to the lung and other sites primarily through the blood vascular system.
The extent of metastasis could be monitored by tumor foci in the lung,
and this could be reduced markedly by either cyclophosphamide, aspirin,
or Corynebacterium parvum treatment (24). This appears to be a primary
effect on the mechanism of metastasis because the primary subcutaneous
lesions were not reduced in size. In contrast, anesthetic agents increased
the extent of metastasis. In addition, the tumors do not appear to be
antigenic.

The tumors can be controlled but not cured with cyclophosphamide (cytoxan) therapy. These tumors may be good models for studying metastasis; furthermore, they can be grown easily in culture which is an asset to metabolic studies. The disadvantages of these tumor models are that they are not hormone sensitive nor well differentiated and they grow very rapidly (doubling time of 18-20 hours in vitro).

PROSTATIC ADENOCARCINOMAS IN THE AGED A X C RAT

Spontaneous prostatic adenocarcinomas were detected in the ventral lobes of 7 of 41 virgin male A x C rats whose ages exceeded 34 months (27, 28). No tumors were observed in the dorsolateral prostate. These adenocarcinomas form proliferating epithelial cells which build up into cribiform patterns which in some cases form secretory products. Treating a group of 33 aged A x C rats with exogenous testosterone increased the incidence of prostatic adenocarcinomas to 70%.

At present three tumors have been successfully transplanted (27).

It is too early to assess the advantages and limitations of these tumor lines. They do, however, represent another case of a high incidence of spontaneous prostatic tumors in rats, a species that has often been assumed to be free of this disease.

OTHER SPONTANEOUS PROSTATIC ADENOCARCINOMAS

Dog: Spontaneous tumors of the prostate gland have been observed in other species. In 1968, Leav and Ling made a comprehensive study of the pathology of adenocarcinoma of the canine prostate (15). In an eleven year period, between 1956 and 1967, they reported on twenty cases of prostatic adenocarcinoma in the dog and compared their finding with 761 cases in an age matched (no tumor) control series. In this study, 90% of the 20 cases of canine prostatic adenocarcinoma occurred in dogs eight years of age or older. Similarities of this neoplasm to the one in man were demonstrated. The included morphologic similarities, a frequency of the tumor in older animals, skeletal metastases, histochemical demonstration of acid phosphatase, and lipids in neoplastic cells, and routes of metastasis similar to those thought to exist in man. The main differences between the neoplasm in man and dog were: 1) The reported absence of latent carcinoma in the canine prostate, and 2) The apparent low frequency of prostatic tumors in dogs, probably less than 1%. In addition, no specific anatomic regions of the canine prostate have been associated with the development of adenocarcinoma.

Mastomy: Snell and Sturid reported in 1965 the observation of an adenocarcinoma of the prostate gland in one female Mastomy and proliferative hyperplasia in four others among a group of 55 untreated virgins (31). Holland (1970) has also reported on spontaneous prostatic adenocarcinomas in two untreated, 26 month old female Mastomys (13). The Mastomy (Rattus natalensis) is a small, African rodent.

Hamster: Dr. Joseph G. Fortner reported that a 21 month old hamster, of an untreated group, died on August 10, 1960, and on autopsy, a large tumor was observed in the pelvic region in the area of the prostate gland. There was invasion of the abdominal wall and of the bony pelvis. Mestastasis was also present on the serosa of the colon and in the lungs. The tumor was a moderately undifferentiated prostatic adenocarcinoma with foci of papillary formation. The tumor was transplanted and grew well in both male and female animals and did not appear to be hormone sensitive. After 67 generations, the tumor retained the morphology similar to the original tumor. Hosts bearing the transplantable tumor developed lymph nodes and pulmonary metastasis. Details of these findings were reported by Drs. Fortner, Funkhaueser, and Cullen in 1963 (9). Karyotype studies indicated that this tumor was composed of several cell lines. It has been reported that this hamster prostatic tumor line was later lost due to a freezer storage failure.

INDUCED TUMORS

Hormone Induction: Dr. R.L. Noble has reported the development of adenocarcinomas of the dorsal prostate of Nb rats following prolonged treatment with testosterone propionate alone or in combination with estrone (19, 20, 21). A few transplantable tumors were obtained and were hormone-independent, but one required estrogens for growth. Following withdrawal of the required estrogen the tumor involuted, and when subsequently treated with androgens became androgen-sensitive. These experiments were more complex than described here; however, Noble believes he has produced tumor progression which is apparently directed by switching from exogenous androgens to estrogens. These are most interesting observations that require further study and elucidation.

HUMAN TUMORS PASSAGED IN NUDE MICE

In the laboratory of Dr. F.H. Schroeder (Rotterdam), Dr. W. Hoehm

216

has been successful in transplanting tissue from a moderately differentiated adenocarcinoma of the human prostate into nude mice. The tumor has been growing with a doubling time of about 3 months. The original tumor has been passaged to other nude mice 3 times; there are now five animals bearing the tumor. The histology of the tumor is unchanged. The presence of prostatic acid phosphatase in the tumor has been demonstrated with the immunofluorescence technique (12).

SUMMARY

There is ample evidence for a need for appropriate animal models for prostatic adenocarcinoma. There are several animal models now available that should be evaluated. This will require a detailed characterization of their biochemical, pathological and pharmacological properties. Appropriate animal models should be selected on the basis of how closely they correlate with our previous clinical experience with the several different types of human prostatic cancer. Several of these models should be studied in detail to develop and evaluate new methods of chemotherapy. Results should be compared with past and future results from well-controlled and randomized clinical studies. With this approach it should be possible to choose appropriate animal models to develop basic principles of tumor biology to derive new modalities of therapy.

REFERENCES

1. Block, N.L., Canuzzi, F., Denefrio, J., Troner, M., Claflin, A., Stover, B., and Politano, U.: Chemotherapy of the transplantable adenocarcinoma (R-3327) of the Copenhagen rat. Oncology 34: 110-113, 1977.
2. Brannen, G., and Coffey, D.S.: Tumor-specific immunity in patients with prostatic adenocarcinoma or benign prostatic hyperplasia. Cancer Treat. Reports 61: 211-216, 1977.
3. Brannen, G., Gomolka, D., and Coffey, D.S.: Specificity of cell membrane antigens in prostatic cancer. Cancer Chemo. Reports 59: 127-130, 1975.
4. Byar, D., and Mostofi, F.: Carcinoma of the prostate: prognostic evaluation of certain pathologic features in 208 radical prostatectomies. Examination of the step-section technique. Cancer 30: 5-13, 1972.
5. Claflin, A.J., McKinney, F.C., and Fletcher, M.A.: The Dunning R3327 prostate adenocarcinoma in the Fisher-Copenhagen F_1 rat; a useful model for immunological studies. Oncology 34: 105-109, 1977.
6. Coffey, D.S., Isaacs, J.T., and Weissman, R.M.: Animal models for the study of prostatic cancer (in press) Prostatic Cancer Today, 1979.
7. Dunning, W.F.: Prostate cancer in the rat. Nat. Cancer Inst. Monog. 12: 351-370, 1963.

8. Engle, E.T. and Stout, A.P.: Spontaneous primary carcinoma of the prostate in a monkey. Amer. J. Cancer 39: 334-337 (1940).

9. Fortner, J., Funkhauser, J., and Cullen, M. A transplantable spontaneous adenocarcinoma of the prostate in Syrian (golden) hamster. Nat. Cancer Inst. Monog. 12: 371-379,(1963).

10. Fraley, E., and Paulson, D.: Experimental carcinogenesis of the prostate. Edited by David Brandes. In Male Accessory Sex Organs: Structure and Function. New York: Academic Press, 1974.

11. Heston, W.D.W., Menon, M., Tananis, C., and Walsh, P.C.: Androgen, estrogen, and progesterone receptors of the R-3327 Copenhagen rat prostatic tumor (in press).

12. Hoehn, W., Foebsis, A.C., and Schroeder, F.H.: (submitted for publication).

13. Holland, J.: Prostatic hyperplasia and neoplasia in female Praomys (Mastomys) natalensis. J. Natl. Cancer Inst. 45: 1229-1236, 1970.

14. Isaacs, J.T., Heston, W.D.W., Weissman, R.M., and Coffey, D.S. (1978). Animal models of hormone sensitive and insensitive prostatic adenocarcinoma: Dunning R-3327-H, HI, and AT. Can Res. 38: 4353-4359 (1978).

15. Leav, J., and Ling, G.V.: Adenocarcinoma of the canine prostate. Cancer 22: 1329-1345, 1968.

16. Lubaroff, D.M., Canfield, L., Feldbush, T.L. and Bonney, W.W.: R-3327 Adenocarcinoma of the Copenhagen rat as a model for the study of the immunologic aspects of prostate cancer. J. Nat. Cancer Inst. 58: 1677-1689 (1977).

17. Markland, F., and Lee, L.: Estrogen receptor characterization of the R-3327 transplantable prostatic adenocarcinoma. Fed. Proc. 36: 513, 1977.

18. Muntzing, J., Kirdani, R., Saroff, J., Murphy, G., and Sandberg, A.: Inhibitory effects of Estracyt on R-3327 rat prostatic carcinoma. Urology 10: 439-445, 1977.

19. Noble, R.L.: The development of prostatic adenocarcinoma in Nb rats following prolonged sex hormone administration. Cancer Res. 37, 1929-1933 (1977).

20. Noble, R.: Sex steroids as a cause of adenocarcinoma of the dorsal prostate in Nb rats, and their influence on the growth of the transplants. Oncology 34: 138-141, 1977.

21. Noble, R., and Hoover, L.: A classification of transplantable tumors in Nb rats controlled by estrogen from dormancy to autonomy. Cancer Res. 35: 2935-2941, 1975.

22. Pollard, M.: Spontaneous prostate adenocarcinoma in aged germ free Wistar rats. J. Natl. Cancer Inst. 51: 1235-1241, 1973.

23. Pollard, M.: Prostate adenocarcinomas in Wistar rats. Rush-Presbyterian St. Luke's Med. Bull. 14: 12-22, 1975.

24. Pollard, M., Chang, C.F., and Luckert, P.H.: Investigations on prostatic adenocarcinomas in rats. Oncology 34: 129-132, 1977.

25. Pollard, M., and Luckert, P.H.: Transplantable metastasizing prostate adenocarcinomas in rats. J. Nat. Cancer Inst. 54: 643-649, 1975.

26. Pollard, M., and Luckert, P.H.: Chemotherapy of metastatic prostate adenocarcinoma in germfree rats. Cancer Treat. Reports 60: 619-621, 1976.

27. Shain, S.A., McCullough, B., Nitchuk, M. and Boesel, R.W.: Prostate carcinogenesis in the AXC rat. Oncology 34: 114-122 (1977).

28. Shain, S.A., McCullough, B. and Segaloff, A.: Spontaneous adenocarcinomas of the ventral prostate of aged AXC rats. J. Nat.

Cancer Inst. 55: 177-180 (1975).

29. Smolev, J.K., Coffey, D.S. and Scott, W.W.: Experimental models for the study of prostatic adenocarcinoma. J. Urol. 118: 216-220 (1977).

30. Smolev, J.K., Heston, W.D.W., Scott, W.W. and Coffey, D.S.: Characterization of the Dunning R3327H prostatic adenocarcinoma: an appropriate animal model for prostatic cancer. Cancer Treat. Rep. 61: 273-287 (1977).

31. Snell, K.C. and Stewart, H.L.: Adenocarcinoma and proliferative hyperplasia of the prostate gland in female Rattus (Mastomys) natalensis. J. Nat. Cancer Inst. 35: 7-14 (1965).

32. Voigt, W., and Dunning, W.F.: In vivo metabolism of testosterone-^{3}H in R-3327, an androgen-sensitive rat prostatic adenocarcinoma. Cancer Res. 34: 1447-1450, 1974.

33. Voigt, W., Feldman, M., and Dunning, W.F.: 5α dihydrotestosterone binding protein and androgen sensitivity in prostatic cancers of Copenhagen rats. Cancer Chemo. Reports 35: 1840-1846, 1975.

34. Weissman, R.M., Coffey, D.S., and Scott, W.W.: Cell kinetics studies of prostatic cancer: adjuvant therapy in animal models. Oncology 34: 133-137, 1977.

35. Weisman, R.H., Scott, W.W., Isaacs, J.T. and Coffey, D.S.: Concepts related to prostatic cancer as revealed by a study of the Dunning R-3327 prostatic adenocarcinoma models. (in press) Proceedings of the 12th International Cancer Congress. Oct. 5-11, 1978, Buenos Aires.

36. Isaacs, John T., Isaacs, William B. and Coffey, Donald S.: Models for development of non-receptor methods for distinguishing androgen-sensitive and -insensitive prostatic tumors. Cancer Res. 39: 2652-2659 (1979).

CHAPTER XIII. NEW CONSIDERATIONS IN THE HORMONAL INDUCTION
AND REGULATION OF ANIMAL TUMORS*

A. INDUCTION OF PROSTATIC ADENOCARCINOMA

Three factors seem to contribute to the development of adenocarcinoma in
the rodent prostate gland. The relevance of genetic background is undeniable,
since tumors have been reported to occur only in susceptible animals such
as the Copenhagen (37), Lobund-Wistar (29), AXC (33,34) and Nb stocks
(27,28). In confirmation of earlier predictions (24), age has emerged as
an important factor as well. Thus, when longevity of the AXC rat extends
to the extreme limits of the normal life span, the incidence of spontaneous
adenocarcinoma of the prostate rises to 70% (33). The third predisposing
factor is hormonal imbalance. Noble has shown that prolonged treatment of
Nb rats with testosterone proprionate increases the incidence of adenocarcinoma from 0.5% to 18.4% (28).

B. HORMONAL SENSITIVITY

There are a number of ways in which the hormonal sensitivity of a tumor
can be evaluated. Ideally the tumor should grow only in the presence of
androgens and regress when androgens are withdrawn. The method of reducing
the circulating level of testosterone, whether it is castration or the administration of estrogens, should not influence the rate or degree of involution.
Much would be offered by any tumor model which facilitates the study of the
growth and regression of different neoplastic lesions simultaneously in
the same animal. During the course of withdrawal therapy the tumor should
progress from a sensitive to a resistant state such that upon reactivation
very few, if any, of the tumors should respond to further endocrine manipulations. Lastly, there should be the opportunity to measure the effects of
therapy not only on direct parameters of tumor growth but also on the
survival of the host.

*Nicholas Bruchovsky and P. S. Rennie; Department of
Medicine, The University of Alberta, Edmonton, Alberta, Canada, T6G 2G3;
Supported by grants from the National Cancer Institute of Canada and the
Medical Research Council of Canada (MRC MT 3729)

The most meaningful results will probably be obtained with tumor models
displaying the variability of therapeutic responses observed clinically.
This implies that the practice of assaying for hormonal sensitivity of
a transplantable tumor by comparing the rates of growth in intact male,
castrated male, and intact female recipients (22,37,40,41) probably is
inadequate for revealing the degree of similarity to human disease.

C. COMPARISON OF ANIMAL MODELS

There are four different prostatic carcinomas which appear to be suitable
for experimental investigation. Particulars are given in Table I, as well
as a description of the Shionogi mouse mammary carcinoma. Functionally,
this breast tumor has much in common with prostatic carcinoma, since it
requires androgens for growth, regresses after castration, and may recur
in a hormone-deficient environment.

D. CLINICAL AND EXPERIMENTAL OBSERVATIONS
ON THE EFFECTS OF HORMONAL THERAPY

Although it is customary to describe a tumor as being hormone-dependent
if it regresses upon withdrawal of hormone, and hormone-responsive if it
regresses upon administration of hormone, the growth patterns observed
clinically and experimentally are unquestionably more varied and complex
than indicated by such definitions. A brief review of clinical responses
will serve to illustrate the fact that the reactions of a human cancer may
be difficult to reproduce even with the currently available and highly
promising tumor models described in Table 1. Knowledge of the effects of
hormonal therapy on the growth patterns of cancer is based mainly on experience with breast and endometrial carcinomas. These cancers give rise to
metastatic deposits in the lung and skin which are easier to observe than
the visceral and skeletal extensions of prostatic carcinoma. Nevertheless,
it is safe to say that in several respects all three neoplasms manifest
similar behaviour when treated by alterations in hormonal balance. The
spectrum of responses for each carcinoma is outlined in Table 2.

E. BASIC RESPONSES OF A HORMONE-SENSITIVE TISSUE

The reduction in size of a tumor in response to hormonal therapy involves
the death of large numbers of individual cells. This process appears to
be related to the fact that the proliferation of epithelial cells which
populate the breast, uterus and prostate is regulated through the expression
of three homeostatic constraint mechanisms very typical of hormone-sensitive
cells (6). The first mechanism initiates cell proliferation in response

221

Table 1. Experimental animal models for the study of prostatic carcinoma

			Animal model		
Tumor characteristic	Copenhagen rat	Lobund-Wistar rat	AXC rat	Nb rat	Shionogi DD/S mouse
1. Anatomical site of origin	dorsal prostate	prostate (lobe not specified)	ventral prostate	dorsal prostate	mammary gland
2. Transplantable	yes	yes	yes	yes	yes
3. Metastatic	yes	yes	no	yes	after i.v. injection
4. Sex hormone dependence	androgen	probably androgen	probably androgen	estrogen and androgen	androgen
5. Resistant lines	yes	yes	uncertain	yes	yes
6. Androgen metabolism	yes	unknown	yes	unknown	low
7. Androgen receptors	yes	unknown	unknown	yes	yes
8. Growth					
A. in males	fast	fast	unknown	moderately fast	fast
B. in castrated males	slow	unknown	unknown	slow	none
C. in females	slow	unknown	unknown	slow	none
9. Regression after castration	partial	unknown	unknown	partial	complete
10. Recurrence after regression	yes	unknown	unknown	yes	yes
11. Progression[a]	yes	unknown	unknown	probably	yes
References	12,21,22,36,37,40,41	11,29,30,31	33,34,35	27,28	4,5,7,23

[a] Stepwise loss of hormonal sensitivity

Table 2. Hormonal responses in carcinoma

Response	Therapeutic considerations	Carcinoma		
		Breast	Endometrium	Prostate
1. Accelerated growth	After replacement therapy	yes	yes	yes
2. Regression	A. After withdrawal therapy	yes	not routine	yes
	B. After replacement therapy	yes	yes	not routine
3. Rebound regression	After cycle of replacement and withdrawal therapy	yes	rare	rare
4. Arrest	A. After withdrawal therapy	yes	not routine	probably
	B. After replacement therapy	yes	yes	not routine
5. Progression		yes	yes	yes
6. Recurrence		yes	yes	yes
References		17,20,38,39	1,9,19,32	10

to hormone. The second stops cell proliferation when a sufficient number
of cells has been generated. The size of the organ is then maintained as
long as hormone is present, but upon its withdrawal the third mechanism,
an autophagic or self-digestion process, is mainfested, causing cell death
and reduction in the number of cells. The three mechanisms have been termed
initiation, negative-feedback and autophagia, respectively (3). Although
an epithelial cell may undergo neoplastic transformation, one or more of
the regulatory processes is likely to be conserved in the cancerous version
of the cell. Understandably, for successful therapy, the most important
of these is the autophagic mechanism (15,16).

F. THEORETICAL BASIC RESPONSES OF NEOPLASMS

The information presented in Table 2 indicates that the reaction of a tumor
in response to alterations in hormonal balance is not limited to regression.
Since autophagia is only one of three homeostatic constraint mechanisms
influencing tumor growth, other responses are theoretically possible, some
of them unfavourable to the host. Various possibilities are shown in
Table 3.

Many tumors show a deficiency in negative-feedback control, accounting for
their continuous growth. In such tumors, growth is accelerated by the
administration of hormone, owing to the fact that initiation control is
intact. Withdrawal of hormone elicits tumor regression since autophagic
control, too, is intact. Where deletion of both negative-feedback and
autophagic controls has occurred, initiation of growth remains responsive
to hormone; however, when hormone is withdrawn, growth simply stops and
the tumor mass remains constant in size. The further absence of initiation
control renders the tumor completely unresponsive; hormone has no effect
on growth because all three constraint mechanisms fail to operate. Other
growth patterns are possible depending upon whether the tumor retains the
capacity to express negative-feedback control or autophagic control in the
absence of the other two constraint mechanisms. Lastly, biphasic control
of the autophagic mechanism, as discussed in the next section, introduces
the chance of effecting the regression of a tumor by administering hormone.
These and other theoretical aspects of hormonal responsiveness in carcinoma
are reviewed in more detail elsewhere (6,8).

G. THE AUTOPHAGIC MECHANISM

Since the primitive cells that reside in an immature or unstimulated hormone-
sensitive organ show no tendency to undergo autophagic death, this capacity

Table 3. Theoretical basic responses of neoplasms

Hormonal status	Homeostatic constraint mechanisms		
	Initiation	Negative-feedback	Autophagia
Normal	+	+	+
Sensitive	+	−	+
Sensitive	+	−	−
Insensitive	−	−	−
Sensitive	−	+	−
Sensitive[a]	−	−	+ (1)
Sensitive[b]	−	−	+ (2)
Sensitive[c]	−	+	+
Sensitive[c]	+	+	−

[a] Regression after hormone withdrawal owing to biphasic control.

[b] Regression after hormone replacement owing to biphasic control.

[c] Possibly invalid combinations.

is gained only during periods of growth and maturation under the influence
of hormones. Acquirement of the property is a commonplace occurrence in
the breast during pregnancy and lactation (18), the uterine endometrium
during the menstrual cycle (14), and the prostate gland during pubertal
development (2). Although these tissues are endowed with the potential
to involute, such potential is not realized in the presence of hormone.
This implies that hormone acts as both an agonist to induce the autophagic
mechanism, and an antagonist to inhibit its activation. Biphasic control
of the autophagic mechanism probably accounts for the paradoxical responses
of breast cancer to opposite hormonal therapies (17,39). Since the cancer
in a premenopausal woman is conditioned by ovarian hormones, their withdrawal precipitates the autophagic reaction by eliminating the antagonistic
function of estradiol. On the other hand, the cancer in a postmenopausal
woman has not been conditioned by hormones. Hence the administration of
estradiol produces an unimpeded surge of agonistic activity and, consequently,
lysis of cells.

In those instances where the agonistic function of a hormone might produce
a lethal effect, cell viability is ensured by the counter-acting antagonistic
effect of the hormone. Most likely the latter is expressed through a blockade mechanism whose development in the cell must precede the earliest
appearance of the lethal process. If a cell matures for a great length of
time in a hormone-deficient environment, the blockade mechanism may fail
to develop. Thus, sudden exposure to a hormone with agonistic activity
may result in rapid killing of cells. Unusual sequences of regression and
rebound regression of tumors, such as those reported by Stoll (39) and
Bruchovsky et al (6), are probably explained on this basis.

H. CONDITIONING OF TUMORS BY STEROID HORMONES AND HINDRANCE OF PROGRESSION

The multiple factors involved in organ homeostasis, the manner in which
these are influenced by hormones (6), and the biphasic control of the
autophagic mechanism together denote a complexity of regulation that might
be expected to protect the cell against sudden conversion to the autonomous state. It follows that a few or many elements of regulation are likely
to be conserved in tumors. Conceivably, by ensuring the function of these,
the rate of autonomous change in a population of malignant cells could be
reduced. Noble (26) conducted experiments along these lines, in which he
studied the effects of fractional hormone-replacement therapy on the pro-

gression of estrogen-dependent mammary tumors in male Nb rats. The experimental protocol and results are summarized in Table 4. In controls, all 41 transplants that regressed after estrogen withdrawal and then exhibited spontaneous regrowth became autonomous. The fractional replacement of 10% estrogen did not alter the response in six animals. However, when fractional replacement was increased to 20-25% of the standard dose, there was a marked reduction in tumor progression. If therapy neither prevented complete regression nor altered regrowth, 40% of 10 tumors became autonomous. If therapy allowed only a partial regression followed by regrowth, 14% of 14 tumors became autonomous. Lastly, in four rats in which it was possible to achieve a stationary growth pattern, none of the tumors became autonomous.

Noble (28) conducted similar studies on an adenocarcinoma of the dorsal prostate in Nb rats, which grows only in estrogenized hosts. Removal of estrogen from animals with growing tumors led to tumor regression, but with progression and eventual regrowth of tumors that were autonomous. Replacement with lower doses of estrogen reduced the extent of regression and prevented autonomous change.

In summing up, Noble (26) concluded that regression per se was not a prerequisite for autonomous change; furthermore, he drew attention to the paradox that progression toward autonomous growth was accelerated with procedures expected to check tumor growth, and was minimal with procedures that accelerated it. Clearly, these observations and statements imply that fractional hormone-replacement therapy is preferable to unmodified withdrawal therapy in controlling tumor progression.

I. SPECIFIC QUESTIONS REQUIRING INVESTIGATION

In view of the variety of animal models available for study, and the numerous responses that can be followed under controlled conditions, the investigator is faced with an awesome number of potential experiments. However, this prospect becomes less formidable in scope with the realization that the therapy of prostatic cancer might be improved if a few practical questions could be answered. In this regard some specific points raised by Catalona and Scott (10) are paraphrased here. Firstly, is hormone withdrawal therapy more effective when orchidectomy is combined with postsurgical administration of estrogen? Secondly, if orchidectomy is refused, what is the preferred daily dose of estrogen? Thirdly, when is the best time to begin endocrine therapy in relation to symptoms

Table 4. Effects of fractional replacement of estrogen on growth and
progression of hormone-dependent mammary tumors in male Nb rats[a]

| No. of rats | Hormonal therapy | | | Effects | |
	Withdrawal	Replacement (% of dose)	Regression	Regrowth	Autonomous change (% of tumors)
41	+	0	+	+	100
6	+	10	+	+	100
10	+	20–25	+	+	40
14	+	20–25	±	+	14
4	+	20–25	–	–	0

[a] Condensed from data of Noble (26).

and signs of advancing disease? Lastly, should the aim of therapy be the hindrance of tumor progression, or simply the reduction of tumor mass? Which approach, if either, increases survival?

Although answers to these questions are undoubtedly long overdue, Noble's findings (26) suggest that the critical experiments are certainly capable of being done.

J. CONCLUSIONS

Several rodent animal models are now available for studying hormonal mechanisms in prostatic carcinoma. The complex growth patterns of neoplasms arising from hormone-sensitive glands and organs are attributed to the function of three homeostatic constraint mechanisms. All of these are required for a normal growth pattern, and any fewer will result in predictable deviations from it. Biphasic control of cellular autolysis introduces a further level of regulation in which the agonist and antagonist functions of a hormone are finely balanced against each other. Tumor progression in the endocrine sense is controlled and delayed by the conditioning effect of a small amount of hormone. In fact, the absence of a conditioning effect mitigates against the long-term survival of the host (25,26,28).

If practiced without regard to the risk of tumor progression, endocrine therapy may compromise the outlook of the patient. Foulds draws attention to this paradox in his monograph on neoplastic development (13). He states, "There is a disturbing possibility that therapy, by suppressing or retarding growth, may favour progression from the responsive to the unresponsive, independent state." The remedy may lie in a revised approach to therapy incorporating the fractional replacement of hormone after ablative surgery. There is little doubt that the animal models described herein are satisfactory for the experimental testing of this and other propositions.

References

1. Bonte, J., Decoster, J. M., Ide, P. and Billiet, G.: Hormonoprophylaxis hormonotherapy in the treatment of endometrial adenocarcinoma by means of medroxy-progesterone acetate. Gyn. Oncol., 6, 60-75, 1978.
2. Brandes, D.: The fine structure and histochemistry of prostate glands in relation to sex hormones. Int. Rev. Cytol., 20, 207-276, 1966.
3. Bruchovsky, N., Lesser, B., Van Doorn, E. and Craven, S.: Hormonal effects on cell proliferation in rat prostate. Vitamin

Horm., _33_, 61-102, 1975.

4. Bruchovsky, N. and Meakin, J. W.: The metabolism and binding of
    testosterone in androgen-dependent and autonomous transplantable
    mouse mammary tumors. _Cancer Res._, _33_, 1689-1695, 1973.

5. Bruchovsky, N. and Rennie, P. S.: Classification of dependent and
    autonomous variants of Shionogi mouse mammary carcinoma based on
    heterogeneous patterns of androgen binding. _Cell_, _13_, 273-280,
    1978.

6. Bruchovsky, N., Rennie, P. S., Van Doorn, E. and Noble, R. L.:
    Pathological growth of androgen sensitive tissues resulting from
    latent actions of steroid hormones. _J. Toxicol. Environ. Health_,
    _4_, 391-408, 1978.

7. Bruchovsky, N., Sutherland, D. J. A., Meakin, J. W. and Minesita,
    T.: Androgen receptors: relationship to growth response and to
    intracellular androgen transport in nine variant lines of the
    Shionogi mouse mammary carcinoma. _Biochim. Biophys. Acta_, _381_,
    61-71, 1975.

8. Bruchovsky, N. and Van Doorn, E.: Steroid receptor proteins and
    regulation of growth in mammary tumors. _Recent Results in Cancer
    Res._, _57_, 121-142, 1976.

9. Carter, S. K.: Clinical trials and avenues of research in the
    chemotherapy of endometrial carcinoma in "_Endometrial carcinoma
    and its treatment_" (Gray, L. A., ed.) pp. 195-204, Charles C.
    Thomas, Springfield, 1977.

10. Catalona, W. J. and Scott, W. W.: Carcinoma of the prostate: a
    review. _J. Urol._, _119_, 1-8, 1978.

11. Celesk, R. A. and Pollard, M.: Ultrastructural cytology of
    prostate carcinoma cells from Wistar rats. _Invest. Urol._, _14_, 95-
    99, 1976.

12. Dunning, W. F.: Prostate cancer in the rat. _Nat. Cancer Inst.
    Monograph_, _12_, 351-369, 1963.

13. Foulds, L.: _Neoplastic Development_, vol. 1, p. 73, Academic Press,
    New York, 1969.

14. Gordon, M.: Cyclic changes in the fine structure of the
    epithelial cells of human endometrium. _Int. Rev. Cytol_, _42_,
    127-172, 1975.

15. Gullino, P. M., Grantham, F. H., Losonczy, I. and Berghoffer, B.:
    Mammary tumor regression. 1. Physiopathologic characteristics
    of hormone-dependent tissue. _J. Nat. Cancer Inst._, _49_, 1333-1348,
    1972.

16. Gullino, P. M. and Lanzerotti, R. H.: Mammary tumor regression.
    II. Autophagy of neoplastic cells. _J. Nat. Cancer Inst._, _49_,
    1349-1356, 1972.

17. Heuson, J. C.: Hormones by administration in "_The Treatment of
    Breast Cancer_" (Atkins, H., ed.) pp. 113-163, University Park
    Press, Baltimore, 1974.

18. Hollmann, K. H.: Cytology and fine structure of the mammary
    gland in "_Lactation 1: The Mammary Gland/Development and
    Maintenance_" (Larson, B. L. and Smith, V. R., eds.) pp. 3-95,
    Academic Press, New York, 1974.

19. Kistner, R. W.: Endometrial and cervical cancer in "_Endocrine
    Therapy in Malignant Disease_" (Stoll, B. A., ed.) pp. 323-337,
    W. B. Saunders Company Ltd., Toronto, 1972.

20. Lee, Y. T. and Spratt, J. S.: Rate of growth of soft tissue
    metastases of breast cancer. _Cancer_, _29_, 344-348, 1972.

21. Lubaroff, D. M., Canfield, L., Feldbush, T. L. and Bonney, W. W.:
    R3327 Adenocarcinoma of the Copenhagen rat as a model for the

study of the immunologic aspects of prostate cancer. J. Nat. Cancer Inst., 58, 1677-1689, 1977.

22. Markland, F. S., Chopp, R. T., Cosgrove, M. D. and Howard, E. B.: Characterization of steroid hormone receptors in the Dunning R-3327 rat prostatic adenocarcinoma. Cancer Res., 38, 2818-2826, 1978.

23. Minesita, T. and Yamaguchi, K.: An androgen-dependent mouse mammary tumor. Cancer Res., 25, 1168-1175, 1965.

24. Moore, R. A. and Melchionna, R. H.: Production of tumors of the prostate of white rat with 1:2-benzpyrene. Amer. J. Cancer, 30, 731-741, 1937.

25. Noble, R. L.: A new approach to the hormonal cause and control of experimental carcinomas, including those of the breast. Ann. Roy. Coll. Phys. Surg. Can., 9, 170-180, 1976.

26. Noble, R. L.: Hormonal control of growth and progression in tumors of Nb rats and a theory of action. Cancer Res., 37, 82-94, 1977.

27. Noble, R. L.: The development of prostatic adenocarcinoma in Nb rats following prolonged sex hormone administration. Cancer Res., 37, 1929-1933, 1977.

28. Noble, R. L.: Sex steroids as a cause of adenocarcinoma of the dorsal prostate in Nb rats, and their influence on the growth of transplants. Oncology, 34, 138-141, 1977.

29. Pollard, M.: Metastatic adenocarcinoma of the prostate. Amer. J. Path., 86, 277-280, 1977.

30. Pollard, M., Chang, C. F. and Burleson, G. R.: Investigations on prostate adenocarcinomas in rats. Cancer Treat. Rep., 61, 153-156, 1977.

31. Pollard, M. and Luckert, P. H.: Transplantable metastasizing prostate adenocarcinomas in rats. J. Nat. Cancer Inst., 54, 643-649, 1975.

32. Reifenstein, E. C.: Hydroxyprogesterone caproate therapy in advanced endometrial cancer. Cancer, 27, 485-502, 1971.

33. Shain, S. A., McCullough, B., Nitchuk, M. and Boesel, R. W.: Prostate carcinogenesis in the AXC rat. Oncology, 34, 114-122, 1977.

34. Shain, S. A., McCullough, B. and Segaloff, A.: Spontaneous adenocarcinomas of the ventral prostate of aged AXC rats. J. Nat. Cancer Inst., 55, 177-180, 1975.

35. Shain, S. A., Nitchuk, W. M. and McCullough, B.: C_{19}-Steroid metabolism by spontaneous adenocarcinoma of the AXC rat ventral prostate. J. Nat. Cancer Inst., 58, 747-751, 1977.

36. Smolev, J. K., Coffey, D. S. and Scott, W. W.: Experimental models for the study of prostatic adenocarcinoma. J. Urol., 118, 216-220, 1977.

37. Smolev, J. K., Heston, W. D. W., Scott, W. W. and Coffey, D. S.: Characterization of the Dunning R3327H prostatic adenocarcinoma: an appropriate animal model for prostatic cancer. Cancer Treat. Rep., 61, 273-287, 1977.

38. Stoll, B. A.: Hormonal management in Breast Cancer, pp. 13-19, Lipincott, Philadelphia, 1970.

39. Stoll, B. A.: Palliation by castration or by hormone administration in "Breast Cancer Management, Early and Late" (Stoll, B. A., ed.) pp. 133-146, Year Book Medical Publishers, Chicago, 1977.

40. Voigt, W. and Dunning, W. F.: In vivo metabolism of testosterone-$3H$ in R-3327, an androgen-sensitive rat prostatic adenocarcinoma. Cancer Res., 34, 1447-1450, 1974.

41. Voigt, W., Feldman, M. and Dunning, W. F.: 5α-Dihydrotestosterone-
    binding proteins and androgen sensitivity in prostatic cancers of
    Copenhagen rats. Cancer Res., 35, 1840-1846, 1975.

CHAPTER XIV. EXPERIMENTAL CONCEPTS IN THE DESIGN OF NEW TREATMENTS
FOR HUMAN PROSTATIC CANCER[*]

The purpose of this chapter is to review briefly some of the recent concepts that are providing new directions for the study and treatment of
prostatic cancer.

Tumor Cell Kinetics

Cell kinetics have provided valuable insights into the treatment of many
types of human cancer (12). A simple mathematical analysis of tumor growth
indicates the magnitude of the problems that the clinician must face in
controlling this disease. For example, the now classic studies of Skipper
and his associates (48) demonstrated, in animal models, that one cancer
cell is capable of continued growth that will ultimately kill the host.
In addition, a drug treatment regimen kills a constant percent of the tumor
cells that are present, irrespective of the total number of cells (47).
Since one cubic centimeter of tumor volume contains about one billion (10^9)
tumor cells, a very effective drug treatment that kills 99.99% of the cells
would still leave 100,000 viable tumor cells and the patient would succumb
ultimately to the continuing growth of these remaining cells. It is apparent from these simple calculations, that have been tested in many model
systems, that strict restraints are imposed on therapeutic approaches that
are governed by cell kinetic considerations. Simplified cell kinetic
calculations provide idealized limits but must be modified by practical
considerations that include such complications as limited growth from
restricted circulation, cell death and turnover, necrosis, and tumor cell
heterogeneity. These limitations usually decrease the calculated therapeutic advantage. Nevertheless the importance of cell kinetic concepts
for tumor growth may be better understood from the following calculations
and discussions.

After a single prostate cell is transformed into a cancer cell it initiates
uncontrolled cell division and growth. At first, each division doubles the
cell number and, thus, doubles the tumor volume. The time required for the

[*] Chapter prepared by Donald S. Coffey and John T. Isaacs, James Buchanan
Brady Urological Institute, The Johns Hopkins University School of
Medicine, Baltimore, Maryland 21205, U.S.A. This work was supported by
Grant No. CA15416, awarded by the National Cancer Institute, DHEW.

tumor to accomplish this is referred to as the doubling time of the tumor. The consequence of 1 cell doubling 40 times is striking because of the exponential nature of cell accumulation (Table 1). When 1 cancer cell

Table 1

The Results of a Single Prostate Tumor Cell Doubling 40 Times[*]

No. Cell Divisions (Tumor Doublings)	Total Number of Tumor Cells	Tumor Vol. (cc)	Comparison
0	1	10^{-9}	Original tumor cell
1	2	2×10^{-9}	
2	4	4×10^{-9}	
3	8	8×10^{-9}	
5	32	3.2×10^{-8}	
10	1,024	1×10^{-6}	
15	32,768	32×10^{-6}	
20	1,048,576 (1 million)	0.001	one milligram wt.
25	33,554,432	0.033	minimal size for visualization
27	134,217,728	0.134	pea size
30	1,073,741,824 (1 billion)	1.0	one gram wt.
40	1,099,511,755,776 (trillion)	1,099	2.2 pounds, 1 liter, 1 kilogram
		Death	

DIAGNOSIS (spanning rows 25–30)

*Maximum number of cells. Does not consider cell death or loss.

divides or doubles 25 times the tumor volume is approximately the size of a match head (0.03 cc); this is about the smallest size that can be detected by direct visualization. By 30 cell divisions it is 1 cc and the 1 cell has now increased to 1 billion cells. Somewhere between 25 and 30 divisions the original tumor cell will have reached a tumor lesion size that can be detected through rectal examination. By 10 additional divisions, to a total of 40 divisions, the tumor mass is 1 liter in volume, weighs more than 2 pounds and could obviously be enough to kill a patient. Thus, it is possible that the majority of the time (1 to 24 divs.) a tumor grows, it cannot be detected at the clinical level by direct visualization or palpation. If one assumes a match head sized tumor (0.03 cc) to be the lower limit of direct visualization then one can predict from the known doubling

234

time how long a tumor would need to grow before it could possibly be detected. Unfortunately, the real tumor doubling time of human prostate cancers is not known. In a study of 530 human cancers of many types, Charbit and associates reported a mean doubling time for human cancer of 58 days (10). The doubling time, of course, varied with the pathological nature and type of cancer but the 58-day value was the overall mean and has been supported by several studies (25, 26). Therefore, for perspective, if one considered 25 doublings at 58 days, it would require 4 years for 1 cell to grow to the size of a match head. If diagnosed at this size the tumor will grow to 2 pounds in only an additional 2 1/2 years, the time required for 15 more doublings (15 divisions x 58 days/365 days = 2.38 years). Therefore, from onset of the first prostate cell to death would be a total of 6 1/2 years. If tumor cells were lost, or cells went out of the growth phase, the times would be longer, therefore this represents minimal time. Table 2 represents a series of theoretical calculations for various doubling times ranging from 15 to 365 days. The time to first possible visualization for diagnosis (0.03 cc) and to a reasonable size for host death (1 liter) is determined.

Table 2. Effect of Tumor Doubling Time on Minimal Time for One Prostate Cell to Progress to Size for Diagnosis and Host Death[*]

Doubling Time of Tumor Vol.[†] (days)	25 Doublings Growth Time to Reach Minimal Size for Visualization - Tumor Vol.,0.03 cc[‡] (yrs)	40 Doublings Theoretical Time to Death - Tumor Vol., 1 liter[§] (yrs)	Survival Time From Diagnosis to Death[+] (yrs)
15	1.0	1.6	0.6
30	2.0	3.3	1.3
60	4.1	6.6	2.5
90	6.2	9.9	3.7
180	12.3	19.7	7.4
365	25.0	40.0	15.0

[*]Minimal theoretical times. Calculated for no cell losses or decreases in growth fraction or rate. These factors, when present, would slow growth and would increase these times. [†]Determined by cell division time. Potential tumor doubling time. [‡]Minimum of 25 cell divisions is required for 1 tumor cell to reach tumor volume of 3/100 cc, that is limiting size for direct visualization and earliest possible time for diagnosis. Doubling time x 25 produces this time value. [§]Minimum time for 1 cell to grow to a tumor volume of 1 liter (2.2 pounds); (doubling time) x (40). This is in the size range to produce host death. [+]Difference in minimal time from diagnosis (25 doublings) to theoretical death (40 doublings).

These values in Table 2 represent minimal times because they do not consider several very important factors, all of which slow the observed growth
rate. First, cell loss and death can be considerable and would remove cells
from the tumor. In a normal steady state cell loss is equivalent to cell
death and the fraction of tumor cells lost to the system can be considerable
in many tumors. In addition, as a tumor grows large,limitations in growth,
vascularization and central necrosis ensue, all slowing the growth fraction
of the tumor and the cell doubling time. These factors are now being resolved in a quantitative manner for many solid human tumors but this has
not been accomplished for human cancer. Since all of these complications
slow the doubling time the values of Table 2 are an underestimate. It
would take longer than the indicated times in Table 2.

The results of one cell doubling at each division are presented in Figure 1.
The analysis of cell growth kinetics can be visualized graphically.

Figure 1.

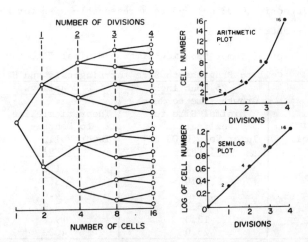

As shown, one cell undergoes four consecutive divisions yielding respectively, 2, 4, 8 and 16 cells. The growth of cell numbers can be plotted
arithmetically which shows the exponential growth as a rapid rise in cell
number with each ensuing division. Clinically the growth in tumor volume
appears to increase rapidly with time but this is actually only the result
of a constant doubling time that yields ever increasing numbers of cells
through the accumulative effects of tumor doublings or divisions. A linear
relationship is observed if the log of the cell number is plotted with time
or divisions. This semi-log plot produces a linear relationship and the

236

slope is related to the tumor growth rate. The tumor doubling time may be derived by measuring the tumor size between two early time intervals and using the following equation:

$$\text{Tumor Doubling Time in Days} = \frac{(\text{days of growth})}{\left[\dfrac{\log(\text{final vol.}) - \log(\text{initial vol.})}{\log 2}\right]}$$

The tumor volume is determined by measuring three diameters in centimeters and using the formula of Janek (23):

[length x width x height x 0.5236] = volume of tumor in cubic centimeters

Precision calipers are used in these measurements. For example, the above methods have been applied in analyzing tumor growth curves of the Dunning R-3327 series of transplantable rat prostatic adenocarcinomas (51, 60).

As the rat prostate tumors grow larger in volume they begin to deviate from a linear relationship in the semi-log plots (60). This decrease in growth rate is often associated with lack of proper vascularization, expulsion of cells and cell death from overcrowding and the presence of toxins or growth inhibitory factors. The effect of these limitations on growth is a progressive slowdown in the observed tumor doubling time. Many factors such as tumor growth rate, angiogenesis and tumor cell types will govern this slowdown with size. The change in doubling times with accumulated cell number is variable and the following example has been presented in a mathematical model (42).

Table 3

Alteration in Tumor Doubling Time

with Increasing Tumor Mass

[Adapted from Salmon (42)]

Tumor Size (Cell number)	Doubling Time (days)
1 to 2	2.34
10^3 to 2×10^3	3.15
10^6 to 2×10^6	4.31
10^9 to 2×10^9	10.2
10^{11} to 2×10^{11}	40.1

The above change in tumor growth rates as a function of increasing tumor volumes is described by Gompertzian kinetics and is discussed in detail elsewhere (42).

Since prostate cancers appear to have a slow growth rate it is probable that few cells are in DNA synthesis at any given time. This can be determined by DNA labeling and may be well below 5% of the total cells. Since most cancer chemotherapeutic agents block DNA synthesis it would be expected that most of these drugs would have very little therapeutic effect against prostate cancer. As these tumors become larger in volume, the growth rate continues to decline at which point the drugs would have even less of an effect.

Several important parameters are required to determine the growth kinetics of tumors, and they can vary with tumor types and sizes. The following are examples of these values that have been reported for four different types of solid human cancers, none of which were prostate cancers (56).

Table 4

Mean Kinetic Parameters of Various Histological

Types of Human Tumors (Non-Prostatic)

Adapted from Tubiana and Malaise (56); Charbit et al. (10);

and Malaise et al. (28)

Type of Human Cancer	Tumor[a] Doubling Time (days)	DNA[b] Labeling Index (%)	Growth[c] Fraction (%)	Cell Loss Factor (%)	Daily turnover rate (%)	Chemosensitivity
Embryonal	27	30	90	93	49	+ +
Malignant Lymphomas	29	29	90	93	47	+ +
Squamous Cell Carcinoma	58	8	25	89	10	+
Adeno- carcinomas	83	2	6	71	2	±

(a) Time in days for tumor to double in volume   (c) % of cells in growth cycle

(b) Percent of total cells labeled, S phase

The data in the above table and the methods by which the values are determined are discussed in more detail in the review by Tubiana (56). This type of cell kinetics information is not available for any prostatic tumor of man or in the several reported animal models.

At present most of the solid human tumors have been very refractory to
chemotherapy and radiation control. This is certainly the case for human
prostate cancer. To circumvent this problem, attention has been given to
adjuvant therapy for the control of other types of solid tumors (43).
A hypothetical approach to how cell kinetic considerations could be applied
to a human prostatic cancer is presented in Table 5. A 25 gram human prostatic cancer would contain about 25×10^9 cells. Surgery could reduce the
total tumor cells by 90% leaving possibly 25×10^8 in metastatic or remaining sites. Effective combination chemotherapy or hormonal therapy could
reduce the remaining tumor cells by 99% leaving 25×10^6 tumor cells.
Following recovery of the immune system from chemotherapy, an immunopoten-
tiating agent might kill the last remaining 25×10^6 cells producing a
tumor free host. Immunotherapy appears to be effective against small tumor
loads of approximately 10^7 cells, therefore, the 25×10^6 cells remaining
would approach a level capable of total eradication by immunotherapy. This
hypothetical therapeutic model would require that the human prostatic cancer
should have antigenic properties allowing it to respond to immunotherapy;
this may be feasible because it has now been demonstrated that human prostatic adenocarcinoma has a tumor associated antigen (4). Furthermore,
since a large cell kill is required through chemotherapy, hormonal therapy,
by reducing the cell mass of many prostatic cancers, is in a sense a potent
form of chemotherapy.

Table 5

Hypothetical Model of Adjuvant Therapy of a 25 g Human
Prostatic Adenocarcinoma

Sequential therapy	Prostatic cancer load		% of tumor cells removed by therapy	Number of tumor cells remaining
	tumor weight	total cell number		
Initial state	25 g	25×10^9	0%	25×10^9
Surgery	25 g	25×10^9	90%	25×10^8
Hormonal and non-hormonal combination chemotherapy	2.5 g	25×10^8	99%	25×10^6
Immuno-therapy	0.025 g	25×10^6	10^7 cell kill potential	0 (cure)

Combinations of surgery, chemotherapy and immunotherapy have been applied to arrest the growth of some rat prostatic adenocarcinomas with some reported success (60). These adjuvant treatments have been developed through theoretical considerations of cell kinetic studies that have provided the basis for a more rational approach to the treatment of cancer (43). Careful studies of experimental models, and well designed and analyzed clinical trials should soon provide some new beneficial treatments that utilize combination and adjuvant therapy.

Heterogeneity of Prostatic Tumors

At present we have available several hormonal therapeutic approaches to retard or to block the growth of androgen-sensitive cells; this includes castration and/or estrogen therapy. The problem is that an androgen-insensitive prostatic growth ensues and this kills the patient. This may be the result of heterogeneity of the tumor. Furthermore, this tumor cell heterogeneity may account for other drug resistant states and may have an important role in the mechanism of metastasis.

1.) Androgen insensitivity: What is the mechanism through which an androgen-sensitive tumor is converted to an androgen-insensitive state? Several models have been proposed to explain this conversion and they include cell adaptation and/or cell selection. Those favoring selection believe that the tumor is heterogeneous and contains a mixed population of androgen-sensitive and -insensitive cells (51, 50, 21, 22).

As discussed in the previous chapter on the Dunning R-3327 rat prostatic adenocarcinomas, it now appears that these animal tumors are heterogeneous in composition. This means that an individual tumor may contain mixed populations of cells (also called clones) that possess different properties. With cell kinetic analysis it has been demonstrated that the R-3327-H tumor is composed of 80% androgen-sensitive cells and 20% androgen-insensitive (51, 50). The hormone-insensitive state that develops during relapse following castration is simply the continued growth of the androgen-insensitive cells (51,50,21,22). The following table illustrates the mathematical principles of this phenomenon in a tumor system that divides or doubles every 20 days.

Table 6

Mathematical Model for the Conversion of Prostatic Cancer
from an Androgen-Sensitive to -Insensitive State

(Tumor Doubles Every 20 Days)

Tumor Composition	Origin	Div. 1	Div. 2	Div. 5	Div. 10		Div. 11	Div. 12	Div. 13
	Day 0	Day 20	Day 40	Day 100	Day 200	Day 200	Day 220	Day 240	Day 260
Androgen	1	2	4	32	1024	C A S T R A T I O N	0	0	0
Sensitive	1	2	4	32	1024		0	0	0
Cells	1	2	4	32	1024		0	0	0
	1	2	4	32	1024		0	0	0
Androgen Insensitive Cells	1	2	4	32	1024		2048	4096	8192
Total Tumor Cells	5	10	20	160	5120		2048	4096	8192

The above illustration (Table 6) is for a single prostate tumor that contains
5 cells at the origin; 4 of these cells require the presence of androgen for
growth and one cell will grow in the absence of androgens. Both the androgen-
sensitive cells and the insensitive cells divide every twenty days. For
example, after ten divisions, that would require 200 days of growth, each of
the original cells would have grown to 1,024 cells. If after this 200 days
of growth, the animal is castrated, the androgen-sensitive cells would involute, leaving only the 1,024 cells that had stemmed from the original cell
which was androgen-insensitive. These cells would continue to grow in the
castrate and by three more divisions (Div. 13) would have grown in 60 more
days to a number exceeding the total tumor size just prior to castration.
This indicates how a tumor may respond to castration and then rapidly relapse
to an androgen-insensitive state. The response to castration would be
dependent on a.) the percent of cells in the total tumor that are androgen-
sensitive and b.) the doubling time of the tumor cells. If there were any
cells present that were androgen-insensitive, one would not anticipate a
cure from castration; this may be the general case in human prostatic cancer.

The example in Table 6 illustrates what is actually observed in an animal tumor model for prostatic cancer (51, 50).

What is the evidence for cell heterogeneity associated with human prostatic cancer? This is supported by microscopic examination of prostatic tumor. Different areas of an individual case of prostate cancer may yield a wide variety of tumor cell types and variable pathology (9). Areas of an individual tumor that are very anaplastic and undifferentiated may also reside with areas of well differentiated tumor cells (9). There may be a wide variety of cell sizes, architecture and tumor cell types within a single tumor. In addition, the amount of DNA or chromosome content can vary in prostate cancer over a wide range of ploidy.

GENETIC INSTABILITY

Figure 2.

Three models for the development of tumor cell heterogeneity. Black and white circles indicate tumor cells with different properties.

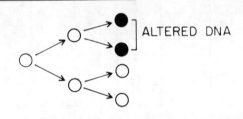

ALTERED DNA

ADAPTATION

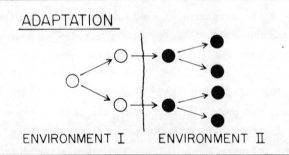

ENVIRONMENT I   ENVIRONMENT II

MULTIFOCAL ORIGIN

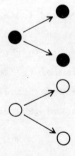

What has not been resolved is the mechanisms that produced this state of cellular heterogeneity. There are several models that might explain this development of tumor cell heterogeneity but at present none have been proven. These models include: (see Fig. 2)

1.) Genetic instability: the original tumor developed in a single cell but as growth continued, progeny cells became unstable and a change occurred in the DNA that was transmitted to subsequent daughter cells. If the genetic instability continued it would soon produce a wide variety of cell types within a tumor. Dr. Peter Nowell has proposed such a model as a general state of cancer (39). It is also recognized that the amount of DNA or chromosome content of a tumor cell can be altered with continued growth often resulting in a state of polyploidy to the more variable aneuploidy. This would indicate a wide variety of genetic compositions within the cells making up these tumors. If this genetic instability were reflected in alteration in tumor cell properties such as drug sensitivity, metabolism, hormone sensitivity, metastatic potential and growth rates, one would face a very difficult therapeutic problem. Since drug resistance is the major reason for therapeutic failure at the present, this potential heterogeneity is not good news and may account for our lack of success in the treatment of many solid human tumors.

At present there is no firm knowledge on what produces genetic instability, although many believe that the process of DNA repair may be altered. It is known that continued cell turnover and renewal can cause some misreading of the genetic code. In addition, random damage to DNA occurs from chemical reactions within the cell and from external chemical and physical events such as carcinogens and mutagens. The cell has an elaborate system of DNA repair to correct or minimize these alterations in the DNA genome. The genetic drift seen in tumors may be either the result of inadequate repair or increased alterations in the DNA.

2.) Adaptation: This type of model proposes that heterogeneous tumor cells are developed from environmental pressures on the cells that produce adaptations in differentiation but not an irreversible change in the DNA. For example, as shown in Figure 2, the prostate cells in environment I might have androgens present and cells stay differentiated requiring androgens for full growth rate. As the cells are then transferred to areas that are androgen deficient, environment II, they then convert to cells with different properties. These states are not irreversible and could be

243

affected by altering the cellular environment. Another chapter in this text by Dr. Nicholas Bruchovsky describes studies with the Nobel rat prostatic adenocarcinoma that might support this type of model, however, the authors recognize that other explanations of their data are also possible.

3.) <u>Multifocal origin</u>: Heterogeneity may be the result of a multifocal origin of prostatic cancer. This model indicates that the original event that transformed the normal prostate cell to the cancer state occurred in more than one cell. Since a single prostate gland contains 25 billion cells, a number more than 6 times the human population of the earth, it is not inconceivable that any carcinogen, virus or random chemical event could occur in more than one cell. Multifocal prostatic cancer has been proposed from careful pathological sectioning (8). Other tumors such as bladder cancer are known to be multifocal.

Even tumors that now appear to be monoclonal could conceivably have originated as multifocal lesions. For example, <u>the tumor cell that has the most rapid growth rate will ultimately out grow the slower cells and in doing so, will enrich the tumor in these rapidly growing cells</u>. As this overgrowth becomes more dominant the tumor will appear as a monoclonal tumor composed only of these rapidly growing cells. This process can be visualized in the following Figure 3.

<u>Figure 3.</u>
Conversion of a Heterogeneous Tumor
Towards an Apparently Monoclonal Tumor

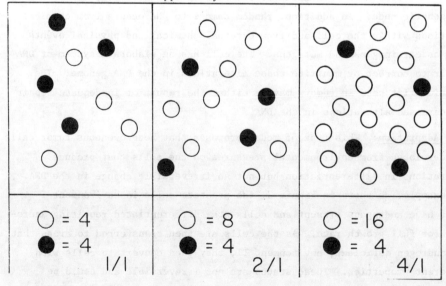

In this example the tumor at some point in time is composed of 50% black cells and 50% white cells. If the white cells could divide twice before the black cells could divide once, the ratio of white to black cells would go from 1/1 to 4/1 in only two divisions. If the growth rates of two cell types were close, but even slightly different, the faster growing cells would dominate by over 90% in just a few divisions. This is demonstrated in Table 7.

Table 7

Enrichment of Multifocal Tumor Towards a Monoclonal State
by Different Growth Rates of Subpopulations of Cells: Hypothetical
Calculations

| | Number of Cells in Tumor | | | Tumor Composition | |
Time of Growth	Cell Type A Divides 10 days	Cell Type B Divides 20 days	Total Cells in Tumor	% A	% B
(days)	(cells)	(cells)	(cells)	(%)	(%)
Start	1,000	1,000	2,000	50	50
10	2,000	1,000	3,000	67	33
20	4,000	2,000	6,000	67	33
30	8,000	2,000	10,000	80	20
40	16,000	4,000	20,000	80	20
50	32,000	4,000	36,000	89	11
60	64,000	8,000	72,000	89	11
70	128,000	8,000	136,000	94	6

For a tumor to possess a series of distinct cell types that are maintained in constant proportion for time, requires similar growth rates for the individual cell types. This is the case for the Dunning R-3327 animal tumor which contains a population of hormone-sensitive cells with an almost identical growth rate (21 day doubling) to the hormone-insensitive cells (51, 50). However, if because of any reason of genetic stability or otherwise, a group of cells develops with a faster growth rate, they will grow out and become the dominant and apparent single type of cell. This proved to be the case in the development of the anaplastic R-3327-AT tumor which divides every 2 days and therefore grows 10 times more rapidly than the R-3327 tumor of origin.

In summary, there appears to be little doubt that human prostate cancer is composed of a heterogeneous group of tumor cells. How this heterogeneity

develops has not been resolved. It is possible that it may develop from
a combination of a multifocal origin combined with a degree of genetic
instability.

While much of the discussion in this paper has focused on the development
of androgen-insensitive state or relapse to drug therapy, it is important
to also realize that heterogeneity can be observed within tumors to a wide
variety of properties. The following properties have been reported to be
heterogeneous in other tumor systems and it will be of interest if these
can be confirmed also in the human prostate. These heterogeneous properties include: metastatic potential (14), drug resistance (19),
antigenic properties (40, 24), growth rates (44), hormone receptor
content (49) and pigment production (18).

Dormant Cancer Cells

The effects of continued growth of heterogeneous cells have been discussed,
but is it also possible for tumor cells to leave the growth state and enter
a quiescent, static or non-growing state? This appears to be the case for
the well known and common form of latent prostate cancer (15, 16). Indeed,
these latent cancers appear in 30% of men over 50 years of age and are found
at the time of autopsy but gave no clinical manifestations; these lesions
are histologically identical to the active prostatic adenocarcinomas and
yet they have not grown or killed the patient (15,16). Do these latent
tumors represent a.) very slow growth rates, b.) growth rates matched by
tumor cell turnover (due to cell loss or death or immunological mediated
control) or c.) tumor cells that have entered a dormant, non-growing
condition produced by cell contact or cellular environment (chalones, etc.)?

Can this development of silent tumor cells also occur in a clinically
manifest prostate cancer by reversing from an active to an inactive form?
This would mean that actively growing and dividing cells would leave the
cell cycle and enter the non-growing state (G_o phase). There are isolated
reports of this having occurred, but the frequency of this event is still
unknown. For example, it has been reported that 20 years following a
total prostatectomy for prostate cancer, that a distant metastasis
appeared. Unless these cells had a doubling time of over 6 months (1 cell
to 1 cubic centimeter is 30 doublings), it would appear that the tumor in
the metastatic area had remained dormant. A review of the general biology
of tumor cell dormancy is available (61).

Prostate Metastasis: The Result of Tumor Heterogeneity?

Prostate cancer, like many other human tumors, appears to have a preferen-
tial site for the development of distant metastasis (1   ). It has long
perplexed clinicians as to why certain types of human tumors prefer specific
sites for metastases (59,62). There is variation of the extent of metastasis even within a single type of cancer that has been difficult to predict.
In prostate cancer osseous metastasis is the most prevalent form of visceral
metastasis. Other common sites include the lung, liver and adrenals and,
of course, lymphatic metastasis, which is most common. The available
evidence would seem to suggest that lymphatic and bone metastasis may occur
independently. Much discussion has ensued regarding blood flow, lymphatic
drainage and other physical methods involved in the transport of prostatic
cancer cells and these concepts have been discussed in more detail in a
recent review (9). Comprehensive reviews of the biology of metastasis are
available (59,62,11).

Several important questions arise: a.) how large does a tumor mass have to be
before cancer cells reach capillaries and venous drainage? b.) are all
cancer cells capable of metastasis? c.) what percent of the cancer cells
which find their way into the hematogenous system are then capable of
establishing distant metastatic lesions? d.) do certain cancer cells within
a tumor have a predisposed tendency for certain visceral organs and is this
mechanism different than simple physical filtration? e.) do all cancer cells
from a single tumor have the ability to grow in any organ in which they are
placed? These and many similar questions are now being answered as other
experimental tumors and our preliminary studies with animal prostatic tumors
seem to indicate that they are applicable to the prostate. Indeed these
new observations appear to be general oncological phenomena and since they
change our view of the mechanism of metastasis, they deserve review and
discussuon. For a detailed discussion of tumor heterogeneity and the
biology of cancer invasion and metastasis, consult the classical reviews
by Isaiah Fidler (14), G. L. Nicolson (37). L Weiss (59), and
R. A. Willis (62). Fidler (14) has pointed out that tumor cells are
heterogeneous and that only some of these variant cells are capable of
metastasis. Very microscopic tumor masses release emboli of cancer cells
into the blood and only a small percent of these cells survive and enter
visceral organs (approximately 0.1% of the cells in the emboli). Specific
cell variants within the tumor are predisposed to grow in certain visceral
organs and these cell types can be cloned from a tumor. Fidler concludes

that metastasis is a selection process of subpopulations of tumor cells from a heterogeneous tumor that favors the establishment of growth in specific organ sites. A successful metastasis requires a large variety of events which is the result of an interplay between the tumor and the host. Prostate tumors have very different malignant and metastatic potential and these properties may involve the heterogeneity and cell kinetic events that were previously discussed. The presence of micrometastasis in prostate cancer has a devastating effect on prognosis and the availability of new animal model systems with a variety of metastatic potentials will assist the study of the control of these events.

New Experimental Approaches for the Future Treatment of Prostatic Cancer

No one knows if there is any real cure rate with our present hormonal treatment (castration and/or estrogen treatment) of disseminated prostatic cancer but if it does exist, it is certainly very low and probably less than 0.1%. So for all practical purposes we must consider a cure with standard therapy as essentially nonexistent. The use of the phrase "cure" has itself been the topic of much debate; what is meant is the long term (>5 yr.) tumor-free state following complete remission from therapy. Cure is even a more elusive term for prostate cancer because it grows very slowly, may remain latent, and in many cases is most difficult to evaluate or detect. In addition, many elderly patients live out the normalized life expectancy with varying tumor loads or succumb to other age associated illnesses. It has been claimed that this standard hormonal therapy increases survival or improves the well being of the patient but the exact extent of this benefit has been debated; the word palliative treatment is best used to describe the present state of therapy. For a discussion of some of these issues see the recent reviews by Catalona and Scott (9), Menon and Walsh (31), and Murphy (35).

Most urologists have witnessed many cases in which there have been dramatic regression of tumor lesions and symptoms of prostatic cancer following castration and estrogen therapy, however, with very few exceptions, these cases are invariably followed by relapse. This has made it difficult to test cancer chemotherapeutic agents prior to standard hormonal therapy because of the general feeling that one should not deprive the patient of the potential benefits of standard hormonal therapy.

Prostate cancer is like most other solid human tumors in being very refractory to most of the common cancer chemotherapeutic agents. However, in honesty, very few of these drugs have actually been tested in a randomized and carefully controlled clinical trial. Efforts to circumvent this have been made through the comprehensive and cooperative clinical trials sponsored by the National Prostatic Cancer Project of the National Cancer Institute, U.S.A. At present, those drugs that have been tested have not been highly effective although most trials have been in very advanced cases that are relapsing from standard hormonal therapy, and have utilized drug dosages that have been reduced to levels consistent with advanced age and outpatient therapy protocols. The results of these trials and how they were conducted and evaluated will be discussed in more detail in a following chapter by Dr. John Horton.

If prostatic cancer is ever to be controlled on a long term basis or eradicated fully, we must first develop some new therapeutic approaches. The following discussion will attempt to outline some current as well as new concepts that may be helpful in approaching this endeavor. We will not attempt a comprehensive review or to give credit to the historical development of these ideas because serious students may find this information elsewhere in the oncology literature. We will only focus on the therapy of prostate cancer, an area that has unfortunately lagged far behind other neoplasias in therapeutic progress. It is also important to develop some new approaches for cancer therapy of solid human tumors; the present situation is not very effective.

OUTLINE OF THERAPEUTIC APPROACHES (OLD, NEW AND THEORETICAL) THAT MAY BE USEFUL IN THE CONTROL OF PROSTATE CANCER

1.) Hormonal therapy: treatment designed to interfere with hormonal requirements for prostate tumor growth. In the early part of the 1940's, when Charles Huggins, Clarence Hodges, William W. Scott and others at the University of Chicago, studied the effects of castration, androgen and estrogens on normal prostatic function it appeared that these hormonal factors might also affect prostatic cancer growth. This logic proved true and the first effective therapeutic treatment of human tumors was initiated in 1943, and for the introduction of hormonal therapy, Huggins was the recipient of a Nobel Prize in 1966. The basic approach was to lower serum androgen levels by castration and/or estrogen treatment. Since then, many approaches have been utilized to further diminish these low levels of serum androgens in the belief that these postcastration levels may still be involved in the almost invariable relapse to castration and estrogen; these additional approaches have included adrenalectomy and hypophysectomy. This has not proven to be very promising or accepted as standard therapy although claims are still made of some benefits. If indeed the relapse following hormonal therapy is due to a clone of androgen-insensitive cells as discussed earlier, it would be apparent why these approaches may have failed.

At present, a clinical approach is to use low estrogen doses (<5 mg) to suppress LH release and to minimize estrogen toxicity. Little is known regarding direct prostate cytotoxic effects of estrogens at higher doses. It is known that estrogen receptors are present in prostate cancer cells and their function is unknown. Many clinicians have claimed that prostate tumors that lack response or relapse to low estrogen treatment may respond to very high estrogen therapy; this needs to be resolved. For example, estracyt, an alkylating analog of estradiol, is administered at very high levels and it is difficult to separate the two functions of this drug. Although it has shown some effects in patients relapsing from low estrogen dosage, it has been proposed by some to function primarily as an alkylating agent (32, 33).

It is also important to realize that estrogens are often administered as non-steroid drugs such as diethylstilbestrol (DES) which is a synthetic compound. Although this drug is under common usage, we have very little insight into its full metabolism and pharmacodynamics, such as the half-life of the levels in blood and tissues. Also, there are some hormonal and clinical differences between 17β-estradiol, the natural steroid estrogen, and DES, the non-steroid synthetic compound. Other derivatives and conjugates of these estrogens (phosphates, polyphosphates, glucuronides, etc.) have been tried, but at present no clear advantage has been established. For more details on the hormonal control of prostate cancer, consult recent reviews (9, 31, 35, 33).

Estrogens not only lower androgen levels through inhibiting LH stimulation of the Leydig cells in testes, but they also have been proposed to block androgen synthesis directly within the Leydig cells. They also stimulate the blood levels of steroid binding globulins and have a wide variety of pharmacological and physiological effects within the male [see recent review (29)].

It is very important to recognize that androgens plus estrogens do not inhibit but on the contrary, can stimulate or synergize prostatic growth and estrogens with androgens have been proposed as a possible agent in the etiology of canine benign prostatic hyperplasia (58). The effects of estrogen and androgen on human prostate cancer has not been determined; however, the only reported induction of prostate cancer in animals has been in the Noble rat tumor that was induced following estrone and testosterone administration (38).

Other growth factors have been proposed to affect prostate growth and these have included prolactin, insulin, and more recently, epidermal growth factors. At present, inhibition of prolactin release has not proven very promising. The role of the other stimulatory factors has proven even more vague. Hypophysectomy should have certainly affected a wide variety of these growth factors.

Natural inhibitory factors of tissue growth, defined as chalones, have not been characterized for the prostate.

Since it now appears that the prostate glands contain androgen, estrogen, progesterone and prolactin receptors that may vary with the pathological state of the gland and that many of these hormones may themselves regulate other hormone receptor levels within the prostate, it therefore should not be assumed that no therapeutic advantage can be developed in androgen-insensitive cells with hormone directed therapeutic agents. This is particularly the case since it has been reported that the androgen-insensitive Dunning R-3327-HI tumor still contains levels of estrogen, androgen and progesterone receptors (20). For these reasons, it would seem important to test further the antiandrogens, antiestrogens and antiprogesterones in the treatment of prostatic cancer. Of these anti-hormones, only the antiandrogens (cyproterone acetate, Medrogestrone and Flutamide) have received limited studies on prostate cancer. The structure of these drugs is somewhat surprising; for example, if one were developing structural steroid analogs to compete with C-19 androgen action such as dihydrotestosterone, they may not anticipate that the C-21 progesterone derivatives which are structurally different from androgens would prove to be the most effective antiandrogens. For example, cyproterone acetate itself is a very potent progesterone (5). There must be some similarity between progesterones and androgens because progesterone itself has some androgenic effects and is one of the most potent competitive

251

inhibitors of the prostate enzyme 5α-reductase which transforms testosterone
to dihydrotestosterone.

Antiandrogens can have several modes of pharmacological actions in suppressing prostate growth and they include: a.) direct competition with androgens
for specific receptors in the cytoplasm and their subsequent translocation
to the nucleus, b.) enzymes metabolizing androgens such as 5α-reductase
and c.) direct inhibition of steroid synthesizing enzymes in the testes
(53, 54).

Since we now have available drugs that are very effective in inhibiting LH
release (e.g. estrogens), steroidgenesis in the testes (Medrogestone)
and androgen action at the enzyme and steroid receptors (cyproterone acetate),
it would seem that a combination therapy approach might be very effective.

This would provide drug action at several physiological stages
of an essential chain of events and would make the combination treatment
more than additive. The combinations of hormonal approaches might also be
combined with other types of inhibitors of growth, as shown in Figure 4.

Figure 4.

Combination Therapy Directed At Sequential Steps

Required for Prostate Growth

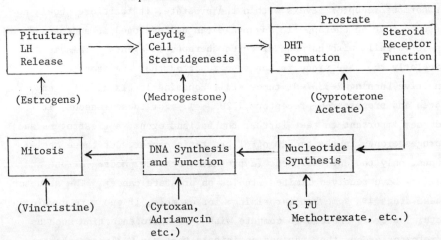

Preliminary tests of such a combination approach to hormonal therapy have been
carried out in animals and appear to have some merit (Heston and Coffey,
unpublished). The effects of such combined therapy on enhancing toxicity and
the induction of gynecamastia have not been determined.

In summary, although we are in urgent need of therapy that may retard androgen-insensitive growth, we should also remember that our rudimentary knowledge of the endocrine nature of prostatic growth as well as the exact mechanism of the development of androgen insensitivity may have limited our insight into some future therapeutic approaches.

2.) Prostate Cytotoxic Steroid Derivatives: These steroid analogs develop cytotoxic compounds when localized within the prostate gland. The development of new types of prostate specific drugs that are transported or become localized in the prostate would seem an appealing approach. Many have proposed to attach cytotoxic drugs to steroids to accomplish this; however, it must be realized that when androgens, estrogens or antiandrogens are administered to an animal, the vast majority of these drugs are not directed to the prostate. From data reported by Fang et al. (13), Bruchovsky and Wilson (6) and Tveter and Attramadal (57), it is possible to calculate that only 0.06% - 0.49% of the total labeled androgen administered to animals was taken up by the prostate gland. Thus, 99% of the androgen given to an animal will appear elsewhere. These steroids are also capable of metabolism in many organs such as liver, lung, adrenals, etc. Berger, Coffey and Scott (3) confirmed the very small distribution of androgens and in addition, found very low fractions of administered estrogens and anti-androgens appearing in the rat ventral prostate. It would therefore appear that administered androgens and estrogens are not localized preferentially to the prostate. This may be seen from the following table.

Table 8. Relative Distribution Two Hours After Tracer Doses of ^{3}H-Testosterone, ^{3}H-Estradiol or the Antiandrogen 3'-^{125}I Flutamide in Rat Tissues

Tissue	^{3}H-Testosterone	^{3}H-Estradiol	Antiandrogen ^{125}I-Flutamide
	(dpm/mg tissue)/(dpm/mg blood)		
Blood	1.0	1.0	1.0
Ventral prostate	1.5	1.2	1.7
Dorsal-lateral prostate	1.3	1.3	1.3
Seminal vesicle	1.5	1.1	0.8
Thigh	0.4	0.9	0.5
Kidney	1.8	2.8	2.0
Adrenal	2.1	3.2	1.6
Stomach	2.6	0.7	7.4
Pituitary	1.2	13.0	1.1
Liver	5.5	7.5	2.2
Urine	9.2	6.1	3.0
Small bowel content	83.0	33.0	6.5

For details see ref. (3).

Although the steroid moiety of a drug may not increase uptake in prostate in comparison to other tissues, it may be argued that binding to specific receptors in the tissue may retain these drugs within the prostate. The absolute amount of specific steroid receptor contained in a human prostate may be very low. If there are 25×10^3 steroid molecules bound specifically in each cell and 10^9 cells per gram then the total amount of receptor in the gland would be only one nanomole (10^{-9} mole) in an entire 25 gram prostate. This would not appear to be a very effective method for concentrating significant amounts of drugs within the prostate. Nonspecific steroid uptake and binding occurs in most tissues, however, prolonged retention is believed to be related to specific binding sites associated with target tissue.

Even though the carrier concept may not appear to enhance transport, it still may be reasoned that small amounts of toxic materials attached to steroid might still be directed via steroid receptor binding to a very critical site within the prostate. This has been some of the reasoning for attaching alkylating moieties to steroids in hopes that they might be carried to the prostate (32, 33). These drugs and the concept have been reviewed recently by A. Mittelman (33) and is the basis for the initial rationale for the mechanism of estramustine phosphate (Estracyt), an estradiol derivative with a phosphate in the 17 position and a nitrogen mustard in the 3 position. It has been reported earlier that Estracyt is effective against hormonally insensitive prostatic tumors (55). The drug is being evaluated by the National Prostatic Cancer Project (36) in clinical trials. It does have activity against the Dunning R-3327 tumor (51,34) which is comparable to that seen with estrogen treatment (51). These are certainly interesting drugs that deserve more study to resolve the specific effects due to the alkylating and estrogen moieties of the congeners.

3.) Enzyme Activated and Directed Drugs: These drugs are activated to a cytotoxic form through serving as substrates for enzymes localized within the prostate tumor.

C. H. Robinson and his colleagues (2) have designed specific steroid like compounds that are inactive until they interact with steroid biotransforming enzymes at which time they become highly reactive and are capable of destroying the activity of the enzyme with which they were a substrate. These types of compounds have been termed suicide-substrates. For example, novel acetylinic and allenic 5,10 secosteroids have been designed to serve as suicide substrates for enzymes involved in androgen synthesis and metabolism.

In this regard, these compounds would be expected to interact in many tissues since liver, lung, vas deferens, pituitary, epididymis, testes and seminal vesicles, as well as other tissues, are all capable of metabolizing androgens. It will be of interest to determine if drug substrates can be made for specific tissue enzymes.

Although the aforementioned suicide-substrates inactivate irreversibly the enzyme with which they reacted, often by alkylation, it is known that they can escape the local enzyme and react with other molecules in close proximity within the environment. Therefore, it is important to develop further this interesting approach to determine the potential for inhibiting critical steps in androgen, estrogen and progesterone reactions, as well as inhibiting other important steps in tumor growth. It is known that androgen-insensitive prostatic animal tumor (R-3327-HI) can still contain considerable levels of 5α-reductase and other enzymes of androgen metabolism (21, 22).

Other prostate enzymes have been proposed as sites for drug activation. Seligman and his associates studied the substrate specificity of prostatic acid phosphatase in hopes that drug-phosphate esters could be synthesized that would be activated by the enzyme. Colchicine like analogs were tested that had little cytotoxicity until hydrolyzed by the enzyme (45). The full potential of this approach has not been determined.

It should be remembered that many of the common cancer chemotherapeutic agents must be activated. Cyclophosphamide is inert until microsomal metabolism converts it into an alkylating agent. 5-FU and 6-MP must undergo synthesis to the nucleotide form before they act as enzyme inhibitors.

At present, we know of no substrate reaction that is specific to the prostate, so some toxicity is to be anticipated. The real goal is to use these methods to improve the therapeutic advantage.

4.) Immunotherapy

Much past excitement has been generated over the promise of immunotherapy but unfortunately at present it has proven disappointing. There are a combination of factors that may have limited this approach and they are in part the following: a.) the use of ill defined and heterogeneous immunostimulants, b.) treatment of large tumor loads in late stages, c.) lack of basic and fundamental knowledge of immunology and the development of anergy, and d.) little understanding of tumor immunology (suppression, blocking, antibodies, etc.) and the heterogenicity of the immunogenicity within the tumor.

255

As our knowledge of immunology expands and better defined immunopotentia-
ting systems are developed, we may expect a revival of interest in this
approach.

The use of immunotherapy as an adjuvant therapy is most difficult. Many
cancer chemotherapeutic drugs themselves produce immunosuppression and the
exact timing of the recovery of the immune system could be very critical to
when immunotherapy is applied. In animal models of prostatic cancer it
appears that the order and timing of chemotherapy, surgery and immunotherapy can be very critical (60).

Human prostatic cancer appears to contain tumor associated antigens (4).
Are these antigens specific for each tumor or crossreactive between individual prostate cancers? One interesting approach stems from the studies of
H. Busch and his associated (7) who report a common nucleolar antigen present
in many types of human cancers including the prostate. The antigen is not
present in BPH. These new tumor antigens have obvious potential in chemotherapy and diagnosis.

Recently a major secretory protein has been identified in prostatic secretion
(29). Can this specific protein product of the epithelial cell be used as
a prostatic specific antigen for developing anti-prostatic antibodies that
interact with both normal and cancer cells?

In summary, four general types of prostate antigens may be utilized: a.)
those specific to proteins or enzymes which are present only in prostate
cells (normal or cancerous), b.) a tumor specific antigen, and c.) an antigen
associated with tumors in general, whether of prostate origin or not, and
d.) the reappearance of embryonic like antigens on the tumors. The development of specific antibodies to these antigens and the identification of new
antigens will be greatly facilitated by the new hybridoma techniques.
In brief, this system allows a crude mixture of unresolved antigens to be
administered to another species such as the mouse. The mouse develops a
mixture of lymphocytes each monospecific to one of the multitude of antigens
to which the animal was exposed. The goal is to isolate in pure culture
each of the specific antibody producing lymphocytes and to grow the cells in
large quantities to produce one specific type of antibody. This goal is
accomplished by collecting the mixture of heterogeneous mouse lymphocytes
and fusing them with myeloma cells. The resulting hybrid cells are now
capable of growing and each line is cloned out to homogeneity. This system

is generally referred to as developing specific hybridomas. It has already provided a very powerful new tool for immunology.

The above system should help to identify antigens and produce specific prostate antibodies which then could be complexed to cytotoxic agents which could be directed toward prostate or prostate tumor cells.

Alternate methods of immunotherapy include reversing the state of anergy or boosting the immune system with macrophage activators or by inhibiting suppressor cell functions. It has long been known that tumors are often rich with macrophages that do not appear to be active. Opsonizing the tumor cells with antibodies and stimulating macrophage function has often been proposed, but as of yet, has not proven effective. Recent insight into the variety of lymphocytes, suppressor cells and macrophages and how lymphokins and growth factors interact between these immune cells, has only enhanced the complexity of tumor immunology; however, these factors must be resolved in part to aid in the rational design of future immunotherapy.

5. Genetic Therapy

For many years investigators have proposed that cancer is not an irreversible state. Recent experiments have indicated that some experimental cancers (renal tumors in frogs) can be reversed if the tumor nucleus, with the genetic complement, is transferred to egg cytoplasm. In these experiments the transplanted cancer cell nucleus in the new egg cytoplasm dedifferentiated further and then after undergoing divisions, developed into a new frog. In addition, experiments of bringing normal and tumor cells together to form a single new cell (hybrids), produced through cell fusion, has provided startling new evidence that the malignant state is not dominant but may be recessive and can be reversed. For more details and credits consult review by Sidebottom (46). This raises the question of whether a brake system has been lost through deletion of genetic information or release of a suppressed phenotypic expression.

New methods are being developed for adding new genetic material to cells. At present the integration of this genetic information from the donor into the recipient cell genome and its ultimate expression in function, is an active area of research in several laboratories.

Special restriction enzymes are being identified and isolated that are capable of clipping out specific areas of genetic information. If these new restriction endonuclease enzymes could be taken up by tumor cells they may

257

provide a very specific approach to cell therapy. Our present knowledge of the uptake of macromolecules, both proteins and nucleic acids, is at a very preliminary level, but once resolved, may provide some new methodology for circumventing one of the major problems in gene therapy.

6.) Other Important New Approaches to Therapy

As a tumor grows it must also stimulate the growth of other supporting elements that originate from the host and not the tumor. These normal components become an integral part of the tumor mass. For example, new blood vessels must be stimulated to grow with the tumor mass and therefore angiogenesis becomes a critical mechanism. Growth factors have been proposed to ensue from the tumor to stimulate the endothelial growth (17). Likewise, stroma components such as connective tissue elements must also develop along with the tumor growth (60). These essential support systems are coupled to tumor growth and may provide new areas for therapy. Folkman and his associates (17) are attempting to produce such an anti-angiogenesis factor. Similar approaches could be taken for other stromal components.

Tumors are also being cycled into synchronized growth states that permits better timing of the use of chemotherapeutic agents specific for certain phases of the cell cycle. This has often been attempted with other tumors by utilizing growth inhibitors (bleomycin, etc.) and then releasing this block in an attempt to approach synchrony. With the prostate this could be accomplished more easily with androgen stimulation, however, this would only affect the synchrony of androgen-sensitive cells.

It is also obvious that the control of metastasis would reduce greatly the devastation of cancer. Pollard, Burleson and Luckert (41) have used three lines of an animal model for prostate cancer (Pollard Tumors I, II and III in Lobund Wistar rats) and have shown marked inhibition of distant metastasis with treatment with Corynebacterium parvus, cytoxan, ICRF 159 [1,2-bis (3,5 dioxopiperazin-1-yl)propane; NSC 129,943], and aspirin. In contrast, inhaled anesthetic agents greatly enhanced the rate of prostatic metastasis to the lung. The mechanisms of these effects are being studied but the phenomenon already demonstrates that the rate of metastasis can be enhanced or retarded in a prostate tumor by drugs and that this is often independent of effects on primary tumor growth.

Metastasis is a complex interaction of host and tumor and the metastatic lesions have survived a multitude of hurdles, all of which may be blocked

258

with more knowledge of the system.

Physical methods such as hyperthermia are also being studied on other tumors and it appears that elevated temperatures (around 41.5°C) may be more lethal to the tumor cells than to normal cells. Furthermore, hyperthermia enhances radiosensitivity and chemosensitivity of the tumor. This general area of hyperthermia has been the topic of a recent review (52).

At present new forms for the delivery of radiotherapy have greatly enhanced the accuracy, safety and specificity of this form of therapy. The effectiveness of these new modes of radiotherapy have improved greatly over the past ten years. Unfortunately, many common opinions are often based on earlier studies before these new improvements were introduced or utilized. Radiosensitizers and hyperthermia have not yet impacted fully on radiotherapy because we are still only in the preliminary phases of these potentially important approaches.

Summary

The purpose of this review has been to provide some rational basis for understanding the present dilemma of prostatic cancer growth and the limitations of the current therapeutic approaches. An overview is presented of new approaches and concepts that may provide new ways of treating this disease.

References

1. Arnheim, F. K.: Carcinoma of the prostate - A study of the postmortem findings in one hundred and seventy six cases. J. Urol. 60, 599, 1948.
2. Batzold, F. H. and Robinson, C. H.: Irreversible inhibition of Δ^5-3-ketosteroid isomerase by 5,10 secosteroids. J. Am. Chem. Soc. 97, 2576-2578, 1975.
3. Berger, B., Coffey, D. S. and Scott, W. W.: Concepts and limitations in the application of radiolabeled antiandrogens, estrogens or androgens as isotopic sca-ning agents for the prostate. Invest. Urol. 13, 10-16,
4. Brannen, G. E., Gomolka, D. M. and Coffey, D. S.: Specificity of cell membrane antigens in prostatic cancer. Cancer Chemother. Reports 59, 127-137, 1975.
5. Bridge, R. W. and Scott, W. W.: A new antiandrogen, SH-714. Invest. Urol. 2, 99, 1964.
6. Bruchovsky, N. and Wilson, J. D.: The conversion of testosterone to 5α-androstan-17β-ol-one by rat prostate in vivo and in vitro. J. Biol. Chem. 243, 2012, 1968.
7. Busch, H., Gyorkey, F., Busch, R. K., Davis, F. M., Gyorkey, P. and Smetana, K.: A nucleolar antigen found in a broad range of human malignant tumor specimens. Cancer Res. 39, 3024-3030, 1979.
8. Byar, P. and Mostof, F.: Carcinoma of the prostate: Prognostic features in 208 radical prostatectomies; examination of the step-section technique. Cancer 30, 5-13, 1972.
9. Catalona, W. J. and Scott, W. W.: Carcinoma of the prostate, in J. H. Harrison, R. F. Gittes, A. D. Perlmutter, T. A. Stamey and P. C. Walsh (eds.), Campbell's Urology, Vol. 2, p. 1085-1117, W. B. Saunders Publishing Co., 1979.
10. Charbit, A., Malaise, E. and Tubiana, M.: Relation between the pathological nature and the growth rate of human tumors. Europ. J. Cancer 7, 307, 1971.
11. Day, S. B., Myers, W. P., Stansly, P., Garattini, S. and Lewis, M. G. (eds.) Cancer Invasion and Metastasis: Biologic Mechanisms and Therapy, Raven Press, N. Y., 1977.
12. Drewinko, B. and Humphrey, R. M. (eds.), Growth Kinetics and Biochemical Regulation of Normal and Malignant Cells, Williams and Wilkins, Baltimore, 1977.
13. Fang, S., Anderson, K. M. and Liao, S.: Receptor proteins for androgens. J. Biol. Chem. 244, 6584, 1969.
14. Fidler, I. J.: Tumor heterogeneity and the biology of cancer invasion and metabolism. Cancer Res. 38, 2651-2660, 1978.
15. Franks, L. M.: Latent carcinoma. Annals of Royal Coll. Surg. 15, 236, 1954.
16. Franks, L. M.: Latency and progression in human tumors. Lancet 2, 1037, 1956.
17. Folkman, J.: Tumor angiogenesis. In, F. F. Baker (ed.), Cancer: A Comprehensive Treatise, Vol. 3, pp. 355-386, Plenum Press, N. Y., 1975.
18. Gray, J. M. and Pierce, G. B.: Relationship between growth rate and differentiation of melanoma in vivo. J. Natl. Cancer Inst. 32, 1201-1211, 1964.
19. Hakannson, L. and Troupe, C.: On the presence within tumors of clones that differ in sensitivity to cytostatic drugs. Acta Pathol. Microbiol. Scand. A. 82, 32-40, 1974.

20. Heston, W. D. W., Menon, M., Tananis, C. and Walsh, P.: Androgen, estrogen, and progesterone receptors of the R-3327-H Copenhagen rat prostatic tumor. Cancer Lett. 6, 45-50, 1979.

21. Isaacs, J. T., Heston, W. D. W., Weissman, R. M. and Coffey, D. S.: Animal model of hormone sensitive and insensitive prostatic adeno-carcinomas: Dunning R-3327-H, R-3327-HI, and R-3327-AT. Cancer Res. 38, 4353-4359, 1978.

22. Isaacs, J. T., Isaacs, W. B. and Coffey, D. S.: Models for development of nonreceptor methods for distinguishing androgen-sensitive and -insensitive prostatic tumors. Cancer Res. 39, 2652-2659, 1979.

23. Janke, P., Briand, P. and Hartmann, N. R.: The effect of estrone-progesterone treatment on cell proliferation kinetics of hormone-dependent GR mouse mammary tumors. Cancer Res. 35, 3698-3704, 1975.

24. Killion, J. J. and Kollmorgen, G. M.: Isolation of immunogenic tumor cells by affinity chromatography. Nature 259, 674-676, 1976.

25. Lameront, L. F.: Tumor cell kinetics. Brit. Med. Bull. 29, 23, 1973.

26. Lameront, L. F.: Cell population kinetics in normal and malignant tissue, In, T. Symington and R. L. Carter (ed.), Scientific Formula-tions of Oncology, p. 119, Year Book Medical Publish., 1976.

27. Lea, O. A., Petrusg, P. and French, F. S.: Prostatein, a major secretory protein of the rat ventral prostate. J. Biol. Chem. 254, 6196-6202, 1979.

28. Malaise, E., Chavaudra, N. and Tubiana, M.: The relationship between growth rate, labeling index and histological type of tumours. Europ. J. Cancer 9, 305, 1973.

29. Mawhinney, M. G. and Neubauer, B. L.: Actions of estrogens in the male. Invest. Urol. 16, 409-420, 1979.

30. McGee, J. O., and Al-adnani, M. S.: Stroma in tumours, In, R. L. Carter and T. Symington (eds.), Scientific Foundationf of Oncology, p. 45-52, Year Bood Medical Publish., 1976.

31. Menon, M. and Walsh, P. C.: Hormonal therapy for prostatic cancer, In, (G. P. Murphy (ed.) Prostatic Cancer, PSG Publishing, Littleton, Mass. 1979.

32. Mittleman, A., Skukla, S. K. Welvaart, K., et al.: Oral estramustine phosphate (NSC-18199) in the treatment of advanced (Stage D) carcinoma of the prostate. Cancer Chemother. Rep. 59, 219-223, 1975.

33. Mittelman, A.: Drug development for carcinoma of the prostate, In, G. P. Murphy (ed.), Prostate Cancer, p. 201-212, PSG Publishing, Littleton, Mass., 1979.

34. Muntzing, J., Kirdani, R., Saroff, J., et al.: Inhibitory effects of estracyt on R-3327 rat prostatic carcinoma. Urology 10, 439-445, 1977.

35. Murphy, G. P.: Current status of therapy in prostatic cancer, In, M. Tannenbaum (ed.), Urologic Pathology: The Prostate, p. 225-239, Lea and Fibiger, Philadelphia, 1977.

36. Murphy, G. P.: Management of disseminated prostatic carcinoma, In, G. P. Murphy (ed.), Prostatic Cancer, p. 213-233, PSG Publishing, Littleton, Mass., 1979.

37. Nicolson, G. L. and Brunson, K. W.: Organ specificity of malignant B16 melanomas: In vivo selection for organ preference of blood-borne metastasis. Gann Monograph Cancer Res. 20, 15-24, 1977.

38. Nobel, R. L.: The development of prostatic adenocarcinomas in the Nb rats following prolonged sex hormone administration. Cancer Res. 37, 1929-1933, 1977.

39. Nowell, P. C.: The clonal evolution of tumor cell populations. Science 194, 23-28, 1976.

40. Prehn, R. T.: Analysis of antigenic heterogeneity within individual 3-methylcholanthrene-induced mouse sarcomas. J. Natl. Cancer Inst. 45, 1039-1045, 1970.

41. Pollard, M., Burleson, G. R. and Luckert, P. H.: Factors that modify the rate and extent of spontaneous metastases of prostate tumors in rats. In, S. B. Day et al. (eds.), Cancer Invasion and Metastasis, p. 357-366, Raven Press, 1977.

42. Salmon, S. E.: Kinetic rationale for adjuvant chemotherapy of cancer. In, S. S. Salmon and S. E. Jones (eds.), Adjuvant Therapy of Cancer, p. 15-27, North Holland Publishing, 1977.

43. Salmon, S. and Jones, S. E. (eds.), Adjuvant Therapy of Cancer, North Holland Publishing, 1977.

44. Schnabel, F. M., Jr.: Concepts for systemic treatment of micrometastases. Cancer 35, 15-24, 1975.

45. Seligman, A., Steinberger, N. J., Paul, B. D. et al.: Design of spindle poisons activated specifically by prostatic acid phosphatase (PAP) and new methods of PAP cytochemistry. Cancer Chemother. Rep. 59, 233-242,

46. Sidebottom, E.: The contribution of cell fusion studies to the analysis of neoplasia. In, T. Symington and R. L. Carter (eds.), Scientific Formulations of Oncology, p. 36-44, Year Book Medical Publishers, 1976.

47. Skipper, H. E., Schnabel, F. M., Mellet, L. B., Montgomery, J. A., Wilkoff, L. J., Lloyd, H. H. and Brockman, R. W.: Implications of biochemical, cytokinetic, pharmacologic and toxicologic relationships in the design of optimal therapeutic schedules. Cancer Chemother. Rep. 54, 431-450, 1970.

48. Skipper, H. E.: Thoughts on cancer chemotherapy and combination modality therapy. JAMA 230, 1033-1035.

49. Sluyser, M. and VanNie, R.: Estrogen receptor content and hormone-responsive growth of mouse mammary tumors. Cancer Res. 34, 3253-3257, 1974.

50. Smolev, J., Coffey, D. and Scott, W.: Experimental models for the study of prostatic adenocarcinoma. J. Urol. 118, 216-220, 1977.

51. Smolev, J., Heston, W., Scott, W. and Coffey, D.: Characterization of the Dunning R-3327-H prostatic adenocarcinoma: An appropriate animal model for prostatic cancer. Cancer Treat. Rept. 61, 273-287, 1977.

52. Streffer, C. (ed.), Cancer Therapy by Hyperthermia and Radiation, Urban and Schwarzenberg, Munich, 1978.

53. Sufrin, G. and Coffey, D. S.: A new model for studying the effects of drugs on prostatic growth: Antiandrogens and DNA synthesis. Invest. Urol. 11, 45-54, 1973.

54. Sufrin, G. and Coffey, D. S.: Differences in the mechanism of action of medrogestone and cyproterone acetate. Invest. Urol. 13, 1-9, 1975.

55. Tritsch, G. L., Shukla, S. K., Mittelman, A. et al.: Estracyt (NSC-89199) as a substrate for phosphatases in human serum. Invest. Urol. 12, 39, 1974.

56. Tubiana, M. and Malaise, E. P.: Growth rate and cell kinetics in human tumours. In, T. Symington and R. L. Carter (eds.), Scientific Formulations of Oncology, p. 126-136, Year Book Medical Publishers, 1976.

57. Tveter, K. J. and Attramadal, A.: Selective uptake of radioactivity in rat ventral prostate following administration of testosterone-1,2-^{3}H. Acta Endocrinol. 59, 218, 1968.

58. Walsh, P. C. and Wilson, J. D.: The induction of prostatic hypertrophy in dogs with androstanediol. J. Clin. Invest. 57, 1093-1097, 1976.

59. Weiss, L. A.: Pathobiologic overview of metastasis. Seminars Oncol. 4, 5-17, 1977.

60. Weissman, R. M., Coffey, D. S. and Scott, W. W.: Cell kinetic studies of prostatic cancer: Adjuvant therapy in animal models. Oncology 34, 133–137, 1977.

61. Wheelock, E. F., Goldstein, L. T., Weinhold, K. J., Carney, W. P. and Marx, P. A.: The tumor dormant state. In, S. B. Daly et al. (eds.), Cancer Invasion and Metastasis, p. 105–116, Raven Press, N. Y., 1977.

62. Willis, R. A.: The spread of tumors in the human Body. London, Butterworths, 1972.

CANCER OF THE PROSTATE - METHODS OF EVALUATING NEW THERAPEUTIC MODALITIES:
RECENT RESULTS OF THE NATIONAL PROSTATIC CANCER PROJECT*

CHAPTER XV

Several clinical models now exist which illustrate how systemic therapy
has been developed to become an integral part of the effective management
of some cancers.

Two examples are pertinent as background. Patients with Hodgkin's Disease
were at one time treated solely with radiation. Their average survival was
approximately two years. During the 1940's and 1950's it became apparent
that nitrogen mustard and other alkylating agents could cause objective
partial remissions in patients with advanced disease. During the following
decade, additional non-cross resistant cytotoxic agents were shown to produce temporary beneficial effects. In the early and mid 1960's, trials of
combinations of these drugs given for long rather than short courses produced a high incidence of complete responses, i.e. the total disappearance
of all manifestations of tumor. Follow-up of these patients indicated that
a significant proportion are cured and chemotherapy now forms a part of the
optimal management of many patients with Hodgkin's Disease (8).

In breast cancer, several single cytotoxic agents and hormonal approaches
were shown to produce a 20-40% incidence of objective partial remission in
patients with advanced and metastatic disease. The development of combinations of these drugs led to an increase in the incidence of these partial
remissions to approximately 60% (2). In contrast to Hodgkin's Disease,
however, complete response and cure of patients with advanced disease is
unusual. Nevertheless, application of some of these agents and combinations
to the patients presenting with localized disease but who have a high risk
of developing systemic metastasis has in some instances reduced recurrences
and prolonged survival (4,2). The progress is not as great as with Hodgkin's
Disease but does demonstrate the validity of the sequence of progression
from demonstration of anti-tumor effectiveness in patients with advanced
disease to utilization of this information in patients with earlier stages
of disease in the hope of producing more or longer responses or even cure.

It is unlikely that the ordered sequence of events can be followed for prostate cancer for two reasons. First, the actual incidence of tumor shrinkage
from cytotoxic chemotherapy in patients with advanced disease will be low
because of the rather general operation of factors adversely influencing
response such as advanced age, debility and pelvic irradiation (17). Second,

*John Horton, M.B., Ch.B.

264

an accurate, objective determination of a positive response is often not possible even though real benefit may occur. An additional impediment for the study of adjuvant systemic therapy is that large pools of patients may not be available since only a small proportion now present with truly localized disease.

Evaluation

Many groups are now performing clinical studies. Each uses different anatomic and pathologic staging systems and criteria for response.

(i) Anatomical Staging

American urologists usually follow the simple alphabetical system summarized as follows:

Stage A: Incidental microscopic focus

Stage B: Localized nodule confined to the prostate

Stage C: Local extension to adjacent structures

Stage D: Distant metastases

This is despite publications of TNM Systems in 1977 by the American Joint Committee for Cancer Staging and End-Results Reporting (10) and in 1978 by the U.I.C.C. (6). The U.I.C.C. system is summarized below:

PROSTATE (ICD-O 185)

Classified 1974. Confirmed 1978

(Approved by CNC, DSK, ICPR, JJC)

RULES FOR CLASSIFICATION

The classification applies only to carcinoma.

There should be histological verification of the disease, to permit division of cases by histological type. Any unconfirmed cases must be reported separately.

The following are the minimum requirements for assessment of the T, N and M categories. If these can not be met the Symbol TX, NX or MX will be used.

T categories: Clinical examination, urography, endoscopy and biopsy (if indicated), prior to definitive treatment.

N categories: Clinical examination and radiography including lymphography and urography.

M categories: Clinical examination, radiography, skeletal studies and relevant biochemical tests.

REGIONAL AND JUXTA-REGIONAL LYMPH NODES

The Regional Lymph Nodes are the pelvic nodes below the bifurcation of the common iliac arteries.

The Juxta-Regional Lymph Nodes are the inguinal nodes, the common iliac nodes and the para-aortic nodes.

TNM PRE-TREATMENT CLINICAL CLASSIFICATION

T - Primary Tumour

Tis Pre-invasive carcinoma (carcinoma in situ).

T0   No tumour palpable

Note: This category includes the incidental finding of carcinoma in an operative or biopsy specimen.

Such cases should be assigned an appropriate pT category.

T1   Tumour intracapsular surrounded by palpably normal gland

T2   Tumour confined to the gland. Smooth nodule deforming contour but lateral sulci and seminal vesicles not involved.

T3   Tumour extending beyond the capsule with or without involvement of the lateral sulci and/or seminal vesicles

T4   Tumour fixed or infiltrating neighbouring structures

Note: The suffix (m) may be added to the appropriate T category to indicate multiple tumours e.g. T2 (m).

TX   The minimum requirements to assess the primary tumour can not be met.

N - Regional and Juxta-regional Lymph Nodes

N0   No evidence of regional lymph node involvement

N1   Evidence of involvement of a single homolateral regional lymph node

N2   Evidence of involvement of contralateral or bilateral or multiple regional lymph nodes

N3   Evidence of involvement of fixed regional lymph nodes (there is a fixed mass on the pelvic wall with a free space between this and the tumour)

N4   Evidence of involvement of juxta-regional lymph nodes

Note: If lymphography indicates extension to the juxta-regional lymph nodes, a scalene node biopsy is recommended.

NX   The minimum requirements to assess the regional and/or juxta-regional lymph nodes can not be met.

M - Distant Metastases

M0   No evidence of distant metastases

M1   Evidence of distant metastases

MX   The minimum requirements to assess the presence of distant metastases
       can not be met.

p.TNM POST-SURGICAL

HISTOPATHOLOGICAL CLASSIFICATION

pT - Primary Tumour

    pTis   Pre-invasive carcinoma (carcinoma in situ)

    pT0   No evidence of tumour found on histological examination of specimen

    pT1   Focal (single or multiple) carcinoma

    pT2   Diffuse carcinoma with or without extension to the capsule

    pT3   Carcinoma with invasion beyond the capsule and/or invasion of
           the seminal vesicles

    pT4   Tumour with invasion of adjacent organs

    pTX   The extent of invasion can not be assessed

        G - Histopathological Grading

           G1   High degree of differentiation

           G2   Medium degree of differentiation

           G3   Low degree of differentiation or undifferentiated

           GX   Grade can not be assessed

pN - Regional and Juxta-regional Lymph Nodes

The pN categories correspond to the M categories.

pM - Distant Metastases

The pM categories correspond to the M categories.

STAGE GROUPING

No stage-grouping is at present recommended.

SUMMARY

PROSTATE

T0	Incidental carcinoma
T1	Intracapsular/normal gland
T2	Intracapsular/deformed gland
T3	Extension beyond capsule
T4	Extension fixed to neighbouring organs
N1	Single homolateral regional
N2	Contra- or bi-lateral/multiple regional
N3	Fixed regional

267

N4   Juxta-regional.

(ii) Pathology

The histopathology is almost always adenocarcinoma. Grading is especially pertinent in studies of patients presenting with early stages of
disease (1). Several systems are in use in the United States. The Gleason
system (5) is based upon the degree of glandular differentiation and the
growth pattern of the tumor in relation to the prostatic stroma. The pattern
may vary from a well formed and questionably malignant grade 1 to an undifferentiated grade 5. It assigns a histologic grade both to the predominant
primary pattern and to any secondary pattern. A modification of Broders
classification is suggested both by the American Joint Committee (10) and
the U.I.C.C. (6). This is: G1 Well Differentiated; G2 Moderately Well Differentiated; G3-G4 Poorly to Very Poorly Differentiated. Other systems
include those of Mostofi (11) and Gaeta (14). Recent workshops of the
National Prostatic Cancer Project (NPCP) (14) have recommended that Gleason's
system should be employed, at least in conjunction with any other system
utilized since there is still a paucity of data on correlations between
histologic grade, tumor natural history and response to various forms of
treatment.

(iii) Response Criteria

Criteria for response in prostatic cancer vary in several respects
from those commonly used for other tumor types (9). These criteria can be
examined for three major categories, localized, regional and advanced disease.

A. Localized

Careful surgical staging, including laparotomy and pelvic and periaortic
node sampling or resection, has demonstrated that many patients who were
thought clinically to have disease localized entirely to the prostate in
fact had regional spread, first to the pelvic and then to the periaortic
lymph nodes (7). Thus, studies that do not include surgical staging must
be considered separately. Evaluation of response of those patients who have
clearly localized disease can only be performed by study for evidence of
local progression or metastasis. The acid phosphatase, even with recent
modifications that improve sensitivity and specificity, is present in the
blood in only a small proportion of these patients (3). Care must be taken
that the frequency and type of evaluation performed must be similar for
both the treated and control groups. Survival has to be the final criterion
of success but this parameter is difficult to use in clinical trials of

this stage of disease since the expected survival with truly localized disease is measured sometimes in decades rather than years. Thus, any study of systemic therapy may not be completed by the same investigator who started the program.

B. Regional

There are no fully satisfactory parameters that can be used for evaluation of the change of the extent of the disease in regional lymph nodes. Lymphangiography only occasionally will provide specific enough radiographic details to allow evaluation of regional lymphadenopathy. Computerized tomographic scans, ultra sound and some radioisotope techniques are capable of demonstrating large or bulky areas of tumor but are not satisfactory for followup except in documenting progression of previously small or microscopic areas of disease. As in the patients with localized disease, the time from the onset of treatment to the detection of first recurrence or metastasis will be the principal parameter to be used and this is correlated with survival. The prognosis for these patients is not as good as for those with disease involving only the prostate (1), so the duration of the study will be shorter.

C. Advanced

Most patients with advanced, metastatic prostatic cancer do not have accurately measurable components of their disease. The initial chemotherapy studies of the NPCP showed that the incidence of objectively measured tumor regressions was low. It became clear that clinical benefit also ensued to another group of patients in whom the previous progression of the disease was halted but the tumor shrinkage did not fulfill the criteria used for partial or complete response.

This resulted in the definition of "stable" disease. Patients achieving this live longer than those who progress. It must be pointed out, though, that patients with advanced disease who are already in a stable state, cannot be evaluated in this way. Here, perhaps, the duration of the stable state may be a significant factor. The situations where objective response can both occur and be measured are summarized in Table I.

Difficulties abound in the reliability of the measurements used for objective change. First, in evaluation of the local extent of the disease, question arises as to whether digital examination is sufficiently specific and reproducible to be used as documentation of response. Gross changes are capable

269

TABLE I

POSSIBILITIES FOR EVALUATION OF OBJECTIVE RESPONSE IN PATIENTS WITH ADVANCED OR METASTATIC PROSTATE CANCER

Type of Metastasis	Status of disease before treatment	OBJECTIVE RESPONSE EVALUATION POSSIBLE		
		Complete or partial response	Stable	Progression
MEASUREABLE *	Newly diagnosed	YES	NO	YES
	Stable	YES	NO	YES
	Progressive	YES	YES	YES
EVALUABLE **	Newly diagnosed	? YES	NO	YES
	Stable	? YES	NO	YES
	Progressive	? YES	? YES	YES
NON MEASUREABLE ***	Newly diagnosed	NO	NO	YES
	Stable	NO	NO	YES
	Progressive	NO	YES	YES

* e.g.   round, parenchymal pulmonary metastasis

** e.g.   palpable mass on rectal examination

*** e.g.   bone marrow metastasis without radiographic bone change.

270

of being measured but since even experienced urologists are correct in the diagnosis of carcinoma of the prostate only 70% of the time, caution must be used. Prior surgery, radiation, inflammation and non-malignant nodules all complicate this evaluation. There are no hard data to suggest that advances in diagnostic techniques for evaluating the size and extent of the local tumor such as computerized axial tomography, isotope scanning using short-lived isotopes such as O^{15} or ultra sound, even with a rectal probe, (15) will be more accurate and more reproducible. Intravenous pyelography and cystoscopy are only indirect measures. The difficulty of evaluation of pelvic and retroperitoneal lymph nodes has already been discussed and it is unusual that there is a peripheral lymph node containing tumor from prostate cancer that can be measured. Only gross areas of nodal disease are usually demonstrable by isotope scans or lymphangiography and it is often inconvenient or expensive to repeat these studies frequently.

Bone metastasis, the most common evident site, is notoriously difficult to evaluate. The usual radiographic manifestation is osteoblastic change and, even if beneficial effect occurs, normalization of the appearance of the bone occurs infrequently. Certainly, if there are osteolytic areas which heal, this can be construed as indicating benefit. Scintiscans can only document progression and not regression. Bone marrow biopsy has a large sampling error and is not sufficiently reproducible to be reliable. Evaluation of the liver is also rather difficult. Histologic documentation of metastasis must be made. Scans or ultra sound techniques can probably be used sequentially if the size of at least one of the tumor masses measures at least 5 cm. in diameter. Clinical measurements for the size of the liver are rather unreliable and for this reasons the Eastern Cooperative Group (ECOG) insists that a liver enlarged by metastasis must extend at least 5 cm. below the costal margin and xiphoid during quiet respiration before it can be used on a measureable parameter (9).

Liver function tests correlate poorly with response but it seems reasonable to think that any tumor shrinkage of the liver should not be associated with worsening function results if an objective regression is to be claimed. Pulmonary lesions are not common manifestations of prostate cancer but these may be measured using standard radiographic techniques.

Because of the difficulties in finding hard and reproducible criteria, several groups have included consideration of symptomatic change in these evaluation criteria. This is clinically important but underscores the importance of

271

having adequate controls in every study where these criteria are used in order to obviate the very powerful "placebo" effect. Most "pilot" studies of a new treatment for prostate cancer are uncontrolled and use unstated, often very loose criteria for response. Almost always, high response rate claimed in initial studies do not hold up when controlled, comparative trials ensue.

For purposes of comparison, the response criteria used by three study groups, NPCP, ECOG and EORTC follow. It is evident that significant differences exist between these criteria:

(A) NPCP

    (a) Objective Complete Response (all of the following)

        1. Tumor masses, if present, totally disappeared and no new lesions appeared.

        2. Elevated acid phosphatase, if present, returned to normal.

        3. Osteolytic lesions, if present, recalcified.

        4. Osteoblastic lesions, if present, normalized.

        5. If hepatomegaly is a significant indicator there must be a complete reduction in liver size, and normalization of all pre treatment abnormalities of liver function.

        6. No significant cancer related deterioration in weight (>10%), symptoms, or performance status (became or remained ambulatory).

    (b) Objective Partial Regression (all of the following)

        1. At least one tumor mass, if present, is reduced by >50% in x-sectional area.

        2. Elevated acid phosphatase, if present, returned to normal.

        3. Osteolytic lesions, if present, undergo recalcification in one or more, but not in all.

        4. Osteoblastic lesions, if present, do not progress.

        5. If hepatomegaly is a significant indicator, there must be a reduction in liver size and at least a 30% inprovement of all pre treatment abnormalities of liver function.

        6. There may be no increase in any other lesion and no new areas of malignant disease may appear.

        7. No significant cancer related deterioration in weight (>10%), symptoms, or performance status (improved or remained the same).

(c) Objectively Stable (all of the following)

1. No new lesions occurred and no lesions measurably present increased more than 25% in x-sectional area.

2. Acid phosphatase level decreases, though need not return to normal.

3. Osteolytic lesions, if present, do not appear to worsen.

4. Osteoblastic lesions, if present, remain stable.

5. Hepatomegaly, if present, does not worsen by more than 30% and symptoms of hepatic abnormalities do not worsen.

6. No significant cancer related deterioration in weight (>10%), symptoms, or performance status (improved or remained the same).

(d) Objective Progression (any of the following)

1. Significant cancer related deterioration in weight (>10%), symptoms, or performance status (at least one score level).

2. Appearance of new areas of malignant disease.

3. Increase in any previously measurable lesion by greater than 25% in x-sectional area.

4. Development of recurring anemia secondary to prostate cancer – (not treatment related – protocols 500 and 600).

5. Development of ureteral obstruction (protocols 500 and 600).

NOTE: An increase in acid or alkaline phosphatase alone is not to be considered an indication of progression. These should be used in conjunction with other criteria.

(B) ECOG

Patients with measurable disease

Complete response – complete disappearance of all measurable disease and no new lesions developing.

Partial response – 50% reduction in the sum of the products of horizontal and vertical tumor diameters.

No change – less than 25% increase in the sum of the products of horizontal and vertical tumor diameters.

Progression – greater than 25% increase in the sum of the products of two tumor diameters or the development of new lesions. Increase in tumor diameters in first two weeks shall be regarded as due to delayed tumor cell death and is not considered evidence of progression but sets a new baseline for future assessment of drug response.

273

Liver enlargement

Measure distance below costal margin at both mid-clavicular lines
and xiphoid during respiration.

Complete response - 2 of 3 distances must be >5cm before treatment
and recede to 0 and definitely abnormal liver scan must become
normal.

Partial remission - greater than 30% reduction in the sum liver
measurements (distance below costal margin).

No change - less than 25% increase in mean liver measurements.

Progression - greater than 25% increase in mean liver measurements.

Lytic bone lesions not irradiated

Complete response - normalization of bone architecture and no new
lesions.

Partial response - 50% decrease in measured lytic lesions.

No change - less than 50% decrease in measured lytic lesions.

Progression - greater than 25% increase in measured lytic lesions
or appearance of new disease of any site.

Biochemical changes (acid phosphatase, etc.) will be analyzed in
these patients by correlating these with above criteria, biochemical
criteria of response will be developed.

Response in patients with elevated acid phosphatase

Response - A greater than 50% decrease from the pretreatment serum
value and/or a return to the normal range will be considered a
response (Record normal range for your laboratory on flow sheet).

No change - less than 50% decrease or less than 50% increase.

Progression - A greater than 50% increase in acid phosphatase
(excluding values obtained immediately after chemotherapy which
may reflect a "relapse reaction") or the development of measurable
disease will be evidence of disease progression.

Patients with evaluable non-measurable disease

The endpoint of drug assessment in these patients will be survival
time and the following are not criteria of response but rather
guidelines for continuing or discontinuing chemotherapy. All

patients in this category require a minimum of six weeks of treatment to be evaluable.

Performance status

At 6 weeks patients who have worsened one or more levels on the performance scale will discontinue initial treatment. At 12 weeks of treatment patients must have shown an improvement in performance status of at least one level to continue on initial treatment.

Patients who initially improve and then worsen by 2 levels in performance status will cross over to the Phase II arm.

Pain score - must be 2 or more to be evaluable. The following guideline for scoring will be used:

Score	Description of Severity	Frequency of Pain	Analgesic Used	Frequency of Analgesic
0	None	None	None	None
1	Mild	<2 per day	Aspirin, darvon, etc.	<2 x per day
2	Moderate	>2 per day	Codeine 32 1 percodan	>2 x per day
3	Severe	Most of the time	2 percodan 2-4 mg dilaudid po	q 3-6 hr
4	Very severe	All of the time	>4 mg dilaudid or 10 mg morphine, etc.	<q 3 hr

At 6 weeks patients who have worsened by two levels on the pain scale will discontinue initial treatment. Stable, or improved patients will continue initial treatment.

At 12 weeks of treatment patients must have shown an improvement of one level on the pain scale or remain stable at a pain scale rating of 0-1 to continue on initial treatment.

Patients who initially stabilize or improve and then worsen by 2 levels on the pain scale will cross over to the Phase II arm.

Increasing pain must be documented with increasing analgesic requirement or other unequivocal evidence of worsening of pain.

Body weight

If during the first 12 weeks patients lose more than 5% of dry body weight on treatment they will cross over to the Phase II arm.

Patients who stabilize or gain weight then subsequently lose more than 5% of their body weight will cross over to the Phase II arm or go off study.

Extent of bone involvement on bone x-rays

This parameter can be used only as an indicator of progression and not of response. The scaling used is that of Hovespin (Hovespin et al) as follows:

0 - no involvement
1 - less than 25% involvement (meaning less than 25% of radiographic area of given site involved with metastasis)
2 - 25 to 75% involvement
3 - more than 75% involvement

Note that this scaling is based on area not density.

This grading will be done on the following seven sites and the data recorded on form C.

Shoulders (including humeral heads, clavicles and scapulas)
ribs
thoracic spine
lumbo-sacral spine
ilia
pubis-ischia
femora (including both femoral heads and necks as seen on pelvic films)

Evidence of progression will be at least one level increase in grade for 2 sites.

Persistent stable disease or increase of less than above should lead to continuation of initial treatment.

(C) EORTC
(a) Objective Specific Criteria (OSC)
1. Prostatic primary growth.
The size of the prostate will be determined by rectal palpation. Presence or absence of the median furrow will be noted. Presence of localized or generalized induration will be indicated. Extraprostatic spread will be looked for; palpation of the seminal vesicles can be felt. All these data will be reported on a Young's

276

scheme. It is advisable that 2 different investigators carry out the rectal examination at the same time. If more objective methods for determining the actual size of the prostatic tumor are used, either roentgenographic or scintigraphic, caliper, measurements of two perpendicular diameters should be obtained, provided the lesions have sufficiently discrete outlines to permit accurate measurements.

2. Cutaneous and subcutaneous lesions; superficial lymph nodes.

These lesions should be measured very carefully each time the patient is seen by the investigator, because these measurements yield the most objectively quantifiable information. The importance of obtaining 2 or more sets of measurements of such lesions during the initial work-up is stressed. The standard caliper is used and the measurements of 2 diameters, one the greatest diameter, the other the largest diameter perpendicular to the first is to be made. If possible, photographs of the soft parts lesions should be obtained; they must include a legible rule for the comparison of size of lesions and some identifying data and the date of the photograph.

3. Bone lesions.

Quantification of such lesions is made difficult by the fact that the x-ray records not the tumor size but rather the response of the surrounding bone to the tumor; this is a two-dimensional record of a three-dimensional process. Therefore the significant deposition of calcium in previously lytic lesions unaccompanied by progressing lysis is a good criteria of objective improvement of the lesion. Nevertheless most common bone lesions are osteo-plastic. In these cases, objective improvement of the bone lesions will be considered if after starting drug administration, no new formation of abnormal bone occurs when the radioactive strontium bone scintigram shows no further elevation of the radioisotope uptake in the same bone area. If disappearance of osteoplastic bone metastases occurs, this will also be considered as criterion of objective improvement.

4. Distant visceral lesions.

i. Thoracic viscera. Caliper measurements of nodular lung parenchymal lesions are to be attempted at each evaluation. The measurements should be carried out on all such lesions that have sufficiently discrete outlines to permit accurate measurements. If a patient with lung metastases has fever or expectoration, start first with 2 weeks antibiotic treatment. The technique of measurement is to be the same as that outlined above and the roentgenographic technique employed must be comparable from one film to the next. Similar measurements are to be made of hilar masses. Pleural effusions do not lend themselves readily to quantitation. However, accurate records concerning the frequency of and the quantity of fluid aspirated from thoracenteses are to be obtained to roentgenographic evidence of decrease or disappearance of effusions.

ii. Abdominal viscera. As accurate measurements as possible of abdominal masses, total height of the liver and distance of the liver edge below the costal margin are to be obtained. Serial liver function tests and scintigram should be carried out in those cases suspected of having liver metastases.

5. Serum acid phosphatase levels (SAP)

Elevation of prostatic acid phosphatase appearing during administration of the therapy will be considered as worsening, even if all the other measurable lesions remain quiescent. Diminution of at least 50% of an elevated value during experimental therapy will be considered as one of the criteria of objective specific improvement.

(b) Objective Non-specific Criteria (ONSC)

1. Degree of dilation of upper urinary tract.
   Determined from intravenous urogram, only in patients without bladder outlet obstruction.

2. Neurological findings.
   Quantification of response of the lesions provoking these signs are difficult, mainly if they are located in the central nervous system. Serial electroencephalograms and ophtalmoscopic examinations can contribute to the evaluation.

3. Serum alkaline phosphatase levels.
   Specific bone and liver isozymes are to be determined; return to normal or diminution of a previously elevated bone isozyme value will be considered as one of the criteria of objective non-specific improvement.

4. Ambulatory status.

This will be evaluated according to Karnofsky's criteria.

(c) Subjective Criteria (SC)

Pain.

This item is included, because marked aggravation of pain or appearance of **excruciating** pain during therapy may cancel the interpretation of an objective regression based partially on modification of indirect or/and non-specific criteria.

Pain has to be classified as follows:

Rating	Comment
1	No pain, or mild pain requiring no medication
2	Pain requiring mild analgesic
3	Pain requiring major analgesic drugs
4	Intractable pain.

Evaluation of Response

(a) General Considerations

1. Responses to therapy are to be classified as follows:
   i. objective regression;
   ii. failure;
   iii. status quo.

2. Cases in which some tumor masses decrease in size while one or several other criteria indicate progression of the disease are to be considered as failure. These criteria are:
   i. progression of other lesions than the ones regressing;
   ii. appearance of new lesions;
   iii. elevation of serum acid phosphatase activity;
   iv. elevation of alkaline phosphatase activity, except if **this** phenomenon is due to recalcification of previous lytic bone lesions;
   v. appearance of hypofibrinogenemia;
   vi. appearance of pain, rate 3.

3. Pathological fracture of a bone is not to be considered as proof of progression.

4. Ideally the objective regression of the tumor masses to therapy would be the sole criterion by which effectiveness of the agent(s) tested is to be evaluated. However, such a method cannot be applied in most cases of prostatic cancer. Therefore some arbitrary rules

have been elaborated to determine the type of response to therapy.

(b) Evaluating Rules

Following criteria are required to consider the response to therapy as a regression:

1. Local prostatic tumor without metastases.

    i.   Marked diminution of the induration and of the size of the local tumor, as revealed by the data of the rectal examination, recorded on the Young's diagrams. If prostate scintigrams are available, they should show objective evidence of this regression.

    ii. Decrease of at least 50% of serum prostatic acid phosphatase (SAP) if previously elevated.

    iii. Objective non-specific criteria (ONSC): unchanged or decreased.

2. Soft-parts metastases alone.

    i.   If no tumor is present in the prostatic region or if no regression of the prostatic tumor occurs, measurable regression of at least half the number of the metastases should be observed.

    ii. If regression of size and induration of the prostatic tumor occurs, regression of at least 1 soft part metastases should be observed provided there is a diminution of at least 50% of an elevated SAP. If such a reduction of SAP is not observed, or if SAP is normal from the start of the therapy, regression of at least half the number of soft part metastases should be observed, despite the regression of the prostatic tumor.

    iii. As well for (i) as for (ii), ONSC unchanged or decreased.

3. Bone metastases alone: an objective regression will be considered only if the following criteria are present:

    i.   Plastic lesions alone: no further calcium deposits visible on bone x-rays or disappearance of at least one plastic lesion, diminution of at least 50% of SAP diminution of bone serum alkaline phosphatase, regression of the prostatic tumor (see Evaluating Rules 1 (i)).

    ii. Lytic lesions alone: recalcification of at least half the number of bone lesions, diminution of at least 50% of SAP, regression of status quo of the prostatic tumor

                or

    recalcification of at least half the number of the bone lesions if there are at least 4 present.

iii. Plastic and lytic lesions: no further calcium deposits visible on bone x-rays, diminution of at least 50% of SAP, diminution of bone serum alkaline phosphatase, regression of status quo of the prostatic tumor

    or

recalcification of at least half the number of the lytic lesions, if there are at least 4 present with no further calcium deposits visible on bone x-rays.

iv. For i, ii or iii, ONSC unchanged or decreased.

4. Bone metastases and/or soft-part and visceral metastases. Evidence for an objective regression will be considered if the following criteria are fulfilled:

i. Plastic bone lesions: No evidence of further calcium deposits on bone x-rays or disappearance of at least one plastic lesion, diminution of at least 50% of SAP, diminution of bone serum alkaline phosphatase, measurable regression of a distant metastase, prostatic tumor regressing or unchanged

    or

no evidence of further calcium deposits on bone x-rays or disappearance of at least one plastic lesion, measurable regression of at least half the number of distant metastases, prostatic tumor regressing or unchanged.

ii. Lytic lesions: Recalcification of at least 1 lytic lesion, diminution of at least 50% of SAP, measurable regression of at least one distant metastase, prostatic tumor regressing or unchanged,

    or

measurable regression of at least half the number of the bone and other distant metastases, provided there are at least 4 soft-parts and visceral lesions present,

    or

measurable regression of at least half the number of distant metastases, provided there are at least 4 present, bone lesions remaining unchanged, with diminution of at least 50% of SAP.

iii. Plastic and lytic lesions: No further deposits of calcium visible on bone x-rays or disappearance of at least one plastic lesion, measurable regression of at least 1 bone lytic lesion and 1 non-osseous distant metastase, with diminution of bone

281

alkaline phosphatase,

or

no further deposits of calcium visible on bone x-rays or disappearance of at least one plastic lesion, measurable regression
of at least half the number of distant bone and other metastases,
provided there are at lease 4 different metastases,

or

no further deposits of calcium visible on bone x-rays or disappearance of at least one plastic lesion, lytic lesions
unchanged, measurable regression of at least half the number
of other distant metastases, provided there are at least 4
different such lesions, diminution of at least 50% of SAP,
diminution of bone serum, alkaline phosphatase.

iv.   No bone lesions: Measurable regression of at least half the
number of distant metastases provided there are at least 4
different such lesions, diminution of at least 50% of SAP.

v.   For i, ii, iii or iv; ONSC unchanged or decreased.

In order to be able to accurately evaluate reports of studies performed in
patients with advanced disease, it is necessary to take cogniscence of at
least:

(a) whether or not the disease was objectively measurable.

(b) whether the patient had newly diagnosed, stable or progressing disease
at the onset of the trial.

(c) what characteristics the patients had that relate to expectation of
response. These include age, performance status, prior radiation therapy,
prior hormone or cytotoxic therapy, hemoglobin level, etc.

(d) what criteria for response were used.

(e) what controls were used.

In order to enable results of investigative programs to be compared, it would
be of great value for the groups performing studies on prostate cancer to
agree to a relatively uniform set of criteria that would (a) characterize
the types of patients being admitted into studies and (b) use similar methods
for evaluation of response. At the present time it is not possible to accurately compare results of treatment, even in patients with advanced disease,
between various groups.

Another feature which demands control in prospective trials is the study of
tumor markers such as acid and alkaline phosphatase and their various isozymes.

It is advantageous to have a central laboratory to monitor quality control
among individual institutions and to allow quick correlations to be made
with any advances in chemical or immunologic techniques with the biology of
the tumors. Such a reference laboratory has been of great value to the NPCP
and has allowed the immediate evaluation of several improvements in methodology. (3)

Toxicity from treatment has always to be evaluated to decide where the balance
lies between beneficial and harmful effects of any new treatment. Good monitoring requires the awareness of the potential side effects, using records
on which the side effects can be noted, a grading system to categorize their
severity and a mechanism for reacting to the findings. This is relatively
easily performed for acute toxicities. Table 2 is a description of the
criteria for acute toxicity currently being used by the Eastern Cooperative
Oncology Group. This is now being amended to include such factors as corti-
costeroid toxicity and psychosocial phenomena. Chronic toxicity is of greater
importance in the patients who are being treated on an adjuvant basis. Re-
cording needs to be made of such factors as organ dysfunction, nutrition and
the development of second cancers.

Protocols and Results of the NPCP Studies

The treatment group of the NPCP is a cooperating group of nine urologic centers
in the United States supported by the National Prostatic Cancer Project of
the National Cancer Institute. It was formed in 1973 and examination of the
development of its studies is pertinent since it exemplifies some important
principles for clinical studies in this disease that include:
(i) Tight definition of patients entered.
(ii) Development of appropriate response criteria.
(iii) Consideration of animal model data in conjunction with human data in
      the choice of treatments for study.
(iv) Institution of studies combining hormonal and cytotoxic therapy.
(v) Institution of studies of combination cytotoxic therapy.
(vi) A range of studies from those for the most advanced to the adjuvant
      setting.

The description and current status of each of the studies is summarized in
Table 3. It should be recognized that all these studies have adequate controls.

The initial study (Protocol 100) (18) took patients with "end stage" i.e.
advanced or metastatic disease who had progressed following standard hormonal

Table 2   **ECOG TOXICITY CRITERIA**

		0	1	2	3	4
Leuko-penia	WBC × 10³	≥4.5	3.0−<4.5	2.0−<3.0	1.0−<2.0	<1.0
	Neut × 10³	≥1.9	1.5−<1.9	1.0−<1.5	0.5−<1.0	<0.5
Thrombo-cytopenia	Plt × 10³	≥130	90−<130	50−<90	25−<50	<25
Anemia	Hgb gm%	≥11	9.5−10.9	<9.5		
	Hct %	≥32	28−31.9	<28		
	Clinical			Sx of anemia	Req transfusions	
Hemorrhage		None	Minimal	Mod—Not debilitating	Debilitating	Life threatening
Infection		None	No active Rx	Requires active Rx	Debilitating	Life threatening
GU	BUN mg%	≤20	21−40	41−60	>60	Symptomatic
	Creatinine	≤1.2	1.3−2.0	2.1−4.0	>4.0	uremia
	Proteinuria	Neg	1+	2+−3+	4+	
	Hematuria	Neg	Micro-Cult−positive	Gross-Cult−positive	Gross+Clots	c̄ obst uropathy

Urinary tract infection should be graded under infection, not GU.
Hematuria resulting from thrombocytopenia is graded under hemorrhage.

		0	1	2	3	4
Hepatic	SGOT	<1.5 × nl	1.5−2 × normal	2.1−5 × normal	>5 × normal	
	Alk Phos	<1.5 × nl	1.5−2 × normal	2.1−5 × normal	>5 × normal	
	Bilirubin	<1.5 × nl	1.5−2 × normal	2.1−5 × normal	>5 × normal	
	Clinical				Precoma	Hepatic coma

Viral hepatitis should be recorded as infection rather than liver toxicity.

		0	1	2	3	4
N & V		None	Nausea	N & V controllable	Vomiting intractable	
Diarrhea		None	No dehydration	Dehydration	Grossly bloody	
Pulm	PFT	Nl	25−50% decrease in Dco or VC	>50% decrease in Dco or VC		
	Clinical		Mild Sx	Moderate Sx	Severe Sx-Inter-mittent O₂	Assisted vent or continuous O₂

Pneumonia is considered infection and not graded as pulmonary toxicity unless felt to be resultant from pulmonary changes directly induced by treatment.

		0	1	2	3	4
Cardiac		Nl	ST−T changes	Atrial arrhythmias	Mild CHF	Severe or refract CHF
		Nl	Sinus tachy >110 at rest	Unifocal PVC's	Multifocal PVC's	Ventric tachy
					Pericarditis	Tamponade
Neuro	PN	None	Decr DTR's	Absent DTR's	Disabling sens loss	Resp dysfunction 2° to weakness
			Mild paresthesias	Severe paresthesias	Severe PN pain	Obstipation req surg
			Mild constipation	Severe constipation	Obstipation	Paralysis—confining pt to bed/wheelchair
				Mild weakness	Severe weakness	
					Bladder dysfunct	
	CNS	None	Mild anxiety	Severe anxiety	Confused or manic	Seizures
			Mild depression	Mod depression	Severe depression	Suicidal
			Mild headache	Mod headache	Severe headache	Coma
			Lethargy	Somnolence	Cord dysfunction	
				Tremor	Confined to bed due to CNS dysfunct	
				Mild hyperactivity		
Skin & Mucosa		Nl	Transient erythema	Vesticulation	Ulceration	
			Pigmentation, atrophy	Subepidermal fibrosis	Necrosis	
	Stomatitis	None	Soreness	Ulcers—can eat	Ulcers—cannot eat	
Alopecia		None	Alopecia—mild	Alopecia—severe		
Allergy		None	Transient rash	Urticaria	Serum sickness	Anaphylaxis
			Drug fever ≤38°C (≤100.4° F)	Drug fever >38°C (>100.4° F)	Bronchospasm—req parenteral meds	
				Mild bronchospasm		
Fever		≤37.5°C	≤38°C (≤100.4° F)	>38°C (>100.4° F)	Severe c̄ chills (>40°C)	Fever c̄ hypotension

Fever felt to be caused by drug allergy should be graded as allergy.
Fever due to infection is graded under infection only.

		0	1	2	3	4
Local Tox		None	Pain	Pain + Phlebitis	Ulceration	

. The toxicity grade should reflect the most severe degree occurring during the evaluated period, not an average.
. When two criteria are available for similar toxicities, e.g., leukopenia, neutropenia, the one resulting in the more severe toxicity grade should be used.
. Toxicity grade = 5 if that toxicity caused the death of the patient.
   Refer to detailed toxicity guidelines or to study chairman for toxicity not covered on this table.

Table 2   RESULTS OF THE PROSPECTIVELY RANDOMIZED NPCP TRIALS OF SYSTEMIC THERAPY FOR CANCER OF THE PROSTATE

Protocol	Type of Patient	Prior Radiation	Treatments	Entered/Evaluated		Objective Response			Remarks
						Partial	Stable	Progression	
100 (18)	Stage D endocrine resistant, progressing disease	No	1. 5FU 600 mg/M² i.v. q week	40	33	4	6		A 'crossover' design was used between the two chemotherapy arms for patients who progressed
			2. Cytoxan 1g/M² i.v. q 3 wks	45	41	3	14		
			3. "Standard therapy"	40	37	0	7		
				125	110				
200 (12)	Stage D, endocrine resistant, progressing disease	Yes	1. Estracyt 600 mg/M² daily orally	54	46	3	11	32	A 'crossover' design was used between the two chemotherapy arms for patients who progressed
			2. Streptozotocin 500mg/M² i.v. daily x 5 q 6 weeks	46	38	0	12	26	
			3. "Standard therapy"	25	21	0	4	17	
				125	105				
300 (16)	Stage D, endocrine resistant, progressing disease	No	1. D.T.I.C. 200mg/M² i.v. daily x 5 q 28 days	68	55	2	13	40	*Procarbazine arm discontinued because of excess nausea and vomiting
			2. Procarbazine 100mg/M² orally daily for 3 wks and repeated q 6w	58*	39	0	5	34	
			3. Cytoxan 1g/M² i.v. q 3 wks	39	35	0	9	26	
				165	129				

285

Protocol	Type of Patient	Prior Radiation	Treatments	Entered/Evaluable		Objective Response			Remarks
						Partial	Stable	Progression	
(13) 400	Stage D, endocrine resistant, progressing disease	Yes	1. Prednimustine 30 mg daily orally for 6 days out of 7 2. Estracyt 600 mg/M² daily orally plus prednimustine	71 64	62 54 116	0 1	8 6	54 47	Nausea and vomiting more severe in the combination treated group
500	Newly diagnosed Stage D. No prior hormonal therapy	No	1. Cytoxan 1g/m² i.v. each 3 wks + estracyt 600mg/M² orally daily 2. Cytoxan + DES 3 mg orally daily 3. DES or orchectomy	109 entered by 9/15/78		—	—		—
600	Stage D currently receiving hormonal therapy. i.e. stable disease	Varied	1. DES alone 3 mg orally daily 2. DES + Cytoxan 1 g/M² i.v. every 3 wks 3. DES + Estracyt 600 mg/M² orally daily	82 entered by 9/15/78		—	—		Evaluation will require observation of duration that stability can be maintained.
700	Stage D, endocrine resistant, progressing disease	No	1. Hydroxyurea 3 g/M² orally each 3 days 2. MeCCNU 175mg/M² orally every 6 wks 3. Cytoxan 1g/M² i.v. each 3 wks	87 entered by 9/15/78		—	—		—

Protocol	Type of Patient	Prior Radiation	Treatments	Entered/ Evaluable	Objective Response	Remarks
800	Stage D, Endocrine resistant. Progressive disease	Yes	1. Estracyt 600 mg/M^2 orally daily 2. Vincristine 1 mg/M^2 I.V. q 2 weeks 3. Estracyt plus Vincristine	93 entered by 9/15/78	—	—
900	Biopsy proven stages B$_2$, C or D$_1$ (without distant metastases)	No	1. Estracyt 600 mg/M^2 orally daily 2. Cytoxan 1g/M^2 I.V. q 3 weeks 3. No treatment	14 entered by 9/15/78	N/A	This is an adjuvant study requiring total prostatectomy (or cryosurgery) with lymph node dissection or lymphangiogram and thin needle biopsy. Careful pathology review will be performed.
1000	Biopsy proven stages B$_2$, C or D$_1$ (without distant metastases)	Yes	1. Estracyt 600 mg/M^2 orally daily 2. Cytoxan 1 g/M^2 I.V. q 3 weeks 3. No treatment	7 entered by 9/15/78	N/A	The staging requirements for this adjuvant study are similar to protocol 900. The management of the primary tumor, however, is with radiation of the prostate and regional lymph node bed.

approaches. The two drugs studied, cyclophosphamide and fluorouracil, were chosen because their effects and tolerance in patients with other tumors was well known. For those patients who had previously received radiation therapy (Protocol 200) (12), estracyt and streptozotocin were chosen for study because of suggestion of activity clinically (estracyt) and in model systems (streptozotocin) and because both were known to produce little hematologic toxicity. Both of these studies included a control arm of "standard" therapy which included various other hormonal approaches as well as palliative radiation therapy.

Although the incidence of objective remissions in these two studies was low, the incidence of partial response and stable disease from chemotherapy was significantly greater than from the "standard" treatments. In the more recent studies looking for activity in patients with advanced disease, then, chemotherapy arms serve as more appropriate controls. This is exemplified in protocols 300, 400, 700 and 800.

With the demonstration that chemotherapy was effective in patients with advanced and progressing disease, it became logical to study patients with advanced but either newly diagnosed or stable disease. This will allow a direct comparison of a hormonal therapy in newly diagnosed patients (Protocol 500) and evaluation of whether the addition of cytotoxic therapy to patients who are stable on hormonal therapy is of value (Protocol 600).

A good rationale exists for the recent activation of adjuvant studies for patients with 'early' disease treated surgically (Protocol 900) or with radiation (Protocol 1000) even though the agents used do not produce a high incidence of objective response in patients with advanced disease. Both agents are tolerated well and have a degree of activity in advanced disease that is not dissimilar from that of L-phenylanaline mustard in patients with breast cancer. This latter agent is effective as an adjuvant in premenopausal high risk (2) patients. A "no treatment" control is included in both these studies.

References

1. Bagshaw, M. A. et al.: Evaluation of Extended Field Radiotherapy for Prostatic Neoplasm. Cancer Treat. Rep., 61: 297, 1977.
2. Bonnadonna, G. et al.: Combination Chemotherapy as an Adjuvant Treatment in Operable Breast Cancer. New England Journal of Medicine, 294: 405-410, 1976.
3. Chu, T. M. et al.: Immunochemical Detection of Serum Prostatic Acid Phosphatase. Methodology and Clinical Evaluation. Invest. Urol., 15: 319, 1978.

4. Fisher, B. et al.: L phenylalamine Mustard (L PAM) in the Management of Primary Breast Cancer. New England Journal of Medicine, 292: 117-122, 1975.

5. Gleason, D. F.: Histologic Grading and Clinical Staging of Prostate Carcinoma. In: Urologic Pathology: The Prostate. Lea Febiger, pp. 171-197, 1977.

6. Harmer, M. H. (Ed.): T. N. M. Classification of Malignant Tumours. 3rd ed., 118-121, UICC Geneva, 1978.

7. Horton, J.: Hodgkin's Disease. In Clinical Oncology. Horton and Hill, Eds., pp. 690-700. W. B. Saunders, 1977.

8. Horton, J.: Breast Cancer. Ibid 366-389, 1977.

9. Klaassen, D.: Methods of Determining Response to Treatment. Chemotherapy of Solid Tumors, Proceedings of the 19th Clinical Conference, The Ontario Cancer Treatment and Research Foundation, John O. Godden, Ed., pp. 13-25, 1976.

10. Manual of Staging of Cancer. American Joint Commission for Cancer Staging and End Results, 1977.

11. Mostofi, F. K.: Grading of Prostatic Carcinoma. Cancer Chemotherapy Rep., 59: 111-117, 1975.

12. Murphy, G. P. et al.: A Comparison of Estramustine Phosphate and Streptozotocin in Patients with Advanced Prostatic Carcinoma Who Have Had Extensive Radiation. J. Urol., 118: 288, 1977.

13. Murphy, G. P. et al.: The Use of Estracyt and Leo 1031 Versus Leo alone in Advanced Metastatic Prostatic Cancer Patients Who Have Received Prior Radiation. J. Urol., in press, 1978.

14. Murphy, G. P. and Whitmore, W. F.: A Report of the Workshops on the Current Status of the Histologic Grading of Prostatic Cancer. Submitted to Cancer.

15. Resnick, M. I., Willard, J. W. and Boyce, W. H.: Ultrasonographic Evaluation of the Prostatic Nodule. J. Urol., 120: 86, 1978.

16. Schmidt, J. D. et al.: Comparison of Procarbazine, DTIC and Cyclophosphamide in Relapsing Patients with Advanced Carcinoma of the Prostate. J. Urol., in press, 1978.

17. Schmidt, J. D. et al.: Chemotherapy of Advanced Prostate Cancer: Evaluation of Response Parameters. Urology VII, 602-610, 1976.

18. Scott, W. W. et al.: Chemotherapy of Advanced Prostatic Carcinoma with Cyclophosphamide or 5-Fluorouracil: Results of the First National Randomized Study. J. Urol., 114: 911, 1975.

NOTES

NOTES

Printed in Switzerland
by
Imprimerie Montfort S.A. — Monthey